**POCKET
COMPANION
FOR**

CANCER

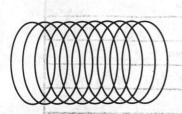

POCKET COMPANION FOR

CANCER NURSING

RUTH McCORKLE, PhD, FAAN

American Cancer Society Professor
School of Nursing
University of Pennsylvania
Philadelphia, Pennsylvania

MARCIA GRANT, DNSc, OCN, FAAN

Associate Research Scientist and Director
Department of Nursing Research and Education
City of Hope National Medical Center
Duarte, California

W.B. SAUNDERS COMPANY

A Division of Harcourt Brace & Company

PHILADELPHIA LONDON TORONTO MONTREAL SYDNEY TOKYO

W.B. SAUNDERS COMPANY

A Division of
Harcourt Brace & Company

The Curtis Center
Independence Square West
Philadelphia, PA 19106

Library of Congress Cataloging-in-Publication Data

Pocket companion for cancer nursing / [edited by] Ruth McCorkle,
  Marcia Grant—1st ed.
     p.   cm.
  ISBN 0–7216–5410–X
  1. Cancer—Nursing—Handbooks, manuals, etc.   I. McCorkle, Ruth.
  II. Grant, Marcia Moeller.
    [DNLM: 1. Oncologic Nursing—handbooks.   WY 39 P738 1994]
  RC266.P63   1994
  610.73`698—dc20
  DNLM / DLC
                                                                94-6847

POCKET COMPANION FOR   ISBN 0-7216-5410-X
CANCER NURSING   WY 156 POC
                                        NORM

Some material in this work was previously published in
CANCER NURSING, copyright © 1991 by W.B. Saunders
Company.

Printed in United States of America

Last digit is the print number: 9   8   7   6   5   4   3   2   1

Graceann Ehlke
Roberta Schofield
Barney Lepovetsky
Linda Arenth

This pocket companion is dedicated to the memory of our friends and colleagues. Their presence, commitment, and professional work contributed significantly to the field of oncology for patients, family members, professionals, and students. They would be very pleased to know that clinicians have access to a quick, convenient, and current resource such as this pocket companion.

Clinical Experts

FRANCES K. BARG, MEd

Program Leader for Cancer Control Education, University of Pennsylvania, School of Nursing, Philadelphia, Pennsylvania

MARIETTA MOSCO BORINSKI, MSN, RN

Oncology Clinical Nurse Specialist, Medical Nursing, Hospital of the University of Pennsylvania, Philadelphia, Pennsylvania

CONNIE LEEK, MSN, RN, C, OCN

Clinical Educator, Department of Nursing Research and Education, City of Hope National Medical Center, Duarte, California; Baccalaureate Instructor, California State University, Dominguez Hills, Carson, California; Clinical Assistant Professor, University of Southern California, Los Angeles, Los Angeles, California

ERIN M. McMENAMIN, MSN, RN, OCN

Adjunct Clinical Instructor, Widener University, Chester, Pennsylvania; Oncology Clinical Nurse Specialist, Memorial Hospital of Burlington County, Mt. Holly, New Jersey

CHARLENE SAKURAI, BA, RN, OCN

Clinical Educator, Department of Nursing Research and Education, City of Hope National Medical Center, Duarte, California

LIZ SULLIVAN, MN, RN, OCN

Assistant Clinical Professor, University of California, Los Angeles, Los Angeles, California; Clinical Educator, Department of Nursing Research and Education, City of Hope National Medical Center, Duarte, California

LINDA SHEGDA YOST, PhD, RN

Assistant Professor, Department of Nursing and Health, Allentown College of St. Frances de Sales, Center Valley, Pennsylvania; Home Care Coordinator, Abington Memorial Hospital, Abington, Pennsylvania

Contributors

ELIZABETH ABERNATHY, MSN, RN, OCN

Adjuvant Faculty, Duke University School of Nursing; Clinical Nurse Specialist, Oncology Research, Duke University Medical Center, Durham, North Carolina.
Biologic Response Modifiers

TERESA ADES, BSN, RN, OCN

Coordinator of Nursing Programs, American Cancer Society, Atlanta, Georgia.
Cancer Organizations

MADALON AMENTA, DrPH, MPH, MN, BA

Associate Professor of Nursing, The Pennsylvania State University, McKeesport Campus, McKeesport, Pennsylvania; Chair, Professional Advisory Committee, Home Health Services of Allegheny County, Pittsburgh, Pennsylvania; Editor of *The Hospice Journal*.
How to Find Hospice Care

PATRICIA S. BRALY, MD

Associate Professor and Director, Division of Gynecological Oncology, Department of Reproductive Medicine, University of California San Diego Medical Center, San Diego, California.
Gynecologic Cancers

NANCY BURNS, PhD, RN

Professor and Director, Center for Nursing Research, School of Nursing, University of Texas at Arlington, Arlington, Texas.
Alterations in Body Image

MARY E. CALLAGHAN, MN, RN

Hematology/Oncology/Bone Marrow Transplant Clinical Nurse Specialist, Green Hospital of Scripps Clinic and Research Foundation, La Jolla, California.
Hematopoietic and Immunologic Cancers

COLETTE CARSON, MN, RN

Nursing Consultant, San Diego Regional Cancer Center, San Diego, California; Consultant, Scripps Memorial Hospital Cancer Center, La Jolla, California.
Hematopoietic and Immunologic Cancers

CYNTHIA CHERNECKY, MN, RN

Doctoral Candidate in Nursing, Case Western Reserve University, Cleveland, Ohio; Clinical Nurse Specialist in Adult Oncology, Marymount Hospital, Inc., Garfield Heights, Ohio.
Complications of Advanced Disease

NESSA COYLE, MS, RN

Clinical Instructor, Columbia University School of Nursing; Director, Supportive Care Program, Pain Service, Department of Neurology, Memorial Sloan-Kettering Cancer Center, New York, New York.
Alterations in Comfort: Pain

KAREN HASSEY DOW, PhD, MS, RN

Assistant Professor, MGH Institute of Health Professions; Nurse Specialist, Beth Israel Hospital, Boston, Massachusetts.
Radiation Oncology

SUSAN DUDAS, MSN, RN

Associate Professor and Acting Associate Dean for Academic Affairs, The University of Illinois at Chicago, Chicago, Illinois.
Alterations in Patient Coping

KARIN DUFAULT, PhD, RN, SP

Clinical Assistant Professor, Oregon Health Sciences University School of Nursing, Department of Adult Health and Illness, Portland, Oregon; Administrator, St. Elizabeth Medical Center, Yakima, Washington.
Alterations in Mobility

GRACEANN EHLKE, DNSc, RN

Education and Training, Row Sciences, Rockville, Maryland.
Gastrointestinal Cancers

SHARON CANNELL FIRSICH, MS, RN

Oncology Clinical Nurse Specialist, Providence Medical Center, Portland, Oregon.
Alterations in Mobility

KATHLEEN M. FOLEY, MD

Professor of Neurology and Pharmacology, Cornell University Medical College; Chief, Pain Service, Department of Neurology, and Attending Neurologist, Memorial Sloan-Kettering Cancer Center, New York, New York.
Alterations in Comfort: Pain

ROSEMARY C. FORD, BA, BS, RN

Clinical Practice Coordinator, Nursing Department, Clinical Division, Fred Hutchinson Cancer Research Center, Seattle, Washington.
Bone Marrow Transplantation

BETTY BIERUT GALLUCCI, PhD, RN

Professor, Department of Physiological Nursing, University of Washington; Staff Appointment, Pathology, Fred Hutchinson Cancer Research Center, Seattle, Washington.
Cancer Biology: Molecular and Cellular Aspects

JOHN GODWIN, MD

Assistant Professor of Medicine, Loyola University Medical School; Attending Physician, and Associate Director, Special Hematology Laboratory, Foster G. McGaw Hospital, Chicago, Illinois.
Blood Component Therapy

MICHELLE GOODMAN, MS, RN

Assistant Professor, College of Nursing, Rush University; Oncology Clinical Nurse Specialist and Teacher Practitioner, Section of Medical Oncology, Rush–Presbyterian–St. Luke's Medical Center, Chicago, Illinois.
Delivery of Cancer Chemotherapy

MARCIA GRANT, DNSc, OCN, FAAN

Associate Research Scientist and Director, Department of Nursing Research and Education, City of Hope National Medical Center, Duarte, California.
Alterations in Nutrition

PATRICIA GREENE, MSN, RN, FAAN

Vice President for Nursing, American Cancer Society, Atlanta, Georgia.
Cancer Organizations

JENNIFER L. GUY, BS, RN

Administrator, Saint Anthony Regional Oncology Center, Franciscan Health System of Central Ohio, Columbus, Ohio.
Medical Oncology—The Agents

DOUGLAS HAEUBER, MSN, RN, OCN

Instructor, School of Nursing, University of Southern Maine, Portland, Maine; Staff RN, Medical Oncology, Massachusetts General Hospital, Boston, Massachusetts.
Alterations in Protective Mechanisms: Hematopoiesis and Bone Marrow Depression

MARILYN D. HARRIS, MSN, RN, FAAN, CNAA

Executive Director, Visiting Nurse Association of Eastern Montgomery County, Abington Memorial Hospital, Abington, Pennsylvania
How to Choose a Home Care Agency

CATHRYN P. HAVARD, BA, RGN, Onc Cert

Former Surgical Manager, Cheltenham General Hospital, Cheltenham, England.
Surgical Oncology

LAURA J. HILDERLEY, MS, RN

Clinical Nurse Specialist in the private practice of Philip G. Maddock, MD, Radiation Oncology, Warwick, Rhode Island.
Radiation Oncology

BARBARA C. HOLMES, MSN, RN, OCN

Oncology Nursing Consultant, San Antonio, Texas
Alterations in Body Image

LINDA EDWARDS HOOD, BSN, RN, OCN

Chemotherapy Head Nurse, Hematology/Oncology Ambulatory Clinic, Duke University Medical Center, Durham, North Carolina.
Biologic Response Modifiers

SUSAN MOLLOY HUBBARD, BS, RN

Director, International Cancer Information Center, and Associate Director, National Cancer Institute, Bethesda, Maryland.
The Biology of Metastases

ANNE M. HUGHES, MN, RN, CFNP

Assistant Clinical Professor, Department of Physiological Nursing, University of California, San Francisco, California; AIDS/HIV Clinical Nurse Specialist, San Francisco General Hospital, San Francisco, California.
AIDS and the Spectrum of HIV Disease

ROBERT J. IRWIN, Jr., MD

Associate Professor of Clinical Surgery, UMD-New Jersey Medical School, Vice Chief, Section of Urology; Chief, Section of Urology, East Orange Veterans Affairs Medical Center, East Orange, New Jersey.
Genitourinary Cancers

RYAN R. IWAMOTO, MN, RN, CS

Clinical Instructor, Department of Physiological Nursing, School of Nursing, University of Washington; Clinical Instructor, School of Nursing, Seattle University, Seattle, Washington; Instructor, Educational Development and Health Sciences Division, Bellevue Community College, Bellevue, Washington; Clinical Nurse Specialist, Radiation Oncology, Virginia Mason Clinic, Seattle, Washington.
Alterations in Oral Status

ANNE JALOWIEC, PhD, RN

Associate Professor, School of Nursing, Loyola University of Chicago, Chicago, Illinois.
Alterations in Patient Coping

PATRICIA F. JASSAK, MS, RN, CS

Clinical Assistant Professor, Medical/Surgical Nursing, Niehoff School of Nursing, Loyola University; Oncology Clinical Nurse Specialist, Foster G. McGaw Hospital, Loyola University Medical Center, Chicago, Illinois.
Blood Component Therapy

M. TISH KNOBF, MSN, RN, FAAN

Assistant Professor, Yale University School of Nursing; Oncology Clinical Nurse Specialist, Ambulatory Service, Yale–New Haven Hospital, New Haven, Connecticut.
Breast Cancer

RUTH L. KRECH, MSN, RN

Clinical Nurse Specialist in Palliative Care, Cleveland Clinic Foundation, Cleveland, Ohio.
Complications of Advanced Disease

MARGARET A. LAMB, MSN, RN

Assistant Professor, Department of Nursing, School of Health and Human Services, University of New Hampshire, Durham, New Hampshire.
Alterations in Sexuality and Sexual Functioning

JULENA LIND, MN, RN

Adjunct Assistant Professor, Department of Nursing, University of Southern California; Executive Director, Southern California Cancer Center, Inc., California Medical Center Los Angeles, Los Angeles, California.
Genitourinary Cancers

ADA M. LINDSEY, PhD, RN, FAAN

Dean and Professor, School of Nursing, University of California, Los Angeles, California.
Lung Cancer

LANCE A. LIOTTA, MD, PhD

Clinical Professor of Pathology, George Washington University, Washington, District of Columbia; Chief, Laboratory of Pathology, Division of Cancer Biology and Diagnosis, National Cancer Institute, Bethesda, Maryland.
The Biology of Metastases

LUCY K. MARTIN, BSN, RN, OCN

Clinical Instructor, City of Hope National Medical Center, Duarte, California.
Gynecologic Cancers

CHRISTINE MIASKOWSKI, PhD, RN, OCN

Assistant Professor, Department of Physiological Nursing, University of California, San Francisco, California.
Oncologic Emergencies

CAROL ANN PARENTE, MSN, RN, CRNP

Hospice Coordinator and Adult Nurse Practitioner, Visiting Nurse Association of Eastern Montgomery County, Abington Memorial Hospital, Abington, Pennsylvania.
How to Choose a Home Care Agency

BARBARA F. PIPER, DNSc, MS, RN

Oncology Staff Nurse, Mt. Zion Hospital of the University of California, San Francisco, California.
Alterations in Energy: The Sensation of Fatigue

JEAN L. REESE, PhD, RN

Associate Professor, College of Nursing, University of Iowa, Iowa City, Iowa.
Head and Neck Cancers

CONNIE R. ROBINSON, PhD, RN, FAAN

Associate Professor, Boston College, Boston, Massachusetts.
Central Nervous System Tumors

MARY E. ROPKA, PhD, RN, FAAN

Chair and Associate Professor, Medical College of Virginia, Richmond, Virginia.
Alterations in Nutrition

Sr. CALLISTA ROY, PhD, RN, FAAN

Professor, Boston College, School of Nursing, Boston, Massachusetts; Neuroscience Nursing Staff Privileges, Beth Israel Hospital, and Beth Israel Center for the Advancement of Nursing Practice, Boston, Massachusetts.
Central Nervous System Tumors

MARGARET L. SEAGER, BA, RN

Clinical Nurse III, University of California and San Francisco Hospitals, San Francisco, California.
Central Nervous System Tumors

AMY SMITH-BRASSARD, MS, RN

Former Associate Professor, University of Vermont School of Nursing, Burlington, Vermont.
Soft Tissue and Bone Sarcomas

JUDITH A. SPROSS, MS, RN, OCN

Assistant Professor, MGH Institute of Health Professions, Boston, Massachusetts.
Alterations in Protective Mechanisms: Hematopoiesis and Bone Marrow Depression

JEROME SCHOFFERMAN, MD

Assistant Professor, University of California San Francisco School of Medicine, San Francisco, California; Director, Internal Medicine and Chief, Pain Management, Spine Care Medical Group, Daly City, California.
AIDS and the Spectrum of HIV Disease

ANNE E. TOPPING, BSc (Hons), RGN, Onc Cert

Senior Lecturer, School of Human and Health Sciences, The Polytechnic of Huddersfield, Queensgate, Huddersfield, England.
Surgical Oncology

JOYCE ZERWEKH, EdD, RN, CS
Assistant Professor, Community Health Care Systems
School of Nursing, University of Washington, Seattle,
Washington.
Supportive Care of the Dying Patient

Preface

The explosion of information related to cancer etiology, prevention, medical treatment, and nursing management inevitably has had its impact on the size of teaching textbooks, including our own *Cancer Nursing*. To help students and practicing nurses overcome the obstacle to ready access presented by a large textbook, pertinent information in the parent text has been condensed by clinicians with expertise in cancer care to create this *Pocket Companion*.

We feel this *Pocket Companion* will fulfill important needs of nurses by meeting the following goals:

- Provide a readily available pocket resource for immediate reference for clinicians in the clinical arena.
- Facilitate the use of the parent book *Cancer Nursing* by cross-referencing with specific page numbers all presentations in the pocket companion with their origins in the text.
- Serve as a guide for nurses who wish to review the large-volume material in *Cancer Nursing*.

It is important that the reader understand that we are not recommending this *Pocket Companion* as a substitute for our parent book *Cancer Nursing*. Instead, it is intended to be a companion to the definitive text. Although they contain essential facts, the condensed presentations do not enrich and expand the knowledge base. In addition, much of *Cancer Nursing* that deals with the theory of practice and issues related to the delivery of cancer care across settings is not included in this companion. We are eager to know whether nurses find this condensed version helpful in their practice, and we welcome your comments and recommendations.

Ruth McCorkle
Marcia Grant

Contents

1 Cancer Biology: Molecular and Cellular Aspects

BETTY BIERUT GALLUCCI

AN OVERVIEW

Often an understanding of the disease known as cancer begins with defining the word. Pitot distinguishes between *cancer* and *neoplasm*, referring to the clinical entity as a cancer and using neoplasm (or neoplasia) to emphasize the basic biologic processes underlying the disease. Pitot's definition, a modification of Ewing's, is as follows: "A neoplasm is a heritably altered, relatively autonomous growth of tissue."

This physiologic definition proposed by Pitot emphasizes the concepts of tissue, autonomy, and growth. Autonomy implies that some normal regulatory controls over cell growth and division are lacking. The term *relatively* is included because cancer cells are not completely independent of all regulatory processes. If they were, such tumors as breast and prostate cancers would not respond to hormonal therapies.

Other definitions emphasize, or imply, that *cellular* abnormalities are crucial to the definition of neoplasia. This

---

See the corresponding chapter in *Cancer Nursing: A Comprehensive Textbook,* by Baird, McCorkle, and Grant, pp. 115–129, for a more detailed discussion of this topic, including a comprehensive list of references.

is not surprising because the basic building block of all tissue is the cell. Bonfiglio and Terry defined cancer as "a disease of the cell in which the normal mechanisms of control of growth and proliferation are disturbed. This results in distinctive morphologic alterations of the cell and aberrations of tissue patterns." These morphologic differences and aberrations (in which the cells in the malignant tissue appear immature or less differentiated) are clues for the pathologist, who helps determine the presence or absence of a malignancy.

The Natural History of Cancer

Cancer is a process—not one event or one alteration but a series of events. Tissue alterations were discovered that could not be placed into either normal or neoplastic categories. Instead, these intermediate lesions were considered to represent the sequential changes leading from the normal cell and tissue structure to the neoplastic ones. These forms include metaplasia, dysplasia, and carcinoma in situ.

Studies of metastases provide an example of cancer as a process. Metastasis is possible because cancer cells invade the blood vessels, withstand the natural immune mechanisms while traveling in the vessels, attach to capillary walls, enter tissue, and grow in the new milieu of the metastatic site. Each of these steps listed and perhaps a dozen others may involve genetic changes in the cell. Indicators of genetic changes include the formation of new clones of malignant cells, the activation of new enzymes, and the expression of new molecules on the cell surface and the loss of others.

CANCER: A DISEASE OF CELL DIFFERENTIATION

Differentiation is the process that results in readily observable changes in cellular characteristics. These changes are irreversible, self-perpetuating, and passed on to the daughter cells. Because most cells contain the entire genome, differentiation is the result of expression of certain genes and the repression of others.

Differentiated cells are mature cells that perform the functions of the particular tissues that they comprise. In the adult, *undifferentiated cells* (not totally committed) are known as pluripotent cells, precursor cells, or *stem cells*. Cells with the least amount of differentiation are found in the embryo. As a cell becomes more differentiated, its potential becomes more restricted. Totally differentiated cells often lose their ability to replicate, implying that the fate of the mature cell is death.

Neoplasia can develop at any point in the process of differentiation. A cancer of the cell line leading directly to the red blood cell (at the point of terminal differentiation) is a erythroleukemia, a rare leukemia. During the natural history of many cancers, as the malignant cells grow and divide, they often lose more and more of their mature characteristics.

CLASSIFICATION OF TUMORS

Classification of the tumor type is based on tissue and cellular staining. Differences in cytoplasmic and nuclear staining distinguish one cell type from another and identify their stages of differentiation. A malignant neoplasm, for instance, is classified as a *carcinoma* if the tissue of the tumor origin is epithelium, as an *adenocarcinoma* if the tissue of origin has both epithelial and glandular components, and as a *sarcoma* if the tissue of origin is connective tissue. (For a list of selected characteristics of benign and malignant tumor types and a simple classification system, see Table 1–1.

The grade of the tumor is based on how well differentiated the tissue or the cells appear. A grade of 1 is given to a neoplasm that is well differentiated (that is, one that appears similar to the adult tissue from which it arose). The highest grade of 4 is given to a neoplasm that appears so undifferentiated (anaplastic) that it is difficult to identify the tissue of origin. For many tumors, the higher the grade or the less differentiated the tumor is, the poorer the prognosis.

PHENOTYPIC CHARACTERISTICS OF MALIGNANT AND TRANSFORMED CELLS

What features of a malignant cell distinguish it from a normal cell? And how are these characteristics studied? The characteristic features of the cell—known as its *phenotype*—are the result of the expression of hereditary information. The phenotype of an individual person is described by hair, skin, and eye coloring and other physical features. The cell's phenotype is determined by histologic and cytologic techniques: the quality and type of cytoplasmic and nuclear staining, the presence of mitosis, the number of nucleolar bodies, and the membrane characteristics. The malignant cell is usually basophilic, has a high nuclear/cytoplasmic ratio, and has multiple nucleoli. The hereditary information of the organism or the cell, on the other hand, is the *genotype*.

Cell Culture and Transformation

Normal cells were established in culture (cell lines) and then exposed to carcinogens (chemicals, viruses, or radiation). These cultured cells subsequently developed characteristics of malignant cells; this process was termed *transformation*. Because these cells are not derived from a tumor in a human or an animal, they are termed transformed rather than malignant cells.

Table 1–1. SOME EXAMPLES OF THE DIFFERENCES BETWEEN BENIGN AND MALIGNANT TUMORS

Property	Benign Tumors	Malignant Tumors
Growth	Slow expansile	Invasive
Differentiation	Fully differentiated	Immature, not differentiated
Metastasis	Absent	Present
Cytoplasm	Normal, uniform	Irregular in size and shape, pleomorphic
	Regular in size and shape	Basophilic
Nucleus	DNA content euploid	DNA content euploid to aneuploid
	Infrequent mitosis	Frequent mitosis
		Many nucleoli
Paraneoplastic syndromes	Absent	Present in many cases, for example, anorexia, cachexia

4

Characteristics of Transformed Cells

The physically obvious features of size, shape, and orientation and the growth characteristics of transformed cells distinguish them from normal cell lines. Transformed cells in culture have basophilic cytoplasm, irregular cellular outlines, and large nuclei that contain multiple nucleoli. Mitotic figures are more numerous in transformed cell lines than in a normal cell line. In addition, transformed cells differ from normal cells in such important characteristics as mobility and growth requirements.

The cell surface

The study of the cytoplasmic membrane adds an important dimension in the study of transformation because (1) loss of contact inhibition is linked to changes in the cell surface, (2) establishment of metastatic deposits depends on the ability of the tumor cells to invade and move, (3) hormones and growth factors often act at the surface, and tumor cells often lose the ability to be regulated by these factors, and (4) it is at the surface that the immune system will or will not recognize the cell as altered.

The cytoplasmic membrane is the interface between the cell and the extracellular medium. It consists of lipids (phospholipids), proteins, and carbohydrates bound to either the lipid or the protein components. The bilipid layer of the membrane is capable of movement. Molecules in the membrane can move or rearrange themselves. Tumor cells have a greater fluidity, perhaps owing to changes in the lipid composition.

The plasma membrane proteins are involved in transport of metabolites, as receptors, and in enzymatic activity. Some of the proteins are located at the surface, others span the whole bilipic leaflet layer, and some of these integral membrane proteins are linked to the cytoplasmic skeletal structures. Some proteins serve as receptors for hormones, growth factors, and antibodies. It is estimated that a single cell could have 100,000 or more specific membrane receptors.

Proteins can transport ions and metabolites across the osmotic barrier of the cytoplasmic membrane. Transformed cells often have higher transport activities than normal cells. For instance, some sugars and amino acids are transported into the cell at a faster rate. Higher transport activities, in turn, may alter the ratios of cyclic nucleotides in the cytoplasm. These nucleotides serve as intracellular messages, altering the metabolic state of the cells and perhaps DNA synthesis.

The cell surfaces of transformed cells often will contain new antigens not present in the normal cell type. Some of these antigens are called tumor-associated antigens in animal models. In human cells, they are oncofetal antigens, viral antigens, or tumor-associated molecules.

Cytoplasmic structures

Tumor cells survive in oxygen-poor environments because of oncogenesis rather than the lack of oxygen being the initiator. For every cytoplasmic structure and metabolic pathway, a similar story holds.

1. When the phenomenon is first investigated, it seems to hold for all the cases investigated.
2. It is difficult to determine which alterations in the cytoplasm and cell membrane are primary and which are secondary events in transformation.

Contact inhibition

Normal cell lines in culture exhibit a property known as contact inhibition. That is, when a cell line is plated onto a Petri dish, the cells will keep growing and dividing until the bottom of the dish is covered with cells, and then division stops. These cells in monolayer will orient themselves with respect to one another. Transformed cells, on the other hand, do not stop dividing. Instead, they move over and pile on top of one another until a multilayered culture is formed. This lack of contact inhibition is thought to be the result of two independent properties of the cell, mobility and replication.

First, transformed cells are more mobile and do not adhere to other cells as well as do normal cells. This property is linked to changes in the plasma membrane of the transformed cell as well as to alteration in the cytoplasmic skeletal elements. Normal cells, however, will form tight junctions and other areas of close contact with cells of their own type.

Second, transformed cells do not stop dividing and, therefore, grow to a high density in culture. Because contact inhibition may be the result of either property, the term *density-dependent inhibition of growth* is now considered the more precise term. This ability to grow in conditions unfavorable to normal cell lines often signals when transformation has occurred.

Growth requirements

The environment provided for the cell cultures determines the success of establishing cell lines. Most cell lines require a rigid substrate on which to grow; this requirement is known as substrate dependency. Fibroblasts, for example, can proliferate in plastic Petri dishes. Transformed cells often do not have this requirement. In fact, they can grow in soft agar.

Besides the usual requirements, such as an energy source, normal cell lines require the addition of serum to the nutrient bath. Fetal calf serum, which often is added to the medium, contains many complex substances, among which are polypeptide growth factors, pituitary hormones, insulin, epidermal growth factor, vitamins, minerals, and a variety of other substances, some of which have not been characterized. These substances must be present to stimulate and support cell replication.

Autocrine growth factors

The process by which transformed cells became autonomous of growth factors present in serum was conceptualized as autocrine secretion.

In normal cells, binding of growth factors to membrane receptors initiates a cascade of metabolic events that ultimately leads to cell division. Three mechanisms have been proposed to explain the transduction of the signal from the surface membrane to cytoplasmic and nuclear molecules. The first is the activation of protein kinases, which generate cyclic nucleotides, such as cyclic adenosine monophosphate (cAMP) and cyclic guanosine monophosphate (cGMP). The second involves endocytosis (engulfing and incorporation) of the complexed hormone and receptor. The third mechanism involves the influx into the cytoplasm of small ions, such as calcium and magnesium. These mechanisms then often act at the genetic level, perhaps regulating DNA synthesis and stimulating mitosis.

Malignant and transformed cells are known to have surface receptors for growth factors as well as the ability to release growth factors. This discovery led to the hypothesis of autostimulation.

GENETIC CHANGES IN CANCER CELLS

Cancer is recognized and diagnosed by the phenotypic, functional, and growth requirement changes in cells. However, the evidence is strong that these phenotypic alterations and other changes result from a change in the genetic information of the cell.

Genetic changes are studied from multiple perspectives, including familial, epidemiologic, chromosomal, and oncogenic. All of these areas of research give a slightly different perspective on the linkage of genetic changes with malignancy. Familial disorders are being linked to specific chromosomal defects, chromosomal defects to oncogenes and antioncogenes, and these genes, in turn, to the molecular events that occur in carcinogenesis.

Hereditary Cancers

"Cancer families" were described as early as 1913. In these extremely rare families, cancer is inherited in an autosomal dominant fashion. In familial polyposis coli (FPC), family members have a very high risk of developing colon cancer. The probability of developing colon cancer is 80% by the time the person reaches the age of 40 years unless preventive treatment is initiated. Two other examples are Gardner's syndrome and basal cell nevus syndrome.

Other families appear to have an increased risk of cancer,

but the inheritance pattern is suggestive of a strong familial tendency rather than a simple autosomal dominancy. One example of this type is premenopausal breast cancer. Daughters of mothers with bilateral premenopausal breast disease have close to a 50% probability of developing the disease themselves. Other examples include Bloom's syndrome, Fanconi's anemia, and xeroderma pigmentosum. In xeroderma pigmentosum, the gene that repairs DNA damage created by ultraviolet light is defective.

Characteristic patterns in families with increased risk for the development of cancer include the following.

1. Diagnosis of the cancer in these families occurs at an earlier age than in the general population. A diagnosis of colon cancer in the patient's 30s is indicative of a familial tendency.
2. There is increased risk of having a primary cancer in both sites in bilateral tissues, such as the breast. In organs such as the gut there is an increased risk for having multiple primary sites.
3. In some of the hereditary cancer syndromes, there is a higher incidence of second primaries in other organs.

Chromosomal Studies: Congenital and Noncongenital

The first specific karyotypic change found to be associated with a malignancy was the description of the Philadelphia chromosome in patients with chronic myeloid leukemia by Nowell and Hungerford. The Philadelphia chromosome results from the translocation of material from chromosome 22 to the long part of the arm of chromosome 9. This is represented by the abbreviation t(9;22). Oncogenes have been localized to the sites of translocation in the Philadelphia chromosome (chromosomes 9 and 22). Evidence is accumulating that the alteration in chromosome 9 is the important pathogenic event in leukemogenesis. When the gene from the break in chromosome 9 is positioned at the breakpoint in chromosome 22, a new hybrid gene is formed.

In general, knowledge of cytogenetics is more advanced for the leukemias and lymphomas, and, in comparison, very little is known about the solid tumors. The cytogenic changes in solid tumors appear to be more complex and numerous than those in the leukemias and lymphomas. This may be due to the advanced nature of the solid tumor when studied.

Oncogenic Studies: Studies at the Single Gene Level

In general, three main types of genes are involved in the development of the malignant phenotype. The first type is the oncogene, which actively induces the development of a tumor or transformation in cell culture. The second type is the antioncogene, the loss or the inactivity of which permits development of a tumor. The third type is the modulating genes that are involved in the modification of the tumor–host interactions and, therefore, involved in tumor progression. Because single genes cannot be visualized even by the most sensitive chromosomal banding techniques, transformation studies are used to detect the presence of a gene or an altered form of the gene.

Oncogenes

Oncogenes are studied by introducing a gene into cells growing in culture and noting whether the cells then undergo transformation. The genes causing the transformation can be obtained from two sources, tumor viruses or malignant cells. More than 30 oncogenes have been identified and have provided a great deal of evidence that the critical event in carcinogenesis is a genetic change.

Oncogenes were first studied in the retroviruses. The genetic material of retroviruses is RNA, and once inside a cell the viral RNA is used as a template to form viral DNA. The viral DNA can then induce the formation of more viral particles or become incorporated into the host's genetic material and remain latent.

Cellular oncogenes are likely to be the regulators of normal proliferation and differentiation during embryogenesis, growth, and wound healing. In this sense, the term oncogene does not adequately describe the function of these genes but rather describes how they were first investigated.

The other method used to study oncogenes is termed *transfection*. In this technique, DNA from malignant cells, either human or experimentally induced tumors, is introduced into normal cultured cells. Some of these recipient cells will then undergo transformation and acquire a malignant phenotype.

How do oncogenes differ from their normal cellular counterparts—that is, if they do? Theoretically, two major mechanisms can be responsible for the activation of oncogenes. The first involves the *regulation* of the gene and the second the *alteration of the structure* of the gene itself. Another process, called *gene amplification*, occurs when multiple copies of the gene are made. This could also lead to overexpression of the oncogene. For some oncogenes, it appears that a mutation (structural change) has occurred. Therefore, the oncogene differs from its normal counterpart by one or more DNA bases.

What is known is that (1) families of oncogenes exist, and the actions of one family will be different from those of the others, (2) growth factors, receptors for growth factors, the transduction of the growth factor signal, and inhibition of the growth factor signals are all major candidates for the primary mechanisms of carcinogenesis, (3) carcinogenesis may involve the sequential activation of oncogenes—that is, the activation of more than one oncogene may be necessary to induce a malignancy, and (4) many oncogenes are located at chromosomal breakpoints.

Antioncogenes

Antioncogenes also have been termed *recessive cancer genes* and *tumor suppressor genes*. The significant cytogenetic change appears to be the loss (deletion) of a gene from each of a pair of chromosomes. The term *antioncogene* does not imply that this gene inhibits an oncogene because the functional role of antioncogenes is not yet known. Antioncogenes involve gene deletion or inactivation, as compared with oncogenes, which are involved in gene activation.

2 The Biology of Metastases

SUSAN MOLLOY HUBBARD
LANCE A. LIOTTA

All neoplasms are characterized by a certain degree of autonomy from the host and are detrimental inasmuch as they compete for the nutrients and space required by normal cells. However, because the cells of benign tumors remain encased within a capsular membrane, tissues generally are damaged only when the mass grows large enough to damage vital tissues. Malignant cells are not encapsulated and are characterized by the ability to invade and destroy normal tissues even when microscopic in size. This ability to metastasize is the principal functional characteristic that makes an abnormal cell malignant.

How cancer cells form metastases is one of the most important questions in tumor biology. The development of a metastasis is a dynamic process that occurs as a complex cascade of events whose outcome hinges on anatomic factors, various forces in the host microenvironment, and intrinsic tumor cell properties. Disseminated tumor cells that cannot complete all of the steps in the metastatic cascade are eliminated by host defenses. Experimental evidence indicates that less than 0.01% of cancer cells that disseminate actually become established as metastases.

See the corresponding chapter in *Cancer Nursing: A Comprehensive Textbook,* by Baird, McCorkle, and Grant, pp. 130–142, for a more detailed discussion of this topic, including a comprehensive list of references.

CELLULAR PROPERTIES THAT INFLUENCE INVASION AND METASTASIS
Cell Surface Membrane Determinants

Certain intrinsic physicochemical properties appear to be cellular determinants of metastatic potential. A key component of the cell surface membrane structure is its lipid bilayer, which allows membrane proteins to move freely. Cell membrane proteins, particularly glycoproteins, function as enzymes, transporters, antigens, and cell membrane receptors. The controlled distribution of these cell surface proteins is a key feature of normal differentiated cells. A cytoskeletal apparatus, comprising membrane-associated microtubules and microfilaments, regulates the distribution of cell surface proteins in the lipid bilayer and holds them in patterns that are recognized by receptors on other cells. A wide variety of cellular feedback mechanisms and recognition systems are mediated by molecules on the cell's surface that either interact with or bind to molecules on adjacent cells. Alterations in the cell surface are known to develop during neoplastic transformation and are thought to contribute to loss of growth control, increased cell motility, altered patterns of cell recognition, diminished cell cohesion, and the development of cellular and biochemical properties that enable tumor cells to overcome mechanical barriers to invasion.

Cell-to-cell communication is an important factor in growth control. When normal mammalian cells are grown in culture, they migrate away from the center of the colony in an orderly radial pattern until continued cell contact is made. Then forward motion abruptly ceases. This phenomenon, known as *contact inhibition of movement,* is a feedback mechanism that serves to regulate normal cell growth and to suppress tissue invasion. Other mechanisms regulate parameters, such as adhesive specificity, density-dependent growth inhibition, anchorage-dependent growth, and cell orientation, that enable normal cells to organize into functional tissues. Defects in these feedback mechanisms are thought to contribute to the invasive behavior demonstrated by metastatic cancer cells, a key cellular determinant of metastatic potential.

Although tumor growth may be promoted by loss of the cell's ability to regulate growth, it also may be enhanced by autocrine stimulation. Autocrine (self-stimulatory) growth involves the secretion of and response to endogenously produced polypeptides that serve as growth hormones by a cell. Autocrine growth is mediated by receptors on the cell's surface. Autocrine growth factor expression appears directly or indirectly linked to changes in cellular genes (proto-oncogenes) that cause neoplastic growth when damaged or activated.

Invasion

In its earliest stages, local invasion may occur as a function of direct tumor extension. At some point, however, cells or clumps of cells become detached from the primary tumor and infiltrate the surrounding interstitial spaces. Among the mechanisms believed to play a role in local invasion by neoplastic cells are generation of mechanical pressure by the tumor growth, decreased cell-to-cell cohesion, increased cell motility, and the release of chemotactic substances and matrix-degrading enzymes by neoplastic cells and host inflammatory cells. Physical and biochemical properties that facilitate the invasion of normal stroma also enable tumor cells to penetrate lymphatic channels and blood vessels, promoting their dissemination to distant sites (Fig. 2-1). Once the cells are arrested in the capillary bed of a target organ, these invasive properties enable tumor cells to extravasate from the vasculature and infiltrate the perivascular stroma and the parenchyma of a target organ.

Angiogenesis

Tumor growth is limited by the ability of nutrients and waste products to diffuse into and out of the mass efficiently. Tumor cells secrete a diffusible substance called angiogenin or tumor angiogenesis factor (TAF) that causes the host to make blood vessels for them.

Before vascularization, tumors generally are unable to shed cells into the circulation and have a lower probability of metastasizing than tumors in which vascularization has

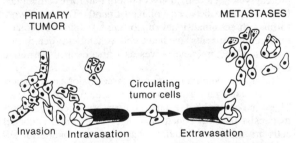

Figure 2-1. Multistep metastatic cascade. Following transition from in situ to invasive carcinoma, tumor cells infiltrate normal stroma and gain access to host blood vessels and lymphatics. Tumor cells enter the bloodstream directly (or indirectly via lymphatic–hematogenous communications) and are carried to a distant site, where they arrest in a vascular bed, extravasate, infiltrate normal stroma, and initiate a metastatic colony. Continued growth of the metastases requires angiogenesis and escape from host defenses.

occurred. As the tumor becomes vascularized, the number of cells released into the circulation increases. The rate of hematogenous spread is also correlated with tumor vascularity in clinical situations.

The growth of metastasis also is dependent on the development of a vascular supply. Therefore, tumor angiogenesis also is critical at the end of the metastatic cascade. However, it may be possible for small populations of tumor to remain in an avascular phase for prolonged periods, a phenomenon that may partially explain dormant metastases. Immunologic defenses that keep tumor growth in check or dependence on exogenous hormones or autocrine growth factors or both also may play important roles in tumor dormancy. These concepts are discussed in greater detail in Chapter 1.

BIOCHEMICAL MECHANISMS OF INVASION AND METASTASIS
Interactions with the Extracellular Matrix

The mammalian organism is composed of a series of tissue compartments separated from each other by two types of extracellular matrix: interstitial stroma and basement membranes. The molecular composition of each extracellular matrix is tissue specific. Each unique set of matrix components identifies the tissue of origin and reflects the organization and physical properties of the tissue. Collagens are the major structural elements in the matrices.

Extracellular matrix exists as a dense latticework composed of collagens and elastin that is embedded in a viscoelastic ground substance composed of glycoproteins and proteoglycan (a modified glycoprotein that forms a hydrated filler substance between collagen fibers). This meshwork forms a three-dimensional supporting scaffold that isolates tissue compartments, mediates cell attachment, determines tissue architecture, and serves as a mechanical barrier to invasion.

Basement membranes contain three major components: type IV collagen, laminin, and a specific proteoglycan. These molecules bind together to form homogeneous sheets that resist physical penetration of cells. Normal epithelial cells are thought to require a basement membrane for anchorage and growth. Three layers of basement membrane have been identified.

Basement membrane loss in invasive carcinoma

Tumor cell interaction with the extracellular matrix occurs at multiple stages in the metastatic cascade. During the transition from in situ to invasive carcinoma, changes in the organization, distribution, and quantity of the epithelial basement membrane occur as tumor cells penetrate the membrane and enter the underlying interstitial stroma. During intravasation and extravasation, tumor cells must also penetrate the vascular subendothelial basement membrane. Following extravasation from the circulation, tumor cells must traverse the perivascular interstitial stroma to establish a metastatic focus in the parenchyma of a target organ.

Invasion of the Extracellular Matrix: A Three-Step Process

A sequence of biochemical events occurs during tumor cell invasion of the extracellular matrix. The first step is tumor cell attachment via cell surface receptors that bind to specific attachment factors in the matrix, such as laminin and fibronectin. The anchored tumor cell then either secretes hydrolytic enzymes or induces host cells to secrete enzymes that degrade the matrix in a highly localized region close to the tumor cell surface. The third step requires tumor cell locomotion into the degraded matrix. During this phase, the pseudopodia of tumor cells attached to blood vessel walls traverse the basement membrane, allowing the cells to extravasate from the vasculature into the interstitial stroma. Continued invasion of the matrix occurs by cyclic repetition of these steps.

The fate of arrested tumor cells also differs according to the mechanism and location of lodgment.

Attachment factors

A major mechanism by which cells attach to the extracellular matrix is through matrix component glycoproteins, which serve as attachment factors. These attachment factors form a bridge between the tumor cell surface and other structural components of the matrix, such as collagen. Attachment factors may be synthesized by the cell that is attaching itself to the matrix, or the cell may use attachment factors already present in the matrix.

In vitro assays developed for evaluating biochemical events that occur during attachment have revealed that type IV collagen and laminin are the matrix components that block cell migration.

Proteolytic enzymes

Proteolytic enzymes secreted by tumor cells are thought to play an important role in the degradation of collagens, which abound in the perivascular basement membrane area and the adjacent connective tissues. Tumor cells can either release collagenases—enzymes that can preferentially digest collagen—or secrete collagenolytic substances in latent forms that are converted to active collagenase by lysosomal proteases, such as plasmin.

A number of other proteases that are bound to or released from the cell surface appear to facilitate tumor invasion through proteolysis. One of the hydrolytic enzymes that is augmented in tumor cells and appears to play a role in invasive behavior is plasminogen activator. Plasminogen activator converts the serum proenzyme plasminogen into the protease plasmin, which can hydrolyze a variety of proteins. A functional role that has been proposed for plasminogen activator is to allow tumor cells to escape the fibrin meshwork associated with tumor emboli.

Locomotion

Like leukocytes, tumor cells possess the organelles necessary for locomotion and can actively migrate through tissues. The motility of tumor cells is increased by a relative lack of cohesiveness in comparison to normal cells. Pseudopodia, cytoplasmic processes formed by microfilament bundles located in the cellular cytoskeleton, enable cells to migrate by diapedesis (the process by which leukocytes pass through unruptured vessel walls into the tissues). Proteins on the surface of these cytoplasmic processes contain receptors for specific substrates. Cell motility occurs as attachments with these substrates are made and broken. Local factors in the host microenvironment influence migratory behaviors by stimulating directional locomotion (chemotaxis). For example, it has been shown that cells move preferentially along continuous gradients of adhesiveness and toward regions of neutral pH.

The movement of neoplastic cells through cellular and connective tissue as well as other biologic barriers may well be influenced by chemotactic factors. It is known that tumor cells can influence the motility of normal cells in a number of instances, frequently to the benefit of the tumor. Tumor cells produce antileukotactic factors, chemotactic factors for the endothelial cells that are responsible for the formation of new blood vessels, and chemoattractants for fibroblasts.

A new class of protein is endogenously produced and profoundly stimulates the intrinsic motility of tumor cells. These *autocrine motility factors* stimulate both random and directional tumor cell motility without affecting leukocyte migration. They exert a recruiting effect on adjacent tumor cells that enables them to move into normal tissues under their own power.

Like autocrine growth factors, the action of autocrine motility factors is dependent on the presence of functional receptors on the tumor cell surface as well as on the production and secretion of a motility-stimulating protein. It is unclear at present whether the production of autocrine motility factor is the result of oncogene activation.

PATTERNS OF DISSEMINATION
Direct Extension

Rapid proliferation of cells within a tumor mass can create intratumoral pressures that force fingerlike projections of tumor cells directly into normal tissues in much the same way plants force their roots through soil. Anatomic routes of direct tumor extension involve infiltration of interstitial spaces, coelomic and epithelial cavities (serosal seeding), and cerebrospinal spaces. Mechanical forces appear to assist invasion rather than serve as the primary mechanism of tissue invasion.

Lymphatic Metastasis

Involvement of the regional lymph nodes draining a cancer is the first clinical sign of metastasis. There is considerable evidence that the immune system has both inhibitory and stimulatory effects on tumor growth, and these effects can be manifested simultaneously. However, data from animal studies suggest that an activated immune system can significantly enhance the development of metastases by selecting out weakly antigenic cell lines, leading to the proliferation of tumor cells that the host's immune system does not recognize as foreign. The lack of antigenicity may enable tumor cells to evade macrophages and other elements of the cell-mediated immune system in the circulation.

Tumors generally lack a well-formed lymphatic network. Communication between tumor cells and lymphatic channels occurs only at the tumor periphery and not within the tumor mass. Initially, regional lymph nodes may exert a barrier effect, impeding the dissemination of tumor cells into the lymphatic system. At some point in the metastatic cascade, lymph nodes lose their ability to filter and destroy tumor cells. Experimental data reveal that within 10 to 60 minutes after tumor cells arrest in a lymph node, a significant fraction of the tumor cells detach and enter the efferent lymphatics.

Regional lymph nodes do not function as true mechanical barriers to tumor dissemination, and it is likely that lymphatic and hematogenous dissemination occur in parallel.

Hematogenous Metastasis

Hematogenous dissemination is a complex process that requires tumor cells to penetrate and leave blood vessels to disseminate to distant organs. Data indicate that vascularized tumors probably shed malignant cells constantly as they grow, often releasing millions of cells without producing metastases. Thus, the mere presence of tumor cells in the bloodstream does not predict metastasis.

Circulating tumor cells use a variety of means to lodge in the vessels of the target organ, where they initiate metastatic colonies. Approximately 80% of the tumor cells circulate as single cells and attach directly to the intact endothelial surface or to preexisting regions of exposed subendothelial basement membrane. Emboli of circulating tumor cells or tumor cells aggregated with leukocytes, fibrin, or platelets can embolize directly in the precapillary venules by mechanical impaction. The formation of a fibrin–platelet complex is thought to protect tumor cells within the emboli from host defenses and to facilitate successful attachment to the vascular epithelium. Growth in the target organ parenchyma requires the development of a vascular network and continued evasion of host immune and non-immune defenses.

Metastases generally do not develop until the primary tumor reaches approximately 1 cm^3 in size (10^9 cells). Although the reasons for this are not completely clear, it is possible that more aggressive tumor cells evolve in larger tumors. Larger tumors may provide a greater antigenic burden that favors the survival of disseminated cells.

Anatomic Location

The most frequent location of distant metastasis in many types of cancer appears to be the first capillary bed encountered by the circulating cells (Table 2–1). Although all blood eventually passes through the heart and lungs, the shunting of tumor cells through different vascular pathways predisposes certain organs to develop hematogenous metastasis.

Organ Tropism for Metastases

Autopsy statistics and modern research models have shown that both the seed and the soil are important. Although 50% to 60% of metastatic sites can be explained by the circulatory anatomy, many cannot be predicted on the basis of anatomic considerations. Clear evidence exists that tumor cells contain organ-specific receptors that can discriminate between various vascular beds and cause preferential homing to certain organs. These data suggest that organ tropism is genetically determined. Indeed, experimental evidence indicates that the metastatic potential of

Table 2–1. INCIDENCE OF METASTASES AT AUTOPSY (%)

Primary Tumor	Site of Metastases			
	Lung	Colon	Breast	Melanoma
Liver	30–50	50–60	40–60	58–70
Lung	20–40	25–40	60–80	66–80
Bone	30–45	5–10	50–90	30–48
Brain	15–43	0–1	15–30	40–55
Adrenal	17–38	14	38–54	40–47
Pituitary	0–2	0–1	20	18
Ovary	0–2	14	15–30	10–15
Kidney	16–23	8	13	31–35
Spleen	9	5	17	31

individual tumor cells in a primary tumor is quite variable and that different patterns of preferential metastasis exist among the cells in an individual tumor.

BIOLOGIC HETEROGENEITY

The generation of biologic heterogeneity in tumors and tumor metastases is attributable to genetic instability that is either inherent in malignant cells or acquired during tumor growth. Genetic instability predisposes them to undergo spontaneous somatic mutations at random intervals, which produce permanent and irreversible changes in cellular DNA that are inherited by all the cell's progeny. Genotypic and phenotypic variations are clinically manifested by heterogeneity with regard to growth rates, karyotypic abnormalities, cell surface receptors, marker enzymes, a variety of cellular and biochemical properties, and responsiveness to radiotherapy and chemotherapy.

3 Surgical Oncology

CATHRYN P. HAVARD
ANNE E. TOPPING

A HISTORICAL PERSPECTIVE

Malignant disease in humans has been traced back to the ancient Egyptians and beyond. Hippocrates realized that fundamentally he was unable to treat malignant disease and cautioned against interfering with hidden cancers within body cavities. However, many of his disciples experimented with surgical techniques, particularly on breast and limbs. John Hunter, father of scientific surgery, believed that cancer was a local disease, but he also was aware that it could appear in other parts of the body.

Developments in anesthesia, antibiotic therapy, and critical care technology have enabled surgical resections to exceed anatomic boundaries not dreamed of by the early pioneer surgeons. Surgery alone, however, can effect a cure only when malignant disease is confined to its primary site. It is increasingly used, therefore, in conjunction with other treatment methods as part of a multidisciplinary approach to cancer therapy. Moreover, there is an increasing recognition that it is not enough to remove the cancer without making every attempt to repair defects and restore function.

THE SCOPE OF CANCER SURGERY

Developments in complementary fields of medicine and patient care have increased the scope of surgery. Advances

See the corresponding chapter in *Cancer Nursing: A Comprehensive Textbook*, by Baird, McCorkle, and Grant, pp. 235–245, for a more detailed discussion of this topic, including a comprehensive list of references.

in critical care, nutritional support, anesthesia, pain management, and antibiotic coverage have all helped improve the potential outcome from surgery. Increasingly, it is becoming the norm for surgery to be used in combination with other treatment methods.

An influence that has promoted multimodality treatment has been the general acceptance of the concept that a tumor is not confined to the primary site at diagnosis and that micrometastases will be more than likely to have disseminated. Table 3–1 gives examples of the variety of interventions currently in use within cancer care.

DIAGNOSIS

A cancer diagnosis may be suspected from physical examination or from radiologic examination. Confirmation, however, needs to be established from a sample of tissue. A number of techniques may be used. These are described in greater detail in Table 3–2.

STAGING

Staging is undertaken to establish stage and extent of disease. A diagnostic laparotomy may be performed before radical surgery to ascertain whether occult metastases are present, which may affect the ultimate extent of resection.

Table 3–1. SURGICAL APPROACHES TO CANCER CARE

Intervention	Example
Diagnosis	Breast biopsy
Staging	Staging laparotomy
	Second-look laparotomy
Treatment of primary tumor	Curative resection (abdominal perineal resection)
Reconstruction, rehabilitation	Breast reconstruction
	Continent urostomy or ileostomy
Palliative	Endocrine ablation
	Pericardial window
Adjuvant	Paraaortic node dissection
	Hickman line insertion
Complications of other methods	Excision of bowel stricture
	Excision of radionecrotic tissue
Resection of metastases	Partial hepatectomy
	Pulmonary resection
Cytoreductive	Abdominal soft-tissue sarcomas
	Ovarian peritoneal carcinoma
Emergencies	Obstruction
	Hemorrhage
Cancer prevention	Colectomy (familial polyposis)
	Orchidopexy (testicular tumors)

Table 3–2. SURGICAL BIOPSY TECHNIQUES

Technique	Method	Example
Incisional	Removal of small portion of tissue, performed under a general or local anesthetic	Punch or shave biopsy
Excision	Removal of complete tumor with little or no margin of surrounding tissue	Lump biopsy
Needle	Aspiration of fluid or actual tissue	Aspiration of breast lump
Exfoliative	Direct smear or scrape or examination of shed cells	Papanicolaou smear
Endoscopy	Removal of tissue from normally inaccessible sites using a rigid or fiberoptic instrument	Laryngoscopy Cystoscopy Bronchoscopy

Alternatively, a laparotomy may be used to obtain tissue specimens and as a basis for treatment planning.

A second-look procedure may be performed to confirm the absence or presence of disease after other treatments. Staging laparotomies are becoming less common with the widespread availability of advanced diagnostic procedures, laboratory tests, and assessment of tumor markers as a means to evaluate response to treatment.

COMPLICATIONS OF OTHER TREATMENT METHODS

Surgery may be deemed appropriate to treat the complications of other treatment methods used in oncology.

RESECTION OF METASTASES

In selected cases, there is a place for resection of isolated metastases. This usually is performed when cure will be effected and when the cancer is controlled at the primary site.

CYTOREDUCTIVE SURGERY

The place for this type of surgery is controversial. In theory, cytoreductive surgery should be beneficial in reducing tumor cell mass to a level that will render chemotherapy, immunotherapy, and host defenses more effective.

SURGERY FOR ONCOLOGIC EMERGENCIES

The decision to intervene surgically in oncologic emergencies is often highly controversial and something of an ethical dilemma. Whatever the procedure, the end result should optimally relieve symptoms and improve the quality of the patient's life.

PROPHYLACTIC SURGERY

In the area of cancer prevention, there are certain clinical settings in which the use of surgery can be effective. Surgery is used in the management of certain familial diseases. For example, certain women with a very high risk may become candidates for prophylactic mastectomy as a treatment alternative to surveillance.

THE SURGICAL EXPERIENCE: IMPLICATIONS FOR THE PATIENT AND FOR NURSING MANAGEMENT

To provide optimal perioperative care for the patient undergoing surgery for malignant disease, nursing care needs to be based on psychosocial as well as biologic factors. Managing pain, meeting nutritional requirements, and attending to wound care often present real problems for the surgeon, nurse, and patient.

Pain-relieving measures, such as epidural analgesia and patient-administered analgesia, are being used increasingly in cancer care to reduce the negative aspects of surgical pain.

Wound management in the cancer patient can present many problems. Healing rate and progression can be severely hindered by a patient's nutritional status, immunologic response, age, drug therapy, and prior exposure to radiotherapy. Care of all wounds should be directed toward providing the ideal microenvironment to effect successful healing.

Products come with varying claims, and nurses must recognize that they have a responsibility to their patients to evaluate and investigate thoroughly all products before using them in the clinical setting.

Considerable investigation of surgery-related anxiety and stress has been conducted, and the patient's need for information has been pinpointed as a highly significant factor in reducing perioperative anxiety.

The general implications of surgery and potential nursing interventions are presented in Tables 3–3 and 3–4 in a sequential manner from diagnosis to rehabilitation. The points illustrated in tabular form should be interpreted as guidelines.

REHABILITATION AND SUPPORTIVE CARE

The diagnosis and treatment of malignancy assault many facets of a person's identity. It usually produces feelings of vulnerability and a heightened awareness of the patient's

Table 3-3. PREOPERATIVE CARE

Patient Needs	Nursing Implications or Interventions
Care Relating to Diagnosis and Biopsy	
Preparation for procedure	Have knowledge of and initiate appropriate preparation (e.g., bowel preparation, skin preparation, positioning)
Information and learning	Identify and provide appropriate information
	Use written and verbal material to assist in reinforcement
Emotional support	Promote a nurse–client relationship that encourages patient to voice fears and anxieties
	Provide information
	If appropriate, involve family or significant others so they can be supported and supportive
Care Relating to Surgical Intervention	
Specific preparation	Have knowledge and initiate appropriate preparation
	Take nursing history, which should include patient profile and assessment of baseline physiologic parameters

24

Physical comfort	Assess of needs or deficits (e.g., skin integrity, nutritional status, mobility, fluid balance, pain assessment)
	Implement care to maintain and prevent complications of surgery
Self-care	Assess patient's abilities and deficiencies and implement care to fulfill patient's needs
	Encourage patient involvement in care planning.
Emotional support	Promote discussion to explore fears and anxieties
	Explore understandings and perceptions of disease and planned surgical procedure
	Explore implications of the disease to the patient and the anticipated outcome from the surgery
	Assess if patient is realistic
	Provide written and verbal information according to client's needs
	Involve family or significant others in discussions if appropriate
Information and learning	Teach skills to promote expectation shaping and postoperative recovery (e.g., deep breathing exercises)
	Explain use of equipment (e.g., antiemboli stockings)
	When possible, allow patient to see or handle equipment to be used postoperatively
	Explain operation and expected status after surgery

25

Table 3–4. POSTOPERATIVE CARE

Patient Needs	Nursing Implications or Interventions
Care relating to diagnosis and biopsy	
Specific care relating to procedure	Have understanding of procedure and implement appropriate care (e.g., wound and dressing care, positioning, medication)
	Assess patient's status and recovery, including physiologic status
	Observe for complications
Emotional support	Provide suitable environment for discussion of results
	Provide support for patient and significant others
	Refer to appropriate resource agencies (e.g., support programs, self-help groups, counselors)
Maintenance of physiologic status and prevention of complications	Monitor important parameters (e.g., shock, hemorrhage, wound dehiscence, infection)
Physical comfort	Monitor efficacy of pain control and implement alteration if necessary
	Give assistance with positioning and movement
	Encourage activity and rest as needed
	Provide adequate nutrition and supplement if appropriate
	Assist with elimination, ensuring patient privacy and hygiene needs are met
	Monitor fluid and electrolyte balance
	Monitor wound healing and provide skilled wound management

Self-care	Assess deficiencies in self-care abilities and implement care to fulfill needs
Information and learning	Provide information regarding specific problems or complications of the procedure
	Teach use of equipment and dressings if required
	Provide support, information, and reinforcement for future treatment plan
	Provide information and planned teaching to assist patient to adapt to altered function, physical status, etc.
	Involve family or significant others and provide information and teaching where appropriate
Emotional support	Facilitate opportunities for client to explore feelings and responses to altered health status
	Organize appropriate support agencies in liaison with client and family
	Provide information as required
	Provide environment for privacy and interaction when necessary

own mortality. It is the primary responsibility of the nurse in the period after physical recovery from surgery to discover the particular needs of the persons being cared for.

ALTERED FUNCTIONING

After surgery, all patients will experience a degree of alteration in their normal bodily functions and in their ability to care for themselves.

Any period of illness or psychologic stress may affect libido or potency in any person, even those without cancer. However, for those who undergo radical surgery of the abdomen or pelvis, sexual activities may be profoundly affected by both anatomic changes and changes in self-esteem and body image.

The nurse can be of enormous assistance in helping patients to "work through" their feelings about how they perceive themselves and what problems they anticipate in the future. Watson found that patients who had received counseling interventions demonstrated positive alterations in self-concept and self-esteem compared with subjects who were not counseled. Patients may require counseling, advice, training, and support from many different sources to achieve successful rehabilitation.

The process of rehabilitation extends well beyond the period of hospitalization, and plans must be made to ensure that progress is maintained beyond discharge. Here the nurse's main function is to act as a coordinator for continuity of care at home and, when appropriate, to provide information about voluntary services and self-help groups that may be useful.

SUMMARY

It is our hope that this chapter has demonstrated the complexities of modern cancer surgery and the wide-ranging implications for the patients, their significant others, and health care professionals. It was our intention to propose that quality patient care can be delivered only when that care is a reflection of planning, when it is based on sound knowledge and expertise, and when it is constantly reappraised by the assessment of patients' needs.

It is our belief, based on our experience, that the ultimate goal of successful adaptation to the surgical experience can only be achieved by the promotion of a patient-centered philosophy of care, education, and support to acquire optimum self-care and control.

CHAPTER

4 Radiation Oncology

LAURA J. HILDERLEY
KAREN HASSEY DOW

Radiation therapy is the use of high-energy, ionizing radiation or x-rays to treat diseases.

PRINCIPLES OF RADIATION PHYSICS

The therapeutic goal of radiation oncology is to deliver a precise dose of ionizing radiation to a specific tumor volume while sparing the surrounding healthy tissue. Ideally, this procedure will result in eradication of tumor, repair of

---

See the corresponding chapter in *Cancer Nursing: A Comprehensive Textbook*, by Baird, McCorkle, and Grant, pp. 246–265, for a more detailed discussion of this topic, including a comprehensive list of references.

healthy tissue, and a reasonably high quality of life for the patient.

The penetrating power of ionizing radiation depends on the energy of that radiation and the composition of the tissue being traversed. Thus, radiotherapy equipment of varying energies is needed to meet particular needs.

Target Theory

Target theory proposes that radiation damage is the result of both direct and indirect hits. A *direct hit* refers to damage to DNA, the critical target. Results of a direct hit are (1) change or loss of a base (thymine, adenine, guanine, or cytosine), (2) breakage of the hydrogen bond between the two chains of the DNA molecule, (3) breaks in one or both chains of the DNA molecule, and (4) crosslinking of the chains after breakage.

An *indirect hit* refers to the ionization of water, the medium surrounding the molecular structures within the cell.

The Four Rs of Radiobiology

Although the goal of treatment is to destroy tumor tissue, healthy tissue must be preserved. Fractionation of dose is based on the following four Rs of radiobiology: repair, repopulation, redistribution, and reoxygenation.

Repair

The dose should allow repair of sublethal damage. Between daily treatment fractions, the normal tissue is able to repair radiation injury, whereas tumor cells are less likely to be able to do so.

Repopulation

Repopulation of normal cells through mitosis after repair of radiation injury allows continued proliferation of normal tissue. Tumor cells are less likely to undergo mitosis because of inability to repair sublethal damage.

Redistribution

Ionizing radiation is believed to be most effective during the mitotic stage of the cell cycle. With each successive dose of radiation, more cells are likely to be in actual mitosis through cycle delay, therefore increasing the effectiveness of each dose. Normal cells are much less likely to be delayed or redistributed in their cycle than tumor cells.

Reoxygenation

Well-oxygenated cells are more sensitive to radiation effect than are hypoxic cells. Protracted fractionation of dose allows reoxygenation and, therefore, enhances radiosensitivity of tumor cells, which may have been hypoxic.

Biologic Response to Radiation

Response to radiation occurs at the cellular level, triggering a sequence of biologic events that result in tissue injury, destruction, or ultimate repair.

Radiosensitivity

Radiosensitivity refers to the degree and speed of response to radiation of any given tissue, whether tumor or normal healthy tissue. Within the cell cycle, radiosensitivity also varies, and, according to Hall (1) cells are most sensitive at or close to mitosis, (2) resistance is usually greatest in the latter part of the S-phase, (3) if G_1 has an appreciable length, a resistant period is evident early in G_1, followed by a sensitive period toward the end of G_1, and (4) the G_2-phase is usually sensitive, perhaps as sensitive as the M-phase, to radiation.

Radiosensitivity varies with the type of tumor as well as with its size and location.

Radiocurability

Radiocurability is a term used to describe the ability to eradicate tumor at the local or regional site. Unfortunately, radiosensitivity does not necessarily equate with radiocurability.

RADIATION TECHNIQUES

Two means of delivering radiation therapy are used: teletherapy and brachytherapy.

Teletherapy

Teletherapy (from *tele*, Greek prefix meaning at a distance) is external radiation treatment given with a machine or source at some distance from the target site.

GOALS OF RADIATION THERAPY IN CANCER MANAGEMENT

Radiation therapy has multiple applications in cancer treatment.

Curative radiation therapy generally refers to a situation in which this modality is the primary treatment, as in treating skin cancers or early-stage breast, laryngeal, or prostate cancers. When the intent is curative and radiation is the primary method being used, the treatment course is generally longer and the dose is higher than in a palliative situation.

Radiation therapy is also used to *control* local disease and often is combined with chemotherapy and surgery in achieving local and regional control.

Adjuvant therapy is given to enhance or assist the primary method of treatment. For example, radiation is used in an adjuvant manner when it is given preoperatively for early colorectal cancers.

Approximately one half of all patients treated with radiation therapy are treated for *palliation* of symptoms. Treatment to sites of bone metastases is very effective in relieving pain as well as in restoring mobility in some situations. Pain attributable to pressure or obstruction of a hollow viscus by bulky lesions can be palliated with radiotherapy. Other situations requiring palliation include bleeding, necrosis, ulceration, superior vena caval (SVC) syndrome, central nervous system metastases, and functional obstruction (respiratory, gastrointestinal, genitourinary). Principles of palliative treatment include use of a short, sometimes intensive course of treatment to achieve a rapid result. This is especially important if quality of life is diminished or disturbed more by the daily travel to the treatment facility than by the symptoms being palliated.

STEPS TO DELIVERY OF RADIATION THERAPY
Consultation

The patient's initial visit to the radiation therapy facility is for consultation, assessment, and discussion of the role of radiation in his or her treatment. During this visit, a complete history is taken, a physical examination is performed, and a plan of radiation is described.

Treatment Planning

Before radiation treatments can be started, a series of steps is taken to define the treatment target, ensure the accuracy of daily setups, and protect healthy tissues from radiation injury. The radiation technologist, physics staff members, and radiotherapist are involved in a process termed *simulation*. In simulation, the target volume is localized and defined by using x-rays, scans, and physical landmarks.

Immobilization devices, such as casts (or other molded materials), head holders, or restraints, may be needed to ensure accurate positioning.

Skin markings are needed to define the target or portal. During simulation, ink marks are placed to indicate the area of treatment as well as to mark the coordinate points as a guide to proper positioning. At a later point, permanent tattoos are placed to identify the field and coordinate points, at which time the ink markings may be removed.

Lead blocks often are needed to help shape the radiation beam and block radiation from reaching organs and tissues adjacent to the tumor site.

Computerized treatment plans based on measurements and radiographs taken during simulation as well as on beam characteristics are now a routine part of treatment planning.

RADIATION TREATMENTS

When simulation and treatment planning are complete, the patient begins a course of therapy, which ranges from 2 to 8 weeks, with the average course lasting 5 weeks. Treatments are given on a daily basis, 5 days per week. Altered fractionation regimens (such as two treatments per day, fewer than five treatments per week, or single hemibody treatments of very large doses) may be employed in special situations.

Treatment Process

Teletherapy treatments take only a few minutes of actual radiation exposure and require approximately 10 minutes in the treatment room altogether. Most of this time is spent in positioning the patient and the machine, then repositioning the beam to a second, third, or fourth angle to treat each prescribed field.

During a course of treatment, the patient is usually seen and examined by the radiotherapist or the nurse (or both) at least once per week. This status check (on-therapy review) serves to monitor the progress of treatment, to assess reactions, and to offer supportive physical and emotional interventions.

The Posttreatment Period

When a course of treatment has been completed, the radiation therapy patient is again examined by the radiation oncologist and the nurse. The appropriate physical examination is followed by review of posttreatment instructions and discussion of changes that can be expected in the coming weeks. Posttreatment evaluation varies in scope from a physical examination to multiple radiographic studies.

SIDE EFFECTS AND THEIR MANAGEMENT

Most side effects of radiation therapy are confined to those tissues and organs within the path of the radiation beam. Onset, severity, and duration of reactions can be correlated with the cell renewal characteristics of the target tissue, total dose, fractionation, concomitant therapies, nutritional status, and volume of tissue irradiated.

Side effects, which occur during a course of treatment and up to 6 months afterward, are considered acute reactions. Acute radiation reactions develop as a result of radiation effect on cell renewal tissues of the skin and mucous membranes. Size and number of doses (fractionation) and the length of course (protraction) are the factors that influence the severity of acute side effects. Acute effects usually resolve fairly quickly when treatment is completed as the rate of new cell proliferation returns to normal and cell destruction ends.

Late or chronic effects of ionizing radiation—which persist or occur 6 months or more after treatment—frequently are unrelated to the occurrence or severity of acute reactions. Late effects appear to be closely related to *total* dose of radiation and *size* of dose fraction. Table 4–1 lists major site-specific early and late effects of radiation therapy.

Common Acute Side Effects of Radiation Therapy: Symptom Management
Skin reactions

Regardless of body site, radiation must penetrate skin to reach its target within the body. Skin reaction varies from very mild erythema to moist desquamation, and some patients exhibit no skin changes at all. An example of skin care instructions for the patient is shown in Table 4–2.

Alopecia

When the head is irradiated, alopecia (either partial or complete) will occur. Doses between 30 and 35 Gy cause temporary hair loss, with regrowth starting approximately 1 month after treatment. Rate of regrowth varies, but most patients will have a reasonable regrowth in 6 to 9 months. At higher doses (40 Gy and above) to the scalp, alopecia is usually permanent.

Radiation-induced alopecia is not preventable. However, care of the hair and scalp is important in minimizing skin reaction. Use of a mild shampoo, followed by thorough rinsing and gentle towel drying, is recommended. Patients should avoid hair dryers, curling devices, chemicals (for coloring or curling), and even vigorous brushing of the hair. Areas particularly susceptible to erythema and desquamation include the forehead and periauricular tissues.

Mucositis

Intraoral and pharyngeal reactions include xerostomia, taste alterations, mucosal erythema, and mucositis. Severity is dose related, with onset of symptoms occurring at doses of 20 to 25 Gy. Oral care includes use of a soft toothbrush and frequent rinsing with water, saline solution, or nonalcohol-containing oral care preparations. Elixir of benadryl and water in a 1-ounce to 1-quart solution makes a mild, soothing rinse. Inspection of the oral cavity and assessment for candidiasis should be done regularly. Nystatin (Mycostatin) (tablets or suspensions) or ketoconazole tablets can be suspensions prescribed for candidiasis.

Dental consultation before treatment is essential for patients who will be having treatments to the oral cavity. Salivary changes can lead to late radiation caries, particularly after high doses to the mouth or oral cavity. Dental prophylaxis, fluoride treatments, and coverage with antibiotics before any dental extractions or other oral surgery procedures are recommended after treatment.

Table 4–1. MAJOR ACUTE AND CHRONIC SIDE EFFECTS OF RADIATION THERAPY

Site	Acute Effect	Chronic Effect
Skin	Erythema (3000–4000 cGy); dry desquamation, moist desquamation (4500–6000 cGy)	Fibrosis, atrophy, telangiectasia, permanent darkening of skin
Oral cavity	Change and loss of taste, dryness, mucositis (3000–4000 cGy)	Permanent xerostomia, permanent taste alterations, dental caries
Esophagus	Pain, esophagitis	Fibrosis
Stomach	Nausea and vomiting (125 cGy)	Obstruction, ulceration, fibrosis
Intestines	Diarrhea (2000–3000 cGy)	Malabsorption strictures, necrosis (6000–7000 cGy)
Kidney		Radiation nephritis
Bladder	Cystitis (3000 cGy)	Fibrosis, contracted bladder (6500–7000 cGy)
Bone marrow	↓ White blood cells and platelets	May be chronic anemia especially with combined modality treatment
Respiratory system	Pneumonitis (2500–3000 cGy)	Fibrosis

Continued

35

Table 4-1. MAJOR ACUTE AND CHRONIC SIDE EFFECTS OF RADIATION THERAPY *Continued*

Site	Acute Effect	Chronic Effect
Cardiovascular system	Rare reports of pericarditis, myocarditis	Fibrosis
Central nervous system	Edema and inflammation	Infarction, occlusion, necrosis
Brain and spinal cord		
Peripheral nerves		
Eyes		Cataracts
Bone and cartilage (child)		Growth disturbances if growth plate of bone is in field (2000–3000 cGy)
Gonads		
Spermatogonia	↓ Sperm count after 90–120 days; temporary sterility (100–300 cGy)	
Ovary	Sterility (500–1000 cGy) depends on age	

From Strohl, R. (1988). The nursing role in radiation oncology: Symptom management of acute and chronic reactions. *Oncology Nursing Forum, 15*(4), 431. Reprinted by permission.

Table 4–2. SKIN CARE DURING RADIATION

Skin over the area where you are receiving radiation therapy needs to be treated with gentle care. During your course of radiation treatment, please follow these guidelines.

KEEP THE TREATED AREA DRY AND FREE FROM IRRITATION

- Do not wash the treated area until the technologist tells you to. This may not be until 2 or 3 days after the start of treatments.
- Do not remove the lines or ink marks that have been placed on your skin until the technologist or doctor tells you to.
- When permitted, wash the treated skin gently, using a mild soap, and rinse well before patting dry. Always use warm or cool water, *not* hot water.
- Do not apply any lotions, creams, alcohol, aftershave, perfume, deodorants, or other preparations in the treated area.
- Heating pads and hot-water bottles should not be used on treated skin.
- Avoid friction, that is, avoid clothing that is tight or may rub over the treated skin, such as tight shirt collars, ties, undergarments, belts, and so forth.
- Men should use an electric razor if they are receiving treatment to the face or neck area. Do not use aftershave.
- If treated skin becomes reddened or tender, you may apply a thin layer of vitamin A and D ointment. Be sure to tell us when this happens. If further irritation develops, we will give you special instructions or medications for skin care.
- Protect the treatment area from exposure to direct sunlight. While you are receiving a course of therapy, do not sunbathe or spend more than a few minutes in the bright sun if the treated area is exposed. We will give you special instructions about future sun exposure when you finish your course of treatment.

Reproduced by permission from Philip G. Maddock and Laura Hilderley, Radiation Oncology, Warwick, Rhode Island.

Esophagitis

Esophagitis can occur when the chest is irradiated. Onset of symptoms is usually marked by a sensation of a lump in the throat or an object stuck in the esophagus. This can be due to edema or to spasm of the esophageal musculature, triggered by the presence of food attempting to pass the irritated mucosa. Within a few days, true esophagitis with dysphagia develops, and the patient experiences pain, particularly when attempting to eat.

Antacids and mild anesthetic agents may be helpful in relieving symptoms. However, until treatment is completed and healing takes place, the discomfort remains.

Dietary adjustments are necessary when intraoral or esophageal mucositis occurs. Protein and calorie requirements may be met with the use of liquid food supplements and soft foods. In addition, the diet should be bland to avoid further local irritation.

Nausea and vomiting

Treatment to the abdomen, particularly to large fields, can cause nausea and vomiting. Patients receiving spinal irradiation (especially to the thoracic and lumbar vertebrae) also may have nausea, and occasionally patients will experience nausea after lower abdominal or pelvic field radiation. Nausea and vomiting are not, however, an inevitable side effect of radiation therapy. Even when treatment is expected to produce these distressing symptoms, reaction can be minimized or prevented with the use of antiemetics. The prescribed medication should be taken before treatment and repeated as necessary. In addition, a light diet should be consumed before treatment and for several hours afterward.

The new patient may have an element of anxiety, which enhances the potential for radiation-induced nausea.

Diarrhea

Patients at risk for radiation-induced diarrhea include those receiving treatment to the abdomen or pelvis. Normal cell loss coupled with radiation-induced cell injury results in flattening or loss of the villi. This, in turn, decreases the absorptive surface area of the intestine, leading to diarrhea. The diarrhea is usually dose related and occurs after doses of 18 to 30 Gy.

Diarrhea is usually controlled with dietary modification (low-residue diet) and various antidiarrheal medications.

Fatigue

Fatigue is a common occurrence in the person receiving radiation therapy. Theories presented to explain the occurrence of fatigue include (1) increased metabolic rate, (2) the presence of toxic breakdown products as a result of cell injury or death, (3) energy expenditure required for tissue repair, and (4) the tiring effects of travel to and from the radiation facility on a daily basis.

Patients should be told they may experience fatigue as treatment progresses. If not forewarned, they may become concerned that their fatigue is an indication of tumor progression.

BRACHYTHERAPY

Brachytherapy is the form of internal radiation therapy in which a radioactive isotope is used for surface, interstitial, or intracavitary application. Brachytherapy techniques provide for a high dose of radiation to be delivered to the treated tumor volume and a rapid fall-off in radiation dose in adjacent normal tissues.

Brachytherapy techniques may be used as the sole method for delivering radiation therapy dose. In most instances, however, this therapy is combined with external beam radiation (teletherapy) to improve local control of disease, preserve vital function, and spare normal surrounding tissues from damage.

Repair

Brachytherapy provides for a continuous low-dose rate of radiation. Sublethal damage accumulation decreases at a low-dose rate. Thus, repair of cells in the radiated volume is less likely after continuous low-dose radiation.

Redistribution and Repopulation

With continuous low-dose rate radiation, a greater percentage of cells are blocked in G_2 and are damaged by the radiation. The repopulation of the tumor during continuous low-dose rate radiation results in cells that progress to late G_2, are blocked in their progression through the cell cycle, and are likely to be destroyed by the radiation.

Reoxygenation

With a dose of radiation delivered continuously at a low rate, there is a decreased requirement for oxygen to eradicate the tumor. Thus, brachytherapy techniques may be more effective in treating anoxic tumors than techniques using conventional, fractionated external beam radiation.

Modes of Radioactive Emission and Decay

The process in which an unstable isotope transforms to a stable one is known as radioactive decay or disintegration. Decay products are alpha and beta particles and gamma rays.

Mechanism of Radiation Injury

Alpha and beta particles and gamma rays produce damage by transferring energy to living matter. They ionize molecules in cells to cause physical and chemical changes that affect the biologic processes responsible for reproduction. Irradiated cells are either destroyed or rendered incapable of reproduction.

Other Radioactive Properties

Sealed or Unsealed Sources. A sealed radioactive source is one in which the radioactive isotope is contained within an outer sheath of material, such as platinum. An unsealed source is contained in a colloidal suspension and placed in direct contact with tissues.

Half-life. The half-life of a radioactive isotope refers to the time it takes for it to decay to 50% of its activity.

General Nursing Care Guidelines

Nursing care may differ slightly depending on the type of radioactive isotope used, whether it is a sealed or unsealed source, and whether it is a temporary or permanent implant.

Sealed, temporary sources include radium-226, cesium-137, and iridium-192. Because they are sealed sources, they do not present a potential contamination problem. Owing to their long half-lives, these sources are inserted into body tissue or cavities for a specified time period and are then removed. Once the implant is loaded, time spent in the room should be minimized and distance maximized. Patients with radioactive implants must have a private room with private bath.

Dose limits for the public are 500 millirems (5 mSv) per year. Therefore, each visitor should be limited to approximately one-half hour per day. A distance of at least 6 feet is to be maintained between the visitors and the source of radiation. Pregnant women and children under the age of 18 are prohibited from visiting.

A pair of long-handled forceps and a lead container should be present in the patient's room. In the extremely unusual—but still potential—event that a source becomes dislodged from the patient, forceps must be used to retrieve the source, which should then be placed in the lead container. The radioactive source should never be touched with bare hands.

Sealed, permanent implants, such as gold-198 and iodine-125, seeds have a short half-life, so they may be inserted permanently into tissues, such as the prostate. Because these sources decay rapidly, patients may be discharged home within a few days after implantation. However, radiation dose levels must be less than 30 millicuries (111×10^7 Bq) of activity before patients may be discharged from the hospital.

Use of unsealed sources, such as iodine-131 in the treatment of hyperthyroidism, requires special precautions because it presents a potential contamination hazard. As iodine-131 is systemically administered, the isotope is excreted in feces, urine, vomitus, saliva, sweat, and other body fluids. One half of the radioactive iodine is excreted in the first 2 days. During this time, rubber gloves should be worn while providing direct care. Patients must flush the toilet several times after each bowel movement or urination.

Because linen and patient gowns may be contaminated, they must be kept in separate isolation bags. Other articles in the room, such as telephone, call light, and floors, must be covered with plastic. Disposable plastic or paper products should be used for dietary trays and utensils.

Standards for Radiation Safety

Regardless of maximum limits, occupational exposure should be "as low as reasonably achievable," or ALARA.

Principles of Time, Distance, and Shielding

The way in which nurses can keep radiation exposure limits as low as reasonably achievable is to follow three key principles of time, distance, and shielding.

Time

The longer the time of exposure, the greater the amount of absorbed radiation. Generally, nurses are limited to one-half hour per shift of direct time with the patient.

Distance

Radiation exposure and distance are inversely related. That is, the intensity of radiation decreases as the square of the distance from the source increases.

Shielding

The type of shielding device used in brachytherapy depends on the type of particle or gamma ray. Alpha particles are not an external hazard. Most beta particles are not external hazards because they cannot penetrate the outermost layer of skin. Gamma rays are indirectly ionizing, and a percentage of gamma rays can pass through any shield. The percentage of radiation that can penetrate decreases as the thickness of the shield increases.

Personnel Monitoring Devices

Personnel monitoring devices, which are required by law, offer a measure of radiation safety and protection. Devices do not protect the individual from radiation but only provide a record of exposure.

Nurses must always wear a monitoring device when caring for patients with implants. Monitoring devices are intended to provide an accurate record of occupational exposure and should not be worn outside the hospital. The film badge is the most widely used personnel monitor because it is accurate, reliable, and inexpensive to use. A film badge should not be shared.

Summary of Brachytherapy

Safety and protection are essential in providing care for patients with radioactive implants. Radiation safety and protection require basic knowledge of the physical properties of the radioisotopes and application of the principles of time, distance, and shielding.

Intraoperative radiation therapy is accomplished by surgically exposing the tumor-bearing organ, excising the diseased portion, and then delivering a single high dose of radiation directly to the tumor bed. Because noninvolved organs, such as the intestine, can be packed out of the pathway of the radiation beam, little or no radiation effect is seen except in the target site.

After the radiation dose has been delivered, the incision is closed, and the patient is transferred to the recovery unit. Once the patient recovers from surgery, a further course of external beam therapy usually is given.

Hyperthermia

The use of controlled hyperthermia *combined* with radiation therapy has been shown to achieve tumor cell killing without excess toxicity to normal tissue.

Several factors combine to produce the desired biologic effect of hyperthermia plus radiation therapy.

1. Hyperthermia is known to be most effective during the S-phase of the cell cycle, when radiation is *least effective*.
2. Hypoxic cells that are generally radioresistant are heat sensitive.
3. Heat inhibits repair of radiation injury.

Nurses caring for patients receiving hyperthermia therapy may have multiple responsibilities, including surgical assistance with probe implantation, monitoring treatment tolerance, and assessing posttreatment response for research protocols.

Chemical Modifiers of Radiation Effect

Radiosensitizers and radioprotectors are chemical compounds used to modify the effect of radiation on cells and tissues. The rationale for the use of radiosensitizers is based on the knowledge that many tumors have hypoxic portions that are highly radioresistant (oxygen effect). Chemical radiosensitizers are drugs that take the place of oxygen in hypoxic cells in order to enhance radiation effectiveness. Compounds in current use include SR-2508, RO-03-8799, metronidazole, misonidazole, and desmethylmisonidazole.

Pyrimidine analogs (BUdR, IUdR) also are useful as radiosensitizers. These substances are very readily incorporated into DNA and subsequently inhibit the repair of sublethal damage. Perfluorocarbons are a third group of chemical modifiers that absorb high amounts of oxygen when exposed to hyperbaric conditions, then release oxygen when environmental oxygen is low.

Thiol depletors, such as diethyl maleate (DEM) and butionine sulphoximine (BSO), act to deplete intracellular glutathione (GSH) before irradiation. The presence of GSH tends to protect against radiation damage and decreases the radiosensitivity of tumor cells.

Protection of normal tissue while enhancing tumor radiosensitivity is a therapeutic challenge. Compounds that serve as radioprotectors must be selective to the healthy tissue to obtain the desired results. Sulfhydryl compounds are the major group of radioprotectors currently under investigation and are described as scavengers in their affinity for the products of irradiated water.

Whenever therapies are combined to produce greater cytotoxicity, side effects also are increased. In addition, radiosensitizers characteristically have their own specific side effects of neurotoxicity and affect both the central and peripheral nervous systems. Prominent among these effects are peripheral neuropathy, somnolence, confusion, and transient coma. Gastrointestinal effects (nausea and vomiting) also are frequently seen.

Patient and family education in preparation for treatment with chemical modifiers is essential.

SUMMARY

Radiation therapy, whether used alone as the primary treatment of cancer or combined in a multimodality approach, has a major role in oncology. Nurses caring for oncology patients in all settings have a responsibility to assist the patient and family by providing accurate information about radiation therapy.

5 Medical Oncology— The Agents

JENNIFER L. GUY

Medical oncology focuses on the systemic management of malignant disease by the use of antineoplastic medications, commonly referred to as *chemotherapy*. Chemotherapy is "the treatment of disease by chemical agents; first applied to the use of chemicals that attack the causative organisms unfavorably but do not harm the patient." Chemotherapy administered to patients for the management of confined or disseminated malignant disease is the focus of this discussion.

Today, many diseases are curable with chemotherapy. Prolonged disease-free intervals and increased survival times have been documented with chemotherapeutic intervention for a number of tumors. For other tumors, chemotherapy can help to control pain and ease suffering.

The clinical management of medical oncology patients is based on an understanding of the principles of chemotherapeutic intervention and of the host factors that determine the choice of drugs, dose, route, and schedule, as well as knowledge of the agents and their acute and delayed toxicities.

HISTORICAL PERSPECTIVES

The concept of using chemicals to treat malignant disease dates to the sixteenth century, when heavy metals were used systemically to treat cancers. They were mostly ineffective and extremely toxic, and thus they were discarded until the resurgence of the use of arsenic in 1865 in the treatment of chronic leukemias.

Chemotherapy evolved from the unlikely province of

See the corresponding chapter in *Cancer Nursing: A Comprehensive Textbook*, by Baird, McCorkle, and Grant, pp. 266–290, for a more detailed discussion of this topic, including a comprehensive list of references.

chemical warfare. During World War I, soldiers were observed to suffer severe bone marrow suppression, aplasia, and death after exposure to sulfur mustard gas. World War II fostered the recognition of the therapeutic application of alkylating agents to the treatment of malignancy. In the 1960s and early 1970s, multidrug chemotherapy regimens were found to improve remission rates without inducing undue toxicity. The use of chemotherapy in combination with other methods of cancer treatment also came into clinical practice at this time.

The 1970s and 1980s were dedicated to the synthesis and clinical testing of available agents, alone and in combination, and the continued screening and synthesis of new agents. The antineoplastic effects of biologic response modifiers were identified in these decades and are currently under investigation to define their role in oncologic therapeutics.

PRINCIPLES OF CHEMOTHERAPY ADMINISTRATION

Chemotherapy may be administered as a single agent, but combinations of antineoplastic agents are more effective than single agents in tumors that are responsive (i.e., sensitive) to multiple agents. The basic principle of combination chemotherapy regimens is to administer simultaneously multiple drugs that do not have overlapping toxicities.

Chemotherapy may be administered as the primary curative modality. Control of malignant disease may be accomplished with chemotherapy when improved survival can be demonstrated. Palliation may be accomplished with chemotherapy.

As an adjunct to curative surgical resection, chemotherapy has been shown to improve the disease-free interval and survival in breast cancer. The success of adjuvant chemotherapy depends on effective agents.

Chemotherapy may be employed preoperatively in an attempt to convert nonresectable disease to resectable disease. Preoperative chemotherapy is sometimes referred to as neoadjuvant therapy.

CLASSIFICATION OF ANTINEOPLASTICS

Cancer chemotherapy agents are classified into several categories on the basis of their mechanism of action, derivation, and chemical structure.

Alkylating Agents

Alkylating agents, the oldest class of antineoplastics, act by substituting an alkyl group ($R-CH_2-CH_2$) for a hydrogen atom in organic compounds. The ultimate effect is an abnormal crosslinking of DNA base pairs that results in cell death or mutation by altering the decoding and replication process. Alkylating agents are most active in the G_0 or resting cell; they are noncell cycle specific.

The selection of alkylators for clinical use must consider

the patient's hepatic function (biotransformation), renal function (excretion), bone marrow reserves (myelosuppression), and inherent alkylator sensitivity of the tumor. Because of the mutagenic, teratogenic, and carcinogenic capabilities of alkylators, patient age and childbearing capability also should be considered.

Plant Alkaloids

The plant alkaloids are so named because they are extracted from foliage. The vinca alkaloids are extracted from the periwinkle plant *(Vinca rosea)*. These cell cycle-specific, phase-specific compounds arrest mitosis (M).

Antimetabolites

This group exerts its effect by interrupting cellular metabolic function. These agents are structurally similar to intracellular substances. The cell incorporates them into essential sites of cellular metabolism and then is unable to continue to divide. Antimetabolites are classified by the compounds with which they interfere.

Antimetabolites are phase specific in the S-phase. They are most effective in tumors with a high growth fraction.

Miscellaneous Antineoplastics

A few agents with clinical use exist whose mechanism of action is poorly defined or unique.

HORMONALLY ACTIVE AGENTS

Many tumors arise from hormonally active tissues. Manipulations of the hormonal milieu are used to inhibit their growth. Hormonal manipulations are based on the observation that tumor cells contain surface receptors for specific hormones, which are then transported intracellularly and are required for cell growth. Antineoplastic hormonal manipulations include obliterating host production of the required hormone, blocking the hormone receptors with competing agents, and substituting chemically similar agents for the active hormone, which cannot be used by the tumor cell.

Adrenocorticosteroids have direct antineoplastic effects in hematologic malignancies. Agents that block the production of adrenocorticosteroids also are used in the treatment of hormonally active cancers.

NEW HORIZONS

The 1980s saw the initiation of investigations into alternative delivery mechanisms of chemotherapy. High-dose chemotherapy with autologus bone marrow transplantation, regional chemotherapy, such as arterial infusions in the treatment of liver metastasis and brain tumors, and limb perfusions in the treatment of melanoma are under investigation.

Additional approaches to combined therapy, such as hyperthermia and perioperative (neoadjuvant) chemotherapy, doubtlessly will be explored through the end of the century. Hyperthermia is used to increase the core temperature of the tumor before treatment with radiation therapy or chemotherapy in an effort to enhance cell kill. Perioperative or neoadjuvant chemotherapy is administered preoperatively, during, or immediately after the surgical procedures.

Chemotherapy is a mainstay of cancer treatment. It is a continually and constantly changing modality whose role is well established in some malignancies and evolutionary in others. As the predominant systemic therapy for malignant disease, chemotherapy will continue to play a major role in oncologic therapeutics.

6 Delivery of Cancer Chemotherapy

MICHELLE GOODMAN

At no other time in the history of medical oncology have the schedule, method, and route of administration of chemotherapy been so varied. Although most drugs are given systemically, regional drug therapy is gaining prominence. Currently, antineoplastic agents are being administered directly into the peritoneal cavity to treat metastases of ovarian carcinoma and colon cancer, into the bladder intravesically to treat early bladder cancer, into the central nervous system to treat meningeal carcinomatosis, and into the arterial system for more direct organ or limb perfusion, which may be the treatment for metastatic colon cancer to the liver or osteogenic sarcoma.

The clinician who administers chemotherapy should have a thorough knowledge of the drugs, their modes of administration, distribution, and elimination, and the technical skills of venipuncture and management of vascular access devices (VADs).

This chapter discusses issues pertinent to chemotherapy administration. These issues include determining the qualifications of the clinician who administers chemotherapy, safe handling of chemotherapy, prevention and management

See the corresponding chapter in *Cancer Nursing: A Comprehensive Textbook,* by Baird, McCorkle, and Grant, pp. 291–320, for a more detailed discussion of this topic, including a comprehensive list of references.

of extravasation of vesicant agents, VADs, and systemic and regional drug delivery.

CHEMOTHERAPY ADMINISTRATION
Professional Qualifications

Chemotherapy drugs are administered to patients in a variety of health care settings, including the hospital, the outpatient facility, and the home. To ensure optimal quality of care and patient safety, antineoplastic agents are administered by professional nurses who have received specialized training in chemotherapy administration.

Preparation and Handling of Antineoplastic Agents

With more than 500,000 patients receiving antineoplastic agents for cancer treatment, it is estimated that thousands of health care employees (e.g., pharmacists, nurses, physicians, housekeeping and maintenance personnel) are potentially at risk for adverse health effects from exposure to these drugs. Although exposure levels during preparation, administration, and disposal are much lower than the pharmacologic doses received by the patient, health care workers' exposure can be additive over many years. In addition, these is no known maximal safe level of exposure below which there is no risk. It is believed that the extent of health risk to employees who handle antineoplastic drugs is a combination of exposure time, amount and method of exposure, and class of drug. The main routes of exposure are inhalation of drug aerosols or droplets, absorption through the skin and mucous membranes either during preparation and handling or during exposure to the patient's body fluids and linens, and ingestion through contact with contaminated food or cigarettes.

The potential hazards of chemotherapy exposures are many and varied when health care personnel do not follow recommendations for safe handling of these drugs. Physical complaints, such as skin, mucous membrane, and eye irritation, lightheadedness, facial flushing, hair loss, nausea, and headache, may be experienced.

A study by Rogers and Emmett found that the association between exposure to antineoplastic agents during pregnancy and spontaneous abortion was statistically significant, with a risk factor of 2.5 for those handling antineoplastic agents without the use of personal protective equipment.

Current evidence suggests that if appropriate safety measures are employed, potential health hazards will be minimized. The Occupational Safety and Health Administration (OSHA) recommendations and the Oncology Nursing Society's cancer chemotherapy guidelines are offered as standards to be incorporated into institutional policies and procedures.

The nurse often is the central figure in establishing appropriate policies and procedures for chemotherapy drug administration. Applying the aforementioned recommendations and guidelines to one's practice setting requires that the nurse remain informed of current issues in drug handling safety and establish a means of sharing that knowledge with other members of the health care team.

Chemotherapy Administration: The Setting

Chemotherapy is administered in various physical settings, including the ambulatory setting, outpatient clinic, physician's private office, hospital setting, and patient's home. Whatever the setting, certain precautions must be taken to ensure a safe environment for the patient and the health care worker. Emergency drugs and resuscitation equipment, including suction tubes and oxygen tanks, should be available and in good working order. Emergency drugs may be needed to take care of fluid overload, heart attack, or respiratory distress as a result of aspiration or anaphylaxis. Policies and procedures for the management of such complications should be known to all concerned. An extravasation kit should be available in the event that a vesicant agent is infiltrated. Up-to-date procedures for the management of extravasation for particular vesicant agents should be included in each kit.

To ensure a safe work environment, a physician should be available in the event of unforeseen complications of therapy. A physician should be present especially when patients are receiving blood, lengthy infusions, or agents that are under investigation. A call light or similar mechanism should be available and within easy reach of the patient.

Chemotherapy Administration: Preparing the Patient and Family

The ideal situation for teaching the patient and family is attained through the collaborative efforts of the medical oncologist, pharmacist, and oncology clinical nurse specialist. The patient should understand that it is normal to feel overwhelmed with information and that opportunities exist for reinforcement of the verbal and written information in the form of drug information cards or similar patient teaching aids. Although the physician has the responsibility of obtaining informed consent, the nurse is usually the member of the team who, during conversations with patient and family, is able to clarify the goals of treatment, restate side effects, and reassure the patient that all efforts will be made to minimize the complications of therapy.

Written or oral consent for treatment is mandatory whether the patient is receiving standard therapy or therapy of an investigational or research nature. The only difference in principle between standard and investigational therapy is that a signature is required for the latter. The purpose of this signature is to demonstrate the individual's understanding of the proposed therapy and voluntary agreement to participate in the investigational study.

Although the patient requires enough information to make a decision regarding therapy, the opportunity to ask additional questions and acquire more information may help the patient feel informed and comfortable with the decision. Five major points should be addressed concerning a patient's consent for treatment.

1. What are the possibilities of treatment-related risks and side effects, both early and delayed?

2. What are the expected benefits of therapy and goals of treatment, and how will the success or failure of the therapy be measured?

3. Is the treatment program research oriented? If so, the patient should be aware of this fact. Likewise, if any other therapy is known to be better, the individual should be offered such therapy. If another kind of therapy has been proved to be better for the individual, he or she is not eligible to participate in the research study.

4. Are there alternate forms of therapy for which the patient would be eligible? Such options are often confusing and should be explained in a straightforward manner.

5. Is the patient aware of the right to refuse therapy or to withdraw from the treatment program at any time?

Written information is not generally identified as a primary factor in a patient's decision-making process. However, written information may serve to supplement verbal information and to help family members, especially those who are not present during the verbal exchange, understand the goals of therapy.

MODES OF ADMINISTRATION

There are two fundamental methods of antineoplastic drug administration: *systemic* and *regional*. The purpose of systemic drug administration is to kill tumor cells from presumed or proven metastatic disease. The goal of systemic chemotherapy is to reach a sufficient drug concentration to achieve a therapeutic cytotoxic effect without causing excessive toxicity to normal tissues. The goals of regional chemotherapy are to deliver the drug or drugs directly into the blood vessel supplying the tumor or cavity in which the tumor is isolated. Regional therapy often permits higher doses of the drug to be delivered to the area of the tumor. Because less of the drug reaches the systemic circulation, toxicities tend to be less severe.

Systemic chemotherapy may be given orally, intravenously, subcutaneously, or intramuscularly. The dose and schedule of drug administration are determined by the effect of the drugs on both normal and neoplastic tissues. The dose usually is increased gradually until the optimal tolerable dose is reached. The major limitations of the use of systemic chemotherapy are its short-term and long-term complications.

Pretreatment Considerations

Before attempting venous access and drug delivery, it is important to consider the following.

1. If the patient is receiving chemotherapy for the first time, make sure he or she has received adequate instruction about the treatment plan and that the patient feels sufficiently informed.

2. If treatment is of an investigational nature, verify that an informed consent form has been signed before initiating therapy.

3. Check the drug dosage against the physician's order. The order should include the patient's name, name of drug or drugs, frequency of administration, and, if appropriate, rate of administration. Most drug doses are based on a calculation of milligrams per kilogram or on body surface area (m²). Body surface area usually is based on a calculation of the individual's ideal body weight and height. Obesity, ascites, or other factors, such as the loss of a limb, are important considerations in dose adjustment. Consider whether the dose and route of administration seem appropriate for the patient.

4. Check the patient's most recent laboratory test results. The complete blood count (CBC), including the platelet count, should be within normal limits or within the limits specified in the research protocol. A dose modification or treatment delay may be needed if the CBC is below normal limits.

5. If the white blood cell count (WBC) is low, calculate the absolute granulocyte count (AGC) to determine the patient's ability to fight infection. The AGC is computed by multiplying the percentages of neutrophils and bands by the total WBC. When the AGC is less than 1200 cells/mm³, treatment with myelosuppressive agents generally is not recommended. An AGC of less than 1000 cells/mm³ is associated with a more severe risk for infection.

6. Consider the way each drug is metabolized and eliminated. If there is any clinical or laboratory evidence of organ dysfunction (e.g., liver or kidney), the pharmacokinetics or pharmacodynamics of the drug may be hindered, leading to excessive toxicity. Dose reductions or treatment delays may be warranted.

7. Consider any pretreatment antiemetics, hydration, or measures to minimize hair loss.

8. Check to see that emergency equipment, including materials to manage an allergic reaction or extravasation, is available. If a vesicant is being injected, review the policy

and procedure on management of an extravasation. Be prepared to manage an allergic or anaphylactic reaction should one occur.

9. Ensure adequate lighting and patient comfort. A call light or similar method of communication should be available if the patient is left unattended or is receiving an infusion.

10. Review the patient's medication history, including over-the-counter drugs. Be alert to drug incompatibilities, drug interactions, and additive toxicities.

Intravenous Drug Administration

Chemotherapy may be given intravenously (1) through the direct push method, also known as the two-syringe technique, (2) through the side port of a freely running intravenous (IV) line, (3) as a mini-infusion, or (4) as a continuous infusion over several hours or days. The method of IV drug delivery often is dictated by the vesicant properties of the drugs, their potential to cause vein irritation, their potential for immediate or delayed complications, such as allergic reactions, hypertension, or hypotension, and the logistics of the specific treatment protocol. In general, the majority of vesicants and nonvesicants are given by the direct push method. The decision to administer a vesicant by the sidearm technique is dependent on whether the patient requires the intravenous infusion for another purpose, for example, for hydration, antiemetics, or antibiotics. The two-syringe technique is the preferred method of administering vesicant agents in that it permits precise and direct control of fluid into the vein without drug backup in the IV tubing. Briskness of blood return and appreciation of any pressure changes (resistance) in the vein are most easily perceived with the two-syringe method. Using the sidearm technique for additional dilution for vesicant agents is unnecessary because the drugs are already optimally diluted according to the package directions. Although either method of drug delivery is considered safe, it is a misconception that the sidearm technique is safer than the two-syringe technique. By way of clarification, the drug—vesicant or nonvesicant—would never be injected directly into a peripheral vein without first flushing with normal saline to ensure adequate blood flow and venous integrity.

Administering the drug as a short-term infusion is generally reserved for agents that produce untoward symptoms or complications when given by the direct push method.

Continuous infusion therapy has gained prominence as a means of overcoming cytokinetic resistance and therapy enhancing tumor response and minimizing toxicities. Prolonged exposure of cancer cells to the drugs may be beneficial because cell cycle times vary and are generally measured in days. Toxicities may be minimized because continuous infusion of chemotherapy avoids the peak plasma levels achieved by bolus administration.

Vein selection and cannulation

Only persons knowledgeable and trained in venipuncture and chemotherapy administration should administer IV chemotherapy. If the patient has a preexisting peripheral IV line, nonvesicant agents may be administered through this line provided there are no signs or symptoms of phlebitis and the blood return is adequate. If the blood return is absent or sluggish or if the IV line has been in place for longer than 24 hours, a new line should be established. If the patient is receiving a vesicant agent and has a preexisting peripheral IV line in place, it is safe to use it provided blood return is adequate and venous irritation or phlebitis is absent. This practice is especially prudent when the patient has small, fragile veins. If any doubt exists as to the integrity of the vein, a new IV line should be established before injecting the drug. The following is a list of some issues to consider in vein selection and cannulation.

1. Selecting the proper site for venipuncture should begin with a careful, systematic assessment of all available arm veins. Full visibility of the arms unencumbered by constricting jewelry or clothing aids in determining venous access, as does good lighting and a firm surface on which to place the arm.

2. All equipment required to achieve venipuncture and secure the line should be assembled before attempting venipuncture. Because this step requires the handling of chemotherapy drugs, in particular, the removal of Luer-Lok caps from the syringes containing the drugs, the nurse should put on any personal protective equipment at this time.

3. During vein selection, the nurse should avoid venipuncture in any arm with possible or proven compromised circulation (e.g., phlebitis, lymphedema due to tumor invasion or axillary dissection, and prior trauma to veins, such as drug extravasation). The risk for drug extravasation is increased when drugs are infused into an arm with evidence of superior vena cava syndrome or compromised circulation or into phlebitic veins that are inflamed and irritated.

4. To preserve venous integrity over time, the nurse should begin distally and alternate venipuncture sites, if possible. In general, veins of the dorsum of the hand are preferred because they are easy to visualize and stabilize. However, the favored site for the administration of vesicant agents is the forearm because this area has more underlying muscle and tissue to protect vital nerves and provide tissue coverage if necessary in the event of surgical management of an extravasation. With the advent of numerous VADs, it is no longer reasonable or safe to resort to administering vesicant agents in the area of the antecubital fossa.

5. If an obvious site for venipuncture is not apparent by observation or palpation following the use of traditional methods of venous distention (tourniquet, vein percussion, heat), a colleague should be consulted before attempting venipuncture. Also, seek assistance after two unsuccessful attempts to secure adequate venous access. Consider whether the patient should have a VAD placed before receiving the drug.

6. A cannula should be selected that is appropriate for both the length of the therapy and the patient's available veins. A 25- or 23-gauge scalp vein needle (butterfly) is ideal for direct push (two-syringe technique) or short-term infusions (30 to 60 minutes). A plastic thin-walled catheter is appropriate for more lengthy infusions, such as for blood components or hydration regimens that last 2 to 3 hours. The site is sterilized by a 1-minute alcohol rub or a povidone-iodine and alcohol rub. To avoid contaminating the area, do not repalpate before venipuncture. Once the scalp vein needle enters the vein and blood return is obvious, release the tourniquet and attach a syringe of saline to the tubing. Tape the phalanges of the needle securely without obstructing the entrance of the needle. Aspirate the air from the tubing and flush the catheter with 7 to 10 ml of saline to ensure that the needle has not punctured the vein. Palpate the site gently and observe for swelling or any evidence of infiltration. If the needle rests securely in the vein with a brisk, full blood return and no evidence of infiltration, the chemotherapy is injected slowly to prevent undue pressure on the vein wall. Check for blood return after every 1 to 2 ml of solution is administered. Flush the vein with 3 to 5 ml of saline between agents and with 5 to 7 ml of saline before removing the needle.

7. If the drug is to be given via the sidearm of a freely running IV line, any dressing hindering visualization of the site should be removed. The size of the needle attached to the syringe must be smaller than the size of the needle in the patient's vein to permit the IV solution to drip while the drug is being injected.

8. When injecting a vesicant into the sidearm of a peripheral IV line, the line should not be infusing with the aid of an infusion pump because of the increased potential for extravasation and the impossibility of quickly reversing the direction of drug flow in the event of a possible extravasation.

9. If a drug in combination is known to be associated with rapid onset of nausea and vomiting (e.g., high-dose cyclophosphamide or cisplatin), it is generally administered last. If a vesicant is to be given along with an infusion, it should be given first in anticipation of perivenous irritation from movement during the time of the infusion. The order of administration of drugs (vesicant first or last) has not

been shown to have any bearing on long-term venous integrity or risk of extravasation. Regardless of the order of the drugs, the line should be flushed with saline before changing drugs at the end of the treatment.

10. The entire course of the vein should be visible during the injection and infusion. Observe for any evidence of vein irritation. The patient is encouraged to report any feelings of pain, itching, or burning during the treatment.

11. A vesicant agent should not be injected distal to a previous puncture site.

12. Vesicant agents should not be infused as a mini-infusion or continuous infusion into a peripheral vein. Regardless of its dilution, the drug has the potential to cause tissue destruction if infiltration occurs. Given the ease of insertion of the numerous short-term and long-term VADs, infusing a vesicant agent into a peripheral vein places the patient at unnecessary risk for drug extravasation and tissue damage. If an infusion of a vesicant is required to achieve the optimum therapeutic result, a central venous access line, as a tunneled, a nontunneled, or an implanted device, should be inserted before initiating therapy (see Vascular Access Devices).

Management of an extravasation

Extravasation may be defined as the extrusion or passage of caustic fluid, in this case vesicant chemotherapeutic agents, from a vein into the surrounding subcutaneous tissues. Once this occurs, tissue damage of varying degrees ensues. The tissue damage may appear initially to be minimal owing to the indolent course of most extravasations. Gradually, after 3 to 5 days, the area appears obviously inflamed and is painful to the touch, providing evidence of cellular destruction. After 12 to 14 days, the actual extent of damage usually is evident, with frank ulceration, demarcation, and eschar formation. The damage to underlying structures (tendons and nerves) may lead to functional impairment. Infection and cellulitis can result in progressive tissue damage and limb dysfunction. Table 6–1 lists the antineoplastic agents according to their vesicant or irritant properties.

The reported incidence of inadvertent chemotherapy extravasation ranges from 0.45% to 5% of all toxic reactions to chemotherapy. The factors that affect the risk of extravasation are (1) the skill of the practitioner, (2) the condition of the vein, (3) the drug administration technique, (4) the order of vesicant administration, (5) the site of venous access, and (6) the use of a preexisting IV line.

Management of an extravasation depends largely on the drug infiltrated and on whether an antidote exists to inactivate the infiltrated drug. For most vesicant agents, no such antidote exists. For extravasations of these agents, it may

Table 6-1. VESICANTS AND IRRITANTS

VESICANT AGENTS: Capable of producing a blister and gradual tissue destruction with necrosis if extravasated

Commercial

Epirubicin hydrochloride (Pharmorubicin)
Dactinomycin (Cosmegen, Actinomycin, ACT-D)
Doxorubicin (Adriamycin, Rubex)
Mitomycin (Mutamycin, Mitomycin-C)
Mechlorethamine (Mustargen, nitrogen mustard)
Vinblastine (Velban, Velsar)
Vincristine (Oncovin, Vincasar)
Daunorubicin hydrochloride (Cerubidine, Daunomycin)

Investigational

Amsacrine (M-AMSA)
Bisantrene
Maytansine
Vindesine (Eldisine)
Pyrazofurin (Pyrazomycin)

IRRITANT AGENTS: Capable of producing perivenous pain at the site of injection or along the vein during injection or infusion

Commercial

Etoposide (VP-16-213, VePesid)
Carmustine (BCNU)
Streptozocin (Zanosar, Streptozotocin)
Plicamycin (Mithracin, Mithramycin)
Dacarbazine (DTIC-Dome, DTIC)
Teniposide (VM-26)

Investigational

Mitoguazone (Methyl-GAG)

---

be advisable to do nothing more than apply ice locally for symptomatic relief. Currently, two antidotes are recommended by manufacturers as treatment for inadvertent drug extravasation: sodium thiosulfate for mechlorethamine (nitrogen mustard) infiltration and hyaluronidase for vinblastine and vincristine infiltration (Table 6–2). Table 6–3 includes local treatment for vesicant infiltration.

The signs and symptoms of extravasation can be subtle. Pain, stinging, or burning can occur, but these are not always present. Resistance to flow, swelling, or diffuse induration may occur but may be less evident in an individual who is obese or dehydrated. The absence of blood return can indicate that the needle bevel is against the vein wall or that

Table 6-2. EXTRAVASATION MANAGEMENT: KNOWN ANTIDOTES AND LOCAL TREATMENT

Drug	Antidote	Antidote Preparation	Method of Administration
Mechlorethamine (nitrogen mustard)	Isotonic sodium thiosulfate (1 g/10 ml)	Mix of 4 ml of 10% sodium thiosulfate with 6 ml sterile water for injection (1:6 molar solution results)	1. For each mg of drug extravasated, inject 5 ml IV through the existing line and subcutaneously into the extravasated site* 2. Only a single course of sodium thiosulfate is recommended 3. Apply cold compresses 4. Elevate the extremity
Vinblastine (Velban) Vincristine (Oncovin)	Hyaluronidase (150 U/ml)	Add 1–3 ml USP sodium chloride to vial of hyaluronidase	*Note:* Initiate treatment immediately and liberally 1. Inject 1–3 ml of hyaluronidase solution (150 U) into needle or catheter or inject subcutaneously into site 2. Gently apply a heat pack to site for 1 hour 3. Elevate the extremity

*If subcutaneous injections are needed, a topical anesthetic such as ice or ethyl chloride may be applied to the site immediately before injection.

Table 6–3. EXTRAVASATION MANAGEMENT: LOCAL TREATMENT

Drug	Local Treatment	Method of Administration
Anthracycline antibiotics Doxorubicin (Adriamycin, Rubex) Daunomycin	Hydrocortisone solution (100-mg vial)	1. Press diluent stopper into vial to reconstitute 2. Inject 1 ml (5 mg) hydrocortisone through the indwelling IV line or, in the absence of a blood return, remove IV line and inject hydrocortisone in a radical fashion into site 3. Do not repeat dosing 4. Apply sterile bandage 5. Apply cold pack every 2–3 hours for 24 hours (on 50 minutes, off 10 minutes)
	OR	OR
	DMSO* (50%–100%) (topical)	1. Soak a sterile gauze or cotton ball in DMSO solution 2. Apply solution to site, allowing it to become saturated 3. Allow site to air dry 4. Apply a sterile bandage 5. Apply cold pack as above 6. Repeat every 4 hours for 7–10 days

Continued

59

Table 6–3. EXTRAVASATION MANAGEMENT: LOCAL TREATMENT *Continued*

Drug	Local Treatment	Method of Administration
Mitomycin C Mutamycin	DMSO (50%–100%) (topical)	1. Soak a sterile gauze or cotton ball in DMSO solution
		2. Saturate site with DMSO immediately after infiltration
		3. Allow site to air dry
		4. Apply a sterile bandage
		5. Apply ice pack for symptomatic relief only
		6. A single application of DMSO may be sufficient
	OR	OR
	Sodium thiosulfate (1 g/10 ml); mix 4 ml of 10% sodium thiosulfate with 6 ml sterile water for injection	1. Inject 3–5 ml IV through the existing line or subcutaneously into the extravasated site
		2. Cover with a sterile bandage
		3. Apply ice pack for symptomatic relief only
		4. Elevate extremity

*DMSO, dimethyl sulfoxide.

the needle is not in the vein. The presence of blood return does not guarantee that an infiltration has not occurred because the needle may have extended partially through the posterior wall of the vein, allowing for a subtle leakage of the vesicant.

How, then, does one determine whether the drug has actually infiltrated? Even a slight change in the appearance of the tissue surrounding the insertion site is ample reason to restart the injection in another vein. However, in the absence of tissue swelling, a complaint of pain, stinging, or burning or a change in the quality of the blood return is highly suspect and warrants further investigation. The first step is to stop the injection of the vesicant and immediately aspirate the contents of the tubing. Then a syringe of saline is attached to the tubing, and the line is flushed to test the patency of the vein. After an adequate amount of fluid (20 to 30 ml) has been injected without evidence of swelling and a blood return is ensured, the vesicant may again be injected. If the patient subsequently complains of pain or burning, the injection should be stopped despite the absence of any other signs of extravasation (absence of blood return or frank swelling).

The procedure for management of an extravasation of a vesicant agent depends on the drug infiltrated and the recommendations of current research concerning appropriate management. In general, the decision to leave the needle in place depends on whether an antidote is available or whether any fluid can be aspirated from the site. If fluid cannot be aspirated or no antidote exists, the needle should be removed. The following describes basic guidelines for management of a known or presumed extravasation.

1. Stop administration of the drug (note amount remaining in syringe); estimate amount infiltrated.

2. Exchange the syringe of chemotherapy for an empty 20-ml syringe.

3. Attempt to aspirate any residual drug and blood in the IV tubing (up to 20 ml).

4. Note the amount aspirated.

5. Remove the needle if no antidote is available. Otherwise stabilize the syringe and prepare the antidote.

6. Instill the IV antidote via the existing needle or cannula if indicated.

7. Remove the needle, being careful not to apply undue pressure to the site.

8. If unable to aspirate the vesicant drug from the tubing, remove the needle. Apply ethyl chloride locally to numb the site. Inject the antidote subcutaneously into the area using a 25-gauge needle. Multiple (3 to 4) injections may be necessary, depending on the extent of drug infiltration.

9. Remove the needle and apply a bandage without applying pressure to the site. Immobilize the extravasation

site, and elevate the arm for 3 days. Observe regularly for pain, erythema, and induration.

10. Notify physician.

11. Consider plastic surgery consultation if pain persists after 72 hours.

12. Document the occurrence in the patient's chart and complete the extravasation record.

13. Include a photograph of the site in the patient's record once an extravasation occurs, and take a photograph regularly with each visit to document progress.

Most extravasations of vesicant agents resolve spontaneously, especially if only a small amount of the drug is infiltrated (less than 0.5 ml). However, if a large amount (5 to 7 ml) has infiltrated, extensive tissue damage can be expected, and surgical intervention may be warranted. Surgical excision is generally indicated if pain persists after 3 to 7 days. Tissue damage may proceed to necrosis, with the amount of ulceration and infection depending on the concentration of the drug and the amount infiltrated. Vincristine, vinblastine, and vindesine usually are given by IV injection and are considered potential vesicants. If infiltration occurs, hyaluronidase (150 U/ml), 1 to 6 ml injected subcutaneously into the extravasated site, plus heat appears to enhance the absorption and systemic dispersion of the extravasated drug. Should extravasation occur from other plant alkaloids (etoposide or teniposide), the same procedure can be used to minimize local tissue changes even though they are likely to be minor. In contrast, the use of steroids, cooling, or both as local therapy for plant alkaloid infiltrations appears to worsen tissue destruction and should be avoided.

Anthracyclines (Daunomycin and Doxorubicin). When considering the anthracyclines doxorubicin and daunorubicin, it is important to note that no known antidotes are available to inactivate these drugs. There are two distinctly different local skin reactions to doxorubicin injection: a benign skin reaction called *flare* and a severe ulceration and necrosis due to infiltration of the drug. The flare reaction is characterized by a local erythematous streaking and inflammation that persists up to 30 minutes after the drug infusion. The redness and induration usually are accompanied by itching along the course of the vein. This reaction occurs infrequently (3% of cases) and does not preclude subsequent use of the drug. The occurrence of the flare reaction may be related to injecting doxorubicin too rapidly or injecting the drug into a small vein. The flare reaction may also be influenced by the practice of injecting doxorubicin after dexamethasone, which is commonly used as an antiemetic. By giving the doxorubicin first, a 4- to 5-ml saline flush next, and the dexamethasone last, the incidence of flare may be reduced. If flare occurs under any circumstance, the first step is to determine that the local redness is not due to a frank extravasation. After liberal flushing with a 10 to 20 ml of saline, the symptoms generally resolve, permitting the continued slow injection of the doxorubicin and eliminating the need to restick the patient. Local therapy with antihistamines is unnecessary because the flare reaction resolves spontaneously 20 to 30 minutes after the injection.

A severe ulceration is another local skin reaction caused by infiltration of an anthracycline into the subcutaneous tissues. The exact mechanism of anthracycline-induced tissue damage is not known but may be related to a process called *endocytosis*. Once the anthracycline–DNA complex is formed, the cell dies, releasing the anthracycline unchanged and free to attach itself to a neighboring cell. The drug itself persists and accounts for the indolent and progressive nature of the tissue damage. Whatever the exact mechanism may be, clinical and histologic studies have demonstrated that major changes in tissues occur within 3 days of extravasation and persist up to 12 weeks or longer.

One commonly proposed therapy for doxorubicin extravasation has been local injection of a corticosteroid, such as hydrocortisone. Theoretically, the action of a corticosteroid stabilizes the cell membrane, thereby initiating the uptake of doxorubicin. In addition, it acts as an anti-inflammatory agent. However, histologic examination of these doxorubicin lesions fails to demonstrate an inflammatory response, making hydrocortisone less likely to be of benefit. Although the injection of low-dose hydrocortisone (25 to 50 mg) locally into the extravasation site has been recommended, not all studies have reported significant benefit from the use of steroids.

Local instillation of sodium bicarbonate (5 ml of 8.4% solution) through the existing IV line has been recommended as a means of raising the local pH and thereby disrupting cellular uptake, DNA binding, and subsequent damage by doxorubicin. Other studies report no benefit from the use of sodium bicarbonate as a local antidote to doxorubicin extravasation. Sodium bicarbonate is known to cause severe tissue necrosis in higher doses. Dimethyl sulfoxide (DMSO) and alpha-tocopherol are two free radical scavengers that have been tested as potential antidotes to doxorubicin extravasation. Svingen et al. reported that a combination of DMSO and alpha-tocopherol applied topically for 48 hours following doxorubicin infiltration significantly reduced the mean ulcer size in rats. Although some investigators have confirmed these positive effects of topical DMSO, the findings are inconsistent. Dorr and Alberts found that neither intradermal nor topical DMSO with or without alpha-tocopherol administered up to 7 days reduced doxorubicin-induced skin ulcerations.

Another local therapy commonly recommended for

doxorubicin extravasation is the immediate application of ice for 20 to 60 minutes four to six times a day. Cold causes a vasoconstriction that limits concentration of the drug to the infiltrated site. Decreasing the temperature locally also reduces the metabolic rate and mitotic activity of the cells. Larson recommends applying ice to the site of extravasation for 20 minutes four times a day for 3 days. The limb is elevated, and the site is observed closely. Using this treatment, 89% of patients ($n = 175$) required no further therapy following extravasation. The rest required surgical intervention. The major indication for wide excision of all tissues that appear abnormal is pain. Delaying surgery for 3 to 5 days allows for a clear definition of the extent of tissue destruction and a delineation of which lesions are likely to resolve on their own and which require surgical intervention.

In summary, no effective local antidote is available to treat anthracycline extravasation. Although topical DMSO or local infiltration of low-dose hydrocortisone may lessen the local reaction in some situations, the application of ice appears to be the most useful local measure to minimize tissue destruction in the event of an anthracycline extravasation.

Mitomycin. Mitomycin is a severe vesicant that is capable of producing extensive local damage if infiltrated. In addition, mitomycin has been noted to produce delayed ulcerations distant from the injection site. A commonly proposed local therapy for mitomycin extravasation is 1:6 molar sodium thiosulfate. Injecting the 3 to 5 ml of sodium thiosulfate in a pincushion fashion or singly through the existing IV line may effectively inactivate the infiltrated mitomycin.

Dorr et al. tested numerous local pharmacologic interventions for their ability to reduce mitomycin extravasation in mice. Among the agents tested and found to be ineffective were hyaluronidase, fumaric acid, hydrocortisone, heparin, isoproterenol, and vitamin E. Neither topical cooling nor topical heating was found to be effective. Sodium thiosulfate was noted to be somewhat effective in treating small lesions but not larger lesions. Of note is the finding that immediate application of topical DMSO (100%) appears to protect against mitomycin tissue damage in the mouse.

Vascular access devices

The most common avenue for antineoplastic drug delivery is an IV one. VADs have evolved over the past 15 or more years and are designed to enable a patient to safely receive chemotherapy, ease the discomfort of IV drug delivery and blood sampling, facilitate blood component therapy and continuous infusion therapy of vesicant and nonvesicant agents in the inpatient or outpatient setting, and permit multiple drug and fluid therapies to be given concurrently or alternately with the chemotherapy.

The nurse is commonly in a position to recommend the insertion of a VAD. Factors to consider include the frequency of venous access, length of treatment, type of treatment, mode of administration, venous integrity, and patient preference.

When a patient requires only short-term continuous or intermittent administration of chemotherapy, fluids, or blood components, a percutaneous, nontunneled catheter usually is preferred. Central catheters, such as the Cook (Cook, Inc.), are inserted via the subclavian vein by a physician, whereas the single-lumen peripheral nontunneled catheter, such as the Per-Q-Cath (Gesco International) or Intrasil (Baxter Healthcare), is inserted by a physician or a specially trained nurse. A transparent dressing is placed over the exit site that allows the extension tubing to extend beyond the dressing for easy access. These catheters require daily irrigation with heparin and meticulous sterile technique during dressing changes.

The percutaneously placed silicone tunneled catheters are intended for long-term indefinite use. They are usually placed on the anterior chest and tunneled beneath the skin to rest in the cephalic, internal, or external jugular or the subclavian vein. The tip of the catheter rests near the entrance to the right atrium. All tunneled catheters have a Dacron cuff, which serves a dual purpose. After about 2 weeks, fibroblasts form around the cuff, securing the catheter in place and theoretically minimizing the risk of bacterial invasion around the catheter. To further minimize the incidence of infection, especially in the bone marrow transplantation population, an infection-control device called a Vitacuff (Vitaphore Corp.) may be placed around the catheter at the time of insertion. This attachable subcutaneous cuff is composed of a collagen impregnated with silver ions. The collagen induces tissue ingrowth, which stabilizes the catheter. The broad-spectrum antimicrobial activity of the silver ions acts as an additional barrier to organisms migrating into the subcutaneous catheter tract.

These catheters are available as single-lumen, double-lumen, and triple-lumen designs. The medical care needs of the individual patient dictate which catheter is most appropriate. These catheters are primarily indicated for patients who require frequent vascular access for blood sampling and chemotherapy administration. Tunneled catheters are the VAD of choice for continuous infusions of a vesicant agent, especially when it is administered by an ambulatory infusion pump on an outpatient basis. The patient can be taught to disconnect the pump and flush the catheter once the therapy is complete.

Disadvantages of the tunneled catheters are that they are

costly, they require exit site care and frequent flushings, and they may lead to body image changes. Immediately after placement, an occlusive dressing is placed over the exit site, which remains in place for 24 to 48 hours. After this time, the dressing is changed using a sterile technique, and a transparent dressing is placed over the exit site and is changed every week or as necessary. After 2 weeks, a dressing is no longer required, provided the patient is not immunocompromised. However, most patients prefer to wear a dressing of some type or an adhesive bandage over the exit site to stabilize and secure the catheter in place. The catheter should always be taped to the patient to prevent its being inadvertently pulled out.

The tunneled catheter is irrigated every other day or once a week with 3 to 5 ml of heparinized saline solution (100 to 500 units of heparin/ml). The cap is changed once a week or once a month, depending on how often the catheter is irrigated. If the patient is using a Groshong catheter, the care needs vary slightly. This single-lumen or double-lumen catheter has a pressure-release valve that prevents blood from backing up into the catheter unless suction is exerted by a syringe to withdraw blood. Therefore, the catheter does not need to be irrigated with heparin, nor is a clamp required at any time. Indeed, to clamp the catheter could damage it. The Groshong catheter is flushed once a week with 5 ml of saline when not being used and with 20 ml after drawing blood. The Groshong is ideal for the elderly patient who is marginally capable of caring for a VAD but requires short-term or long-term continuous infusion of a vesicant agent. The exit site care and catheter flushing can be provided weekly by a visiting nurse or a trip to the physician's office.

Implanted ports are used primarily for IV therapy but can be used to administer drugs in the arteries and into the peritoneum. The implanted ports are made of various materials, including plastic, stainless steel, and titanium. The port septum consists of a dense silicone that is capable of withstanding 1000 to 2000 needle injections. A specially designed deflected point (Huber) needle is used to gain access to these ports and is designed to prevent damage to the septum with repeated injections. Figure 6–1 depicts the cross-section of a port with the Huber point needle in place. The catheter is tunneled a short distance and then placed into a large vein, usually the subclavian. Similar to the tunneled catheters, these ports can be placed in the groin, with the catheter resting in the iliac or femoral vein for patients in whom anterior chest placement is contraindicated. These ports can remain in place indefinitely and can be used for drawing blood and for administering blood products, total parenteral nutrition, and chemotherapy. Because of the risk of needle dislodgment and drug extravasation, these ports are not recommended for long-term infusions of

Accessing The System

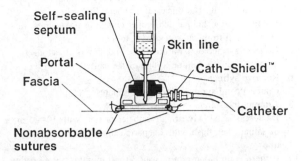

Figure 6–1. Port-A-Cath cross-section with Huber point needle in place. (Courtesy of Pharmacia Deltec Inc., St. Paul, MN.)

vesicant drugs on an outpatient basis. If a continuous infusion of a vesicant into a port is necessary because of prior circumstances, it is advisable to admit the patient into the hospital during the infusion so that proper needle placement can be assured and documented every 8 hours.

Vascular access ports are ideal for patients who have poor veins or who require frequent venous access, such as weekly injections of doxorubicin. To enter the port, the site is sterilized with a povidone-iodine solution, alcohol, or both. A Huber point needle is inserted transdermally through the septum until it meets the back of the port. Proper needle placement is assured with the presence of a blood return. However, it is not uncommon for a blood return to be absent. If a blood return is not obtained, the port can be irrigated with 20 to 30 ml of saline. In the absence of tissue swelling, proper needle placement is assured. If neither irrigation nor aspiration is possible, the catheter may be clotted. Forceful irrigation should be avoided because the catheter may burst. In the majority of cases, the inability to irrigate or aspirate occurs because the needle is malpositioned in the septum itself. Simply advancing the needle farther through the septum generally solves the problem. If the catheter is clotted, however, the procedure for declotting ports is identical to the procedure for declotting tunneled or nontunneled devices (Table 6–4). In the event that there is swelling at the site or pain during the infusion of fluids, the port and catheter should be further evaluated by injecting a radiopaque substance through them and viewing them under fluoroscopy.

Oral Drug Administration

Oral antineoplastic agents are generally considered convenient to administer, economical, and usually less toxic than drugs given IV. However, oral ingestion of antineo-

Table 6–4. MANAGEMENT OF A CLOTTED VAD*

1. Obtain urokinase for catheter clearance†
2. Reconstitute to 5000 IU of urokinase per milliliter
3. Withdraw 1 ml of urokinase in a tuberculin syringe
4. Using sterile technique and proper clamping procedures, disconnect cap from catheter or port tubing
5. Connect syringe of 1 ml urokinase and slowly inject an amount equal in volume to that of the catheter
6. Remove syringe
7. Connect 5-ml syringe; wait 5–10 minutes
8. Attempt to aspirate to remove clot
9. If successful, slowly irrigate catheter or port with 10–20 ml of saline, then flush with a heparin saline solution per routine
10. If there is no blood return, wait 30–60 minutes before trying to aspirate.
11. Repeat steps 1 to 10 if unable to clear catheter

---

*Procedure is the same for tunneled, nontunneled, and implanted devices.
†Urokinase (Abbokinase Open-Cath).
Streptokinase-streptodornase (Varidase).

plastics means that the drugs' availability and concentration are potentially erratic and incomplete for drugs that are poorly soluble, slowly absorbed, unstable, or extensively metabolized by the liver, which is especially a problem in situations of questionable liver or renal function. Oral chemotherapy requires careful patient teaching to ensure compliance and minimize toxicity. Patients are given written instructions concerning their medications and are encouraged to learn the names of their medications and to keep a record of all the prescription medications they are taking, including their schedule and toxicities. In addition, they are cautioned to check with their physician or nurse before taking any nonprescription medications. Because of the nature of antineoplastics and their toxicities, it is advisable to prescribe only enough medication for a single-treatment course to avoid an accidental overdose.

Regional Drug Delivery

The inability to achieve sufficient concentration of the drug at the tumor site without undue toxicity to normal tissues is considered a major factor in the failure of systemic chemotherapy to adequately control disease. Theoretically, regional drug delivery can enhance the dose–response curve by increasing the concentration of the drug at the tumor site and at the same time lower systemic drug exposure, thereby improving the therapeutic index. Drugs most effective by this route are those with a high total body clearance and those that are rapidly bound or inactivated after one pass through the region. The site of delivery, whether in a cavity, such as the peritoneum, or in the central nervous system, should have a low exchange rate so that systemic absorption is minimal. The drug or drugs must be active in their administered form.

The most common methods of regional drug delivery include intraarterial, intraperitoneal, intrathecal or intraventricular, and intravesical bladder chemotherapy. With the development of implantable pumps, ports, and catheters, such therapies are now more technically feasible.

Intraarterial chemotherapy

Intraarterial drugs are administered through a catheter that rests in the vessel supplying the tumor. Intraarterial chemotherapy has been used for osteogenic sarcoma, bladder carcinoma, head and neck carcinoma, cervical carcinoma, melanoma, brain tumors, primary hepatoma, and metastatic disease of the liver. Angiography is employed to demonstrate the blood supply to a particular tumor-bearing area. The artery or vein is then cannulated either during surgery or percutaneously, under radiologic control. Anticoagulation measures are especially important to prevent clotting of the vessel before and during catheterization in patients undergoing infusions that last several days. Patency of the catheter lumen is maintained by continuous pump infusion or intermittent heparinization.

There are basically three methods of arterial catheterization: (1) external rigid, (2) implanted ports, and (3) implanted pumps. The first method involves angiographic placement of a rather stiff catheter for arterial perfusion that lasts minutes to hours. The area is immobilized during the treatment, and the site is assessed regularly for bleeding. The catheter is removed after therapy, and pressure is applied to the site. In the second method, a more flexible (silicone) catheter is surgically placed into the artery, sutured to the skin, or connected to an implanted port for long-term access. These catheters are irrigated regularly to maintain patency. The external catheter is irrigated daily, and the implanted port is irrigated once a week with heparinized saline. Each of these catheters or devices can be connected to an infusion pump for protracted intraarterial infusion chemotherapy. The third method involves surgical placement of a catheter that is connected to a totally implanted infusion pump (the Infusaid 400 or the Medtronics pump). This pump is filled with chemotherapy or saline, and it constantly infuses the involved organ—usually the liver via the hepatic artery. The pumps are refilled by percutaneous injection approximately every 1 to 2 weeks. The toxicities of intraarterial drug therapy relate to the region perfused. Although systemic toxicities may be present, they are often minimal.

Intraperitoneal chemotherapy

Intraperitoneal chemotherapy plays a role in the treatment of ovarian carcinoma, gastrointestinal malignancies, and metastatic disease of the liver. By administering the chemotherapy directly into the abdominal cavity, higher drug concentrations at the tumor site can be achieved. The majority of abdominal cavity fluid is absorbed and detoxified in the portal circulation after one pass through the liver. Because most of the drugs are either metabolized or detoxified in the liver, toxicities are less than when the drugs are given systemically. Cisplatin, a drug commonly used for intraperitoneal perfusion, concentrates in the liver and the kidneys once absorbed. Therefore, a sodium thiosulfate infusion may be given systemically to prevent toxicity.

Patient acceptance is a major concern with this method of drug delivery. Routinely, the Tenckhoff catheter has been used to maintain long-term access to the abdominal cavity to deliver fluid and chemotherapy. The catheter is secured by two Dacron cuffs to prevent dislodgment. Because the catheter exits from the abdomen, it may be uncomfortable, and thus low patient acceptability is common owing to the maintenance required and the body image changes. Sterile technique, including a mask, is used whenever the catheter is manipulated for chemotherapy or irrigations. The Hickman and Groshong catheters also are used for intraperitoneal chemotherapy and are more comfortable and easily tolerated by patients. An alternate method of drug delivery includes the use of the totally implanted port. The port generally is placed over the lower ribcage in the midclavicular line, which provides support for the port during cannulation. Patient acceptance of these ports is generally very good because they are completely implanted, require little maintenance, and do not significantly alter body image.

The port or catheter is accessed using the sterile technique previously described. The chemotherapy is infused in 1 to 2 liters of fluid to ensure adequate drug distribution. The fluid is usually allowed to dwell in the abdomen for 1 to 4 hours, after which it is drained by gravity through the catheter or port. Some protocols do not drain the fluid at all. Fibrous ingrowth can occur around the catheter or the port, creating a one-way valve effect that prevents drainage. This problem occurs in about 30% of patients regardless of the type of access device. The one-way effect occurs whether the catheter is irrigated routinely with saline, heparin, or dextran. Although the patient may be uncomfortable temporarily from abdominal distention, the one-way catheter presents no real problem because the dialysate is gradually absorbed. Occasionally, the catheter can be irrigated vigorously to release a fibrin clot.

Intravesical bladder chemotherapy

The purpose of intravesical bladder chemotherapy is to allow a high concentration of the drug to come in contact with the urothelium over a relatively long period of time. A significant proportion (50% to 70%) of patients with superficial (stage 0 or stage A) transitional cell carcinoma of the bladder have recurrent disease following traditional therapy. Intravesical bladder chemotherapy is intended to destroy any viable cancer cells in the bladder, thereby preventing recurrence of the cancer and the need for cystectomy. Benefits of this therapy include minimal systemic toxicities and preservation of urinary and sexual function. In general, the drug is instilled via a urinary catheter into the bladder and retained for about 1 to 3 hours. The patient changes position about every 15 minutes to ensure optimal bladder exposure. The common side effects of intravesical chemotherapy include dysuria, frequency of urination, hematuria, and bladder spasms. If the drug is allowed to dwell longer than the prescribed time, the patient can experience excessive exfoliation of the bladder epithelium and cystitis.

Intraventricular and intrathecal chemotherapy

Meningeal carcinomatosis is characterized by a diffuse seeding of the surface layers of the brain and spinal cord by tumor. Metastasis to the leptomeninges is often manifested by obstruction of the cerebrospinal fluid pathways and invasion of the nerves within the subarachnoid space, which produces cranial nerve and lower motor neuron dysfunction. The cancers most commonly associated with meningeal metastasis include breast cancer, lung cancer, gastrointestinal carcinoma, leukemia, and lymphoma. The central nervous system is considered a sanctuary for tumor cells because most systemically administered antineoplastic drugs do not cross the blood–brain barrier in sufficient concentrations to be therapeutic. Therefore, intrathecal or intraventricular drug administration provides an amount of drug that is essential to treat presumed or proven leptomeningeal metastases.

Intrathecal drug administration involves the insertion of a needle into the lumbar region and injection of the drug through the dura and the arachnoid into the subarachnoid space. Regardless of positioning, the lumbar puncture technique does not ensure cisternal and ventricular distribution of the drug. In fact, ineffective treatment of meningeal leukemia or carcinomatosis has been related to inadequate drug concentration and distribution into the ventricles.

The large production of cerebrospinal fluid from the ventricles and its outflow generate a pressure that probably inhibits ascent of the drug to the ventricles following lumbar puncture. The Ommaya reservoir is a small, Silastic dome-shaped disc with an extension catheter that is surgically implanted through the cranium into a lateral ventricle. Once placement is verified by radiograph, the scalp flap covering is sutured into place. Twenty-four to 48 hours is generally allowed before gaining access to the reservoir. One of the benefits of an intraventricular reservoir is that the patient is spared the pain and discomfort of repeated lumbar punctures. Injecting drugs directly into the ventricles ensures more consistent drug concentrations and distribution.

The drugs used for intrathecal therapy should contain no preservatives and may be mixed in Elliott's B solution, preservative-free saline, or the patient's own cerebrospinal fluid. The drug is mixed in 10 to 12 ml of diluent and injected over 5 to 10 minutes to ensure distribution and to minimize acute meningeal irritation. Patients are instructed to remain supine or semirecumbent for 20 to 30 minutes. Acute complications include headache, nausea, vomiting, fever, and nuchal rigidity, which usually subside in 48 to 72 hours.

SUMMARY

Over the years, the administration of antineoplastic agents has become the responsibility of the oncology nurse. This responsibility has become more than the actual task of drug delivery and is fast becoming an opportunity for nurses to influence patient care outcomes. It is an opportunity to influence decisions regarding care delivery and to teach patients and their families about the treatment and about how they can minimize the toxicities of the treatment and remain active participants in their own care. The responsibility also exists for the nurse to design and conduct research with other members of the health care team, specifically in the areas of safe handling of antineoplastics, extravasation management, and various issues concerning the management of VADs.

7 Biologic Response Modifiers

LINDA EDWARDS HOOD
ELIZABETH ABERNATHY

It is hoped that the use of biologic response modifiers (BRMs) or biotherapy in cancer treatment will aid researchers in putting together the missing pieces of the cancer puzzle. In 1981, BRMs were defined by the Subcommittee on BRMs to the Division of Cancer Treatment, National Cancer Institute, as "those agents or approaches that modify the relationship between tumor and host by modifying the host's biological response to tumor cells with resultant therapeutic effects." Biotherapy is based largely on the manipulation of the immune system in an effort to control cancer. Immunologic deficiencies are documented in individuals with cancer. If through the use of BRMs the immune system can be modulated to better destroy malignant cells, biotherapy will become a prominent treatment for cancer in the future.

See the corresponding chapter in *Cancer Nursing: A Comprehensive Textbook,* by Baird, McCorkle, and Grant, pp. 321–343, for a more detailed discussion of this topic, including a comprehensive list of references.

MECHANISM OF ACTION

Biologic response modifiers are being researched both clinically and in the laboratory. Even after extensive research, the mechanism of action of many of the agents is not clearly defined. Several of the agents have many known antitumor activities. Thus, for these agents, it is difficult to determine which antitumor capabilities are the most critical.

Biologic response modifiers can be classified into three major divisions: (1) agents that restore, augment, or modulate the host's immunologic mechanisms, (2) agents that have direct antitumor activity, and (3) agents that have other biologic effects (agents that interfere with tumor cells' ability to metastasize or survive, differentiating agents, or agents that affect cell transformation).

There are two major groups of BRMs: lymphokines and monokines (Table 7–1). *Cytokine* is a generic term referring to all BRMs released by any body cell.

CLASSIFICATION

Major technologic advances in the last decade have expanded researchers' ability to study BRMs. Through gene cloning, human genes can be placed inside bacteria or yeast cells in culture to produce large quantities of purified human BRMs, including recombinant human interferons, interleukin 2 (IL-2), and tumor necrosis factor (TNF).

Hybridoma technology has made possible the development of clones of cells that produce specific antibodies against one antigen. *Monoclonal antibodies* (MoAbs), which are antibodies developed to bind with specific types of cancer cells, are used directly in cancer therapy and diagnosis and indirectly in the isolation and purification of other BRMs.

Clinically, interferons have been studied more extensively than any other BRM. Approved by the United States Food

Table 7–1. GROUPS OF BIOLOGIC RESPONSE MODIFIERS (BRMs)

BRM Categories	Cell Origin	BRMs
Lymphokines	Lymphocytes	Interleukin 2
		Interferon-γ
		B-cell growth factor
Monokines	Mononuclear phagocytes	Interferon-α
		Colony-stimulating factor
		Tumor necrosis factor (TNF)
Cytokines	Any stimulated cell	All BRMs

and Drug Administration in 1986 for therapeutic use in patients with hairy cell leukemia, a chronic B-cell malignancy, interferon-α continues to be studied in many phase II and III trials that have examined various indications, dosages, schedules, and routes of administration. Clinical trials of interferon-γ and interferon-β are increasing. Research on the use of interferon in combination with radiation therapy, chemotherapy, and other BRMs also is under way.

In the last 5 years, considerable attention has been focused on IL-2. This BRM, a lymphokine produced by T lymphocytes, is being examined for direct antitumor activity as well as for an exciting approach to immunotherapy: adoptive immunotherapy. *Adoptive immunotherapy* has been defined as a "treatment approach in which cells with antitumor reactivity are administered to a tumor-bearing host and mediate either directly or indirectly the regression of established tumor." With this approach, IL-2 mixes with human peripheral blood lymphocytes and generates cells terms *lymphokine-activated killer* (LAK) *cells* that are capable of killing tumor cells.

Considerable in vitro data but few clinical reports are available on relatively new BRMs, such as colony-stimulating factors (CSFs), antimetastatic agents, and TNF. Multiple clinical trials are under way using CSF, a monokine, in an effort to stimulate production of leukocytes in the stem cells of the bone marrow of cancer patients.

TESTING

With BRMs, the maximum tolerated dose as well as the optimal immunomodulatory dose must be determined because lower doses of some BRMs may be more effective in altering various aspects of the immune response than higher doses, or the agent may be effective by different mechanisms at different doses.

NURSING CONSIDERATIONS

Individuals who receive biologic therapy have many of the same needs as individuals who receive investigational or conventional therapy for cancer (Table 7–2). In the past, nurses caring for individuals receiving immunotherapy were expected to be familiar with basic principles of immunotherapy and to be clinically expert at administering the therapy. Today, the role of the nurse caring for these patients has become quite complex and requires the nurse's understanding of the immune system and the different agents that affect it.

TUMOR IMMUNOLOGY

Tumor immunology is the study of the relationship between tumor development and growth and the immunologic status of the host. An understanding of tumor immunology

Table 7-2. PATIENTS RECEIVING BIOLOGIC RESPONSE MODIFIERS: RISK FACTORS AND NURSING OBSERVATIONS

Symptoms/Organ System Side Effects	Potential Risk Factors	Usual Time Frame	Observations
Constitutional symptoms			
Headache	Age	Acute	Observe for presence and severity of symptoms (acute symptoms generally abate with repeated dosing)
Fever	Poor performance status		
Chills			
Myalgias			
Flu-like symptoms			
Fatigue	Age	Chronic	Monitor use of other medications (e.g., propranolol can contribute to fatigue)
Malaise	Poor performance status		Monitor nutritional status (e.g., weight change)
Weakness	Malnutrition		Monitor hematologic status
	Anemia		
	Other medications		
	Inadequate social support system		
Cardiovascular	Cardiac history	Acute and chronic	Observe orthostatic blood pressure changes with vital signs
	Unstable hypertension		Monitor for potential cardiac symptoms
	Dehydration		
	Age		

Neurologic	History of seizures History of mood swings, depression Age	Acute and chronic	Observe for cognitive and mood alterations Educate family to report subtle changes
Gastrointestinal	History of gastrointestinal disorders	Acute	Observe for symptoms
Hematologic	History of coagulation disorders Leukemia Multiple myeloma Bone marrow suppression	Chronic	Routinely monitor complete blood count, differential, platelets, prothrombin time, partial thromboplastin time
Renal/metabolic	Renal disease	Acute and chronic	Routinely monitor blood urea nitrogen, creatinine, electrolytes Monitor for proteinuria in high-risk patients
Hepatic	History of ethyl alcohol use Other hepatotoxic drugs Malnutrition Preexistent liver disease	Chronic	Obtain baseline liver function tests Routinely monitor lactose dehydrogenase, alkaline phosphatase, serum glutamic oxaloacetic transaminase, serum glutamic pyruvic transaminase, bilirubin Monitor nutritional status Monitor ethyl alcohol and other drug intake

From Irwin, M.M. (1987). Patients receiving biological response modifiers: Overview of nursing care. *Oncology Nursing Forum, 14*(Suppl. 6), 32–37. Reproduced by permission.

and biotherapy is built on a basic knowledge of the immune system. It is necessary to understand the components of the immune system and their function to comprehend this complex new approach to cancer treatment.

Overview of the Immune System

The immune system is a complex network of organs and cells that is responsible for guarding the body against the invasion of harmful elements. When functioning correctly, this system fights off invaders, such as viruses, bacteria, fungi, and parasites, as well as malignant cells and thus provides a safe habitat for the body. When a breakdown in the system occurs, various diseases proliferate.

The defense mechanisms provided by the immune system (immunologic defense mechanisms) can be divided into the first line of host defenses—nonspecific immunity—and the second line of resistance—specific immunity.

Host Defenses

Nonspecific immunity is perhaps the body's most important defense against infection. It is designed to provide immediate protection on the first occasion that the body encounters a foreign invader. Nonspecific immunity is the body's way of protecting itself using the capabilities of its normal anatomy and physiology.

The first line of defense against invaders attempting to enter the body is the physical barrier provided by the intact skin and mucous membranes. However, when the integrity of the skin is broken, for example, from a burn, invasion from foreign cells will occur, thus upsetting the body's homeostasis and allowing disease to flourish. Other examples of nonspecific immunity include the following.

1. The ciliated epithelial lining in the respiratory tract that traps and sweeps away inhaled bacteria
2. The flushing action and composition of urine that help prevent urinary tract infections
3. The large quantities of lysozyme, an enzyme in human tears that destroys bacteria

When these first-line defenses fail to prevent entry of microorganisms into the body, an inflammatory response is activated that attempts to control the infectious growth and systemic invasion. Neutrophils congregate in the area of the invasion and phagocytize the invaders. These are not cells that react specifically with the antigens but are cells that recognize something as foreign and attempt to destroy it.

Specific (acquired) immunity is the immune system's response once an invader (antigen) is recognized as potentially harmful and not belonging to the body. An antigen is anything the immune system recognizes as nonself. Once the antigen is recognized as nonself, an army of cells is activated to destroy and dispose of the antigenic material. Antigens are carried on the cell surface of certain tumor cells, viruses, and bacteria. The cells of the immune system are quite sophisticated and develop a memory response. The immune system must learn about each individual invader to which it is exposed and must develop specific cells (memory lymphocytes and B lymphocytes) that recognize and react to reexposure of the foreign matter. This process is the basis for immunizations.

The antigen is processed by macrophages before the immune response is generated. Antigen receptors on cell surfaces are responsible for the specificity of the reaction. Each antigen reacts only with one lymphocyte receptor in a manner similar to a lock and key. On binding to the antigen, the lymphocyte is activated. It grows and divides and secretes lymphokines that activate other lymphocytes. The cell's clone has the same specificity as the mother cell and facilitates the specific immune response needed to eliminate that antigen.

Acquired immunity may be divided into two subsystems: (1) humoral immunity and (2) cell-mediated immunity. *Humoral immunity* is made of two serum proteins derived from stem cells in the bone marrow: antibody molecules (immunoglobulins or Ig) and complement molecules. Immunoglobulins, by their ability to bind to a specific antigen, are capable of neutralizing that invader. Tumor cells express surface antigens that are capable of being recognized as foreign by the immune system. The antigen-antibody reaction is very specific in that an antibody will react only with one particular type of antigen.

Each immunoglobulin protein consists of two identical heavy chains and two light chains linked by a disulfide bridge (chemical bond). Each of the light chains has a section called the *variable region* that determines to which antigen this particular antibody has binding capability. The heavy chain's amino acid sequences determine the class of the immunoglobulin. The five known classes are IgG, IgA, IgM, IgE, and IgD. The letters that name the heavy chain type of immunoglobulin are from the Greek alphabet (e.g., gamma = IgG). Each of the five classes of immunoglobulins has very specific and independent functions.

The first exposure to an antigen is followed by a latent phase during which no antibody levels are detected. This phase is followed by a primary response, during which a rapid rise in serum antibody is detected, then a plateau, and then a decline in antibody level. This reaction time is not immediate and thus allows the spread of the antigen during the body's first exposure.

After the primary response, an immunologic memory is developed whereby on second exposure to the antigen, the latency period is very short, antibody production is much faster, and higher concentrations of antibody are present, again creating the basis for immunization.

This reaction between the antigen and the immunoglobulin signals the activation of complement, the nonspecific component of humoral immunity. The complement system is composed of a series of proteins circulating in an inactive form in the bloodstream. Complement circulates in a completely inactive form until activated in a cascading fashion by the enzyme above it in the cascade.

Complement destroys the antigen by actually poking holes in cell membranes, allowing the intracellular fluid to leak out. Complement is nonspecific in its destruction of antigen. Thus, normal cells located in the area in which the complement system has been activated also will be destroyed. The destroyed cells are then cleared from the bloodstream by mononuclear phagocytes and monocytes.

Cell-mediated immunity is the key line of defense in fighting viral infections, some fungal infections, parasitic disease, and bacteria that are harbored inside cells. Cell-mediated immunity is responsible for delayed hypersensitivity, transplant rejection, and possibly tumor identification and destruction.

A cell-mediated reaction is activated when an antigen binds with an antigen receptor on the surface of a specialized white blood cell. The nonspecific component of cell-mediated immunity includes other leukocytes (mononuclear phagocytes and natural killer cells) that destroy and ingest a range of antigens. These cells function under the direction of the T lymphocytes. Mononuclear phagocytes and natural killer cells are nonspecific and are capable of destroying and eliminating a variety of antigens.

Immune Surveillance

The hypothesis of immune surveillance is much of the basis for biotherapy. This hypothesis suggests that the immune system is capable of recognizing that cancerous cells are foreign and eliciting an immune response that destroys the cells, thus protecting the host. There are several assumptions from this hypothesis.

1. Cancer cells have surface antigens that are recognizable by the immune system.

2. The immune system through its inherent mechanisms is capable of destroying the cancer cells once they are identified.

3. A failure in the immune system may result in malignancy.

Tumor Antigens

When a cell becomes malignant, the antigens that appear on the surface of the cell are also transformed biochemically. The theory is that tumor cells have distinct antigens that are capable of being recognized by the host as foreign and thus provoke an immune response. In humans, these antigens are called *tumor-associated antigens* or oncofetal antigens.

CLASSIFICATION OF BIOLOGIC RESPONSE MODIFIERS

Monoclonal Antibodies

Mechanism of action

The central issue regarding the future potential of MoAbs is whether tumor-specific antigens exist or whether antigens possessed by tumors are shared with normal tissues. To induce a specific immune response, the tumor cells have to express an antigen specific to or associated with the tumor. But because tumors are derived from normal cells, it cannot be assumed that tumors carry antigens that are different or foreign.

The immune response generated against tumor-associated antigens consists of either the formation of antibodies against the antigens or the attachment of various immune cells (stimulated killer lymphocytes and macrophages) to the antibody that is bound to the tumor, which effects tumor cell death. Tumor cells can shed their surface antigens or alter their appearance within 2 hours of MoAb exposure, an effect that can last up to 36 hours, or circulating tumor antigen may bind with the MoAb, blocking its receptor sites and thus preventing it from reaching the tumor cell. Blocking factors may be released by tumor cells to coat the tumor cell surface antigens, preventing recognition and destruction of the tumor.

Clinical applications

The use of antibodies to mediate specific toxicity for the cancer cell through recruitment of cell-mediated immunity and activation of the complement system is under investigation. Each MoAb has its own unique advantages and drawbacks for use in the localization of tumor. Cancer treatment can be enhanced through the use of MoAbs to target the delivery of drugs, toxins, and radioactive substances specifically to the area of tumor.

The use of MoAbs to detect early or preinvasive tumor by examining serum samples that may reveal the presence of surface antigens that are different from those of normal tissues also holds great promise in the fight against cancer.

Currently, MoAbs are used to purge bone marrow of neoplastic cells before reinfusion for bone marrow transplantation. MoAbs can identify and then disable activated lymphocytes that are responsible for transplant rejection or graft-versus-host disease without causing overall suppression of the immune mechanisms of the host. MoAbs may be used to manipulate the immune system specifically to interfere with the activity of growth factors induced by the tumor and to block other factors secreted by the tumor that induce increased numbers of suppressor lymphocytes to suppress the immune response.

Immunotoxins are created by the linkage of toxins to

MoAbs. The toxin bound to the MoAb attaches to the antigenic receptor on the tumor cell membrane and then penetrates into the cytoplasm by endocytosis through smooth invaginations or coated pits of the plasma membrane. Once this is inside the tumor cell's cytoplasm, protein synthesis is inactivated and cell killing results.

When MoAbs are linked to radioactive isotopes, scanning for areas of MoAb localization on tumor cells can determine if and where tumor recurrence exists.

Side effects

Toxicity to normal cells, although generally mild, must be considered in the use of MoAbs with patients. Side effects related to the administration of MoAbs include fever, chills, flushing, urticaria, rash, nausea, vomiting, headache, and hypotension. Allergic types of reactions that may occur are easily treated with corticosteroids, acetaminophen, and antihistamines. However, immune complexes may stagnate within, causing damage to various organ tissues, for example, liver, lungs, or kidneys.

Toxicities associated with MoAbs have not been major and usually are associated with the initial one or two administrations or with rapid IV infusions. Pulmonary symptoms, such as acute dyspnea and mild wheezing, were noted and are thought to be related to lymphocyte clumping or trapping in the lungs. Such clumping in the lungs and in the kidneys was detected by continued monitoring after administration of MoAbs. These effects were less frequent or were absent with prolonged infusions over 2 to 4 hours.

With some of the human MoAbs, mild erythema at the injection site is the only side effect noted.

Nursing considerations

Patient Safety. Because MoAbs are high molecular weight proteins, they have the potential to induce the production of host antibodies against themselves, and risk of hypersensitivity reactions exists. Resuscitation and intubation equipment should be readily available along with emergency drugs, such as parenteral corticosteroids, diphenhydramine, and epinephrine. Patients should be observed closely for at least the first hour after administration of MoAbs, with assessments of vital signs and pulmonary status taken every 15 minutes and additional assessments taken every hour for a period following completion of administration.

Environmental Safety. When radiolabeled MoAbs are used, the handling and disposal of radioactive substances and body fluids from the patient are important safety issues. Badges that register the amount of radioactivity to which a health care worker is exposed should be worn. Also, radiation safety teams should monitor the emissions of radioactivity from the patient through body fluids, blood samples drawn, and other procedures. Lead shields and lead-lined specimen containers can be used to further minimize individual exposure. The patient's contact with family members, particularly with small children or pregnant women, may be limited for a period of time following the administration of the MoAb.

Documentation. Evaluation of the patient's response and communication with the primary physician about any possible allergic reaction, such as hives, wheezing, urticaria, or rash, should be carefully documented.

Laboratory tests, frequent blood samples of various sorts, multiple scans, and tumor measurements are necessary in the evaluation of response to a new therapy, such as MoAb therapy. Charts, drawings, and printed materials about the immune system and the function of antibodies are useful for the new patient on MoAb therapy.

Health care personnel who will be involved with patients receiving MoAbs need current information to enable them to provide appropriate care.

Interferon

Interferon is a family of cytokines that are glycoproteins produced as part of the cell-mediated immune response by the T lymphocyte after activation by viruses or tumor cells. Interferon is named for its ability to interfere with the spread of viral infection by affecting the synthesis of viral RNA and protein. It has been found to possess antitumor and immunomodulatory potential as well.

Interferon has potent effects on the immune system as an "immunological hormone." It is considered to be the prototype BRM, a natural human protein that can alter the body's immune response to result in detrimental effects to a tumor and, it is hoped, in little toxicity to normal tissues.

Mechanism of action

Antiviral. Interferon was identified originally for its antiviral properties: it is able to induce an antiviral state when a virus attaches to a cell membrane. Interferon stimulates the production of various factors that participate in the events that occur during the immune response to protect cells from a second simultaneous infection. It prevents further viral RNA and protein replication, halting the virus' ability to spread to other body cells.

Interferon is measured in units of antiviral activity based on its ability to inhibit viral multiplication in tissue cultures. One million antiviral units is the common unit for measurement of interferon dosage, also called one megaunit or International Unit (IU).

Antitumor. Direct antitumor effects have been identified that involve inhibition of tumor growth and cell division.

As interferon contacts a tumor cell receptor site, it triggers a number of reactions that arrest or delay the stages of cell division, primarily G_0 to G_1.

Interferon also influences the production of other cellular products, enzymes, and lymphokines. These actions can result in differentiating effects on the malignant cell, alterations in malignant cell phenotype and metabolism, or inhibition of important genes, such as oncogenes.

Immunomodulatory. Interferon causes some indirect effects, influencing various immunomodulatory aspects of both cellular and humoral immunity. Some of these effects include the stimulation of cytotoxic T lymphocytes, macrophages, and natural killer cells as well as phagocytic activity.

Overall, interferon influences a number of immune activities that enhance the body's ability to recognize and rid itself of tumor growth.

Clinical applications

Interferon-α. Interferon-α was approved by the Food and Drug Administration in June 1986 for use against hairy cell leukemia, a rare, chronic form of B-cell leukemia that is highly sensitive to small amounts of interferon. Chronic myelogenous leukemia in the benign or chronic phase has also been found to respond to interferon-α.

Interferon-α is indicated for use against AIDS-related Kaposi's sarcoma. Classic Kaposi's sarcoma is a relatively rare tumor of older men, usually considered to be benign. The incidence of this malignancy in young male homosexuals has increased, which observation, in fact, led to the awareness of the AIDS epidemic. Response to interferon includes the flattening or disappearance or both of the lesions, with no evidence of disease on biopsy of prior Kaposi's sarcoma sites. The response is dose related, with 28% to 35% of the responses occurring with high doses.

Other hematologic disorders that show responsiveness to interferon-α include nodular non-Hodgkin's lymphoma, chronic lymphocytic leukemia, and multiple myeloma. Solid tumors have shown less responsiveness to interferon, but some significant responses have been seen in renal cell carcinoma and superficial bladder cancer, in ovarian carcinoma with intraperitoneal administration of interferon, and in colon cancer, with interferon enhancing the effect of 5-fluorouracil.

Interferon-β. Interferon-β is very similar to interferon-α in both its activity and its toxicities, but it is less potent as an antiviral agent. Intramuscularly administered interferon-β becomes bound to local tissues and is destroyed within the muscle. Therefore, higher doses administered by the IV route have been necessary to attain adequate serum levels.

Interferon-γ. Interferon-γ has several different biologic effects that differentiate it from either interferon-α or interferon-β. Interferon-γ has more of an activation effect on macrophages and demonstrates a much higher cytotoxic effect in vitro through its role in regulating cytotoxic T cells.

Interferon-γ must be administered intravenously to achieve detectable serum levels.

Nursing considerations

Assessment and Administration. Interferon comes in several subtypes and dilutions. The directions on package inserts for different interferons should be followed carefully in preparation of the correct dosage and concentration, route of administration, and procedure for reconstitution and maintenance of stability. Advise the patient not to change brands.

Interferon is a nonvesicant, although soreness and redness can occur at sites of subcutaneous or intramuscular injections. Phlebitis may result from prolonged IV infusions. A common sense approach in handling interferon supplies is recommended by the Oncology Nursing Society's *Biological Response Modifiers Guidelines.*

Constitutional. The acute flu-like syndrome consisting of fever, chills, malaise, and myalgias occurs in 90% of patients. Initially, chills begin about 2 to 6 hours after administration of the interferon dose and include severe, teeth-chattering rigors accompanied by pallor due to peripheral vasoconstriction. Blankets and warm beverages may comfort the patient.

Acetaminophen generally is very effective in controlling the fevers, which may peak at 39° to 40°C (102° to 104°F). The use of aspirin, nonsteroidal anti-inflammatory agents, or steroids to block this acute febrile reaction is generally avoided because of fear that the effects of these drugs on the immune system may block the beneficial results of interferon.

The day following interferon administration is usually free of fever, but a washed-out feeling with muscular aches and fatigue may persist. Patients may become unable to attend to usual daily activities to the extent that they ignore personal care. Patients should be counseled to take planned rest periods and to anticipate some fatigue so that they will not be overly anxious that these symptoms signal the progression of their malignancy. Administration of interferon in the evening results in less fatigue.

Central Nervous System. Dose-related central nervous system toxicities include confusion, inability to perform simple calculations or to concentrate, depression, somnolence, electroencephalogram changes with diffuse slowing as with encephalopathies, and paresthesias. At lower doses, patients may note irritability, lack of patience, low motivation, and depression. Patients may forget appointments and become easily disoriented. Headaches can be relieved with acetaminophen.

Many of these neurologic changes are subtle, and patients tend to try to cover up impairments, such that specific testing and questioning of family members should be a routine element in the assessment of patients.

Gastrointestinal. Fewer than one third of patients experience mild nausea, usually during the first week of treatment. This is a constant nausea, seldom accompanied by emesis, which is managed by the use of antiemetics. Mild diarrhea is reported occasionally, also in the initial stages of therapy.

More common gastrointestinal complaints include chronic taste alteration, early satiety, and cumulative anorexia. Nutritional counseling is important to help patients maintain their strength and to avoid muscle wasting syndrome. Decreased salivary flow may contribute to the occurrence of stomatitis, caries, and candidiasis, which means that good oral care is important.

Cardiovascular. Sudden cardiac deaths and myocardial infarctions are rare, but precautions are given against the use of high doses of interferon in individuals with a strong history of active cardiac disease and for the careful evaluation of the heart and electrocardiogram before initiating interferon therapy.

Orthostatic hypotension is evident during patient monitoring, although most patients are unaware of it. It is managed in most cases by encouraging intake of sufficient fluids and advising patients to avoid sudden changes in position. Hypertensive medications may need to be lowered or discontinued during interferon therapy.

Hematologic, Hepatic, and Renal. These organ toxicities are dose related and disappear when the interferon is discontinued or the dose is lowered. Mild decrease in granulocytes, platelets, and red blood cells is seen during interferon therapy. Transient elevations in serum transaminase levels and mild proteinuria have been reported. Because interferon is cleared via the kidneys, patients with preexisting renal disease should be observed carefully.

Patient Education and Support. Patients need careful explanations, both to educate them regarding their treatment program and to familiarize them with the terminology used with BRM therapies. Patients are taught to self-administer the interferon doses. They learn about preparation of the injection, use of syringes, sterile technique, and proper administration of the injection, including rotation of subcutaneous injection sites. Patients are taught to recognize and report toxicities promptly to the health care team to prevent the development of more severe complications.

Such suggestions as frequent rest periods, evening injections, use of acetaminophen, and hydration to avoid dehydration help patients tolerate longer courses of interferon therapy.

Interleukin 2

Interleukin 2 is a lymphokine that is a BRM (peptide hormone). It is secreted by T lymphocytes, which are capable of directing the function of other cells in the area of an immune response. IL-2 directs the T lymphocytes to multiply into clones capable of performing during an immune response.

Mechanism of action

As a growth factor, IL-2 sustains the proliferation of activated T lymphocytes. T lymphocytes not stimulated by the immune response do not express IL-2 receptors. T lymphocytes activated by antigenic stimulation express IL-2 receptors and will facilitate the multiplication of T lymphocytes under the direction of IL-2. Depending on the subset of activated T lymphocytes that are amplified, IL-2 has several different in vitro immunologic effects.

Clinical applications

IL-2 and LAK cell therapy is known as *adoptive immunotherapy*. This term implies that there is a transfer of active immunologic cells with the potential to directly or indirectly induce an antitumor response in the patient with a tumor. Significant tumor responses in patients with malignant melanoma, colon carcinoma, and metastatic renal cell carcinoma have been reported. Researchers became very optimistic that IL-2 given with LAK cells could be a significant breakthrough in cancer treatment.

Future applications

Tumor-Infiltrating Lymphocytes. The tumor-infiltrating lymphocytes can be infused into the patient, in an effort to mediate tumor regression. Tumor-infiltrating lymphocytes do not require systemic administration of IL-2 to sustain their cytotoxic ability.

Tumor-infiltrating lymphocytes are prepared by surgically removing a portion of the tumor and dissecting it into pieces that are digested in an enzyme solution. The tumor cell suspension is placed in a culture medium. While in culture, the number of lymphocytes increases as the number of tumor cells decreases. Tumor-infiltrating lymphocytes are administered in the same manner as LAK cells, through a central line catheter.

Interleukin 2 and Interferon-β. The combination of IL-2 and interferon-β is being tested in an effort to activate LAK cells and achieve further enhancement of the antitumor response.

Cyclophosphamide and Interleukin 2. In laboratory studies, cyclophosphamide (Cytoxan) given concomitantly with IL-2 inhibits capillary leakage in mice. Cyclophosphamide also may reduce tumor bulk or may remove suppressor cells that interfere with the immune destruction of tumor.

Side effects

Constitutional. Fevers of up to 40.5°C with chills may occur within 2 hours of administering IL-2 and persist until after it has been discontinued. Acetaminophen and nonsteroidal anti-inflammatory drugs control the fever very well.

Headache, malaise, and flu-like symptoms are observed frequently. Nasal congestion, glossitis, and xerostomia have been reported.

Integumentary. The majority of patients develop diffuse erythema that may evolve into a pruritic desquamating rash.

Cardiovascular or Pulmonary. At high doses, systemic vascular resistance drops significantly, producing leaky capillary syndrome with significant hypotension. Intravascular volume depletion occurs, and fluid replacement results in significant amounts of fluid weight gain. Fluid retention is manifested by peripheral edema, ascites, and later by pulmonary interstitial edema that may necessitate intubation.

Gastrointestinal. Some patients experience severe nausea and vomiting and may have significant diarrhea. Mucositis has developed in many of the patients, along with anorexia.

Neurologic. Confusion is observed frequently in patients after receiving several doses of IL-2. Combativeness, disorientation, increased anxiety, and, rarely, psychosis have been reported.

Renal. Oliguria, proteinuria, and elevations of serum creatinine and blood urea nitrogen are exhibited frequently. Restoration of normal renal function usually occurs within 48 hours of discontinuing IL-2.

Hepatic. Most patients develop hyperbilirubinemia to some degree, with liver enzyme changes suggestive of intrahepatic cholestasis.

Hematologic. Progressive anemia, exacerbated by the leukapheresis procedures, thrombocytopenia, and rise in prothrombin and partial thromboplastin times are reported frequently.

Miscellaneous. Several cases of hepatitis A were noted in patients treated with IL-2 and LAK cells. This infection was traced back to the human serum added to the tissue culture medium in which LAK cells were generated. All serum has been routinely screened for hepatitis B and human T-lymphocyte virus III.

After completion of the course of therapy, patients generally recover very rapidly and are discharged within 2 to 3 days.

Tumor Necrosis Factor

Tumor necrosis factor (TNF) was named on the basis of its ability to cause necrosis of established tumors in the mouse. It is a monokine produced by activated macrophages and specialized circulating phagocytic monocytes that selectively kills neoplastic cells.

Mechanism of action

The production of the monokine TNF by mononuclear phagocytes is induced by most infectious agents, including virus particles and some of the other BRMs. TNF is the mediator of general inflammation. Its induction of necrosis appears to be related to its ability to diminish tissue perfusion. It alters hemostatic properties of vascular endothelium, inducing a disseminated intravascular coagulation type of effect at a systemic level with local occlusion of tumor vessels. TNF is directly toxic to vascular endothelial cells, causing the third spacing of plasma water and electrolytes into the extravascular spaces. It also induces the release of interleukin 1 by monocytes and endothelial cells, which may elicit the features of endotoxin poisoning: fever, hypotension, neutropenia, and thrombocytopenia.

Exposure to TNF activates macrophages to release cytotoxic factors that mediate events leading up to hemorrhagic necrosis. The core of the tumor turns blue-black, owing to the extravasation of blood into the tumor, which may then slough off. TNF is effective against established tumors.

Side effects

Considerable toxicity is associated with the administration of TNF.

Thymic Hormones
Historical background

The thymus is located in the chest anterior to the heart and great vessels. It is a rather mysterious lymphoid tissue whose function is still being identified. This organ consists of a dense reticular framework with lymphocytes arranged in the cortex and medulla. The lymphoid tissue receives a rich blood supply.

Mechanism of action

The thymus synthesizes small hormone like polypeptides that differ in chemical structure and circulate in the bloodstream, producing systemic effects similar to those of hormones. The thymus has emerged as the potential master gland of immunity. The thymus secretes an entire family of compounds into the bloodstream that influence a patient's immunologic responses.

Thymic hormones can correct immune function in immune diseases. By increasing numbers and functions of T lymphocytes, by activating other lymphokines with antiviral activity, and by stimulating macrophage populations, thymic hormones help prevent infections in patients with cancer.

Clinical applications

The two best known products—thymosin fraction 5, a partially purified natural compound prepared from the thymus gland, and thymosin-α_1, a potent synthetic component of thymosin fraction 5 that induces helper T cells and lymphokines—are currently in clinical trials with children and adults who have primary and secondary immunodeficiency diseases, including those undergoing cancer therapy, those with pre-AIDS, and those with autoimmune diseases, such as rheumatoid arthritis and multiple sclerosis.

Toxicity

Thymic hormones have been reported to have very mild side effects, only inflammation at the injection site and no organ toxicity.

Nursing considerations

Administration, route, dosage, and stability of the preparations are the primary concerns of the nurse working with thymic hormones. Education of the patient regarding basic immunology and the purpose of thymic hormones involves the nurse in teaching. Representation of the patient who participates in clinical trials with such new agents makes the nurse the patient's advocate.

Growth Factors

Peptide Growth Factors. Normal growth relies on the controlled expression of growth factors. Malignant growth occurs when uncontrolled expression occurs. Platelets, macrophages, and lymphocytes all normally produce peptide growth factors, which in a malignant condition may be stimulated by cancer cell by-products to increase production of peptide growth factors, which mediate further malignant behavior. Peptide growth factors can influence invasiveness and metastasis of tumors by affecting matrix destruction and synthesis and angiogenesis.

A specific peptide growth factor, transforming growth factor-β, is produced by cells of the immune system. Transforming growth factor-β modulates the activity of immune cells, affects matrix syntheses and angiogenesis by cells, and potently inhibits immunoglobulin synthesis by B lymphocytes.

Tumor Growth Factors. Malignant transformation of cancer cells may occur by (1) excessive production, expression, and action of positive autocrine factors or (2) failure of cells to synthesize, express, or respond to specific negative growth factors. Tumor growth factors are substances secreted by transformed cells. Although growth factors secreted by normal cells and tumor growth factors are similar in many ways, normal growth factors do not cause transformation. Growth factors act via a cell surface receptor mechanism, and, in fact, significant similarity has been shown between some growth factor receptors and oncogenic products.

Colony-Stimulating Factors. A number of polypeptide growth factors capable of stimulating the proliferation and differentiation of specific hematologic cell lines have been identified and investigated in the past 15 years.

Granulocyte-macrophage CSF induces colony formation, stimulating a marked response in the total white blood cell count, with particular increments in neutrophils and eosinophils and in lymphocytes and reticulocytes as well.

Erythropoietin was identified in 1906 as the hormone produced primarily by the kidneys that is responsible for the regulation and control of red blood cell production and maturation. Erythropoietin has undergone clinical trials for the correction of anemia related to end-stage renal failure and dialysis. Hemoglobin and hematocrit levels returned to normal without the problems associated with repeated blood transfusions, such as iron overload, development of antibodies, or transmission of infectious viral agents. Patients achieve a sense of well-being and levels of energy that enable them to return to normal lifestyles.

Tumor Vaccines

Another type of adoptive immunotherapy involves removal of patients' lymphocytes, sensitization of lymphocytes immunized against tumor cells from the patients' tumors, and return of the sensitized blood cells to the patient.

Before the initiation of biologic therapy with vaccines, the strength of the patient's immune response must be assessed. An anergic response (weak or nonexistent) would be a poor indicator for the ability of therapy to enhance the host's immune response.

Miscellaneous Factors

Cimetidine (commonly used to treat ulcers) has been shown to have a potent modulating effect on the immune system. Histamines lead to activation of suppressor T lymphocytes and release of suppressor factors. Cimetidine blocks this overall suppression, thereby allowing an increased action of the immune system. Antitumor effects have been noted in patients receiving cimetidine alone or in combination with interferon.

Antimetastatic Agents

Agents with proposed antimetastatic activity include inhibitors of tumor cell invasion (protease inhibitors and disruptors of microtubule function), antagonists of tumor cell–

platelet interactions (prostacyclin thromboxane antagonists, calcium channel blockers), and blockers of tumor cell arrest (laminin fragments).

Anticoagulants

Metastatic cells in the blood have been observed to be associated with platelets or fibrin attached to vessel walls. Platelet aggregation interacting with tumor cells assists in the attachment of tumor cells to the vascular endothelium or in the covering of the tumor cell that prevents its recognition and elimination by the natural killer cells. It has been observed that anticoagulant drugs have substantial antimetastatic effects.

Angiogenesis inhibitors

Interest lies in investigating the idea that if tumors recruit new vessels continuously, inhibition of the angiogenesis factor would lead to tumor atrophy.

Enzymes

Cathepsin B is a lysosomal enzyme that is released primarily by neoplastic tissues. Detection of the activity of this enzyme in serum correlates directly with invasion and metastasis. Attempts to block the activity of this enzyme, such as with an MoAb, may allow interruption of the cascade of biologic events that leads to metastasis.

SUMMARY

Oldham and Smalley suggested that biotherapy would become the fourth modality of cancer treatment, with surgery, chemotherapy, and radiation therapy being the standard three.

Nurses have played and will continue to play an important role in caring for patients receiving BRMs. Now, BRMs are being administered not only in research settings but in community hospitals, physicians' offices, and private homes. Suppers and McClamrock point out that clinical trials with BRMs will demand different nursing approaches than those to which nurses grew accustomed with chemotherapy trials. For example, toxicities may be difficult to determine because they are often subtle, subjective, or cumulative over a period of time. Nurses will need acute observation skills and a systematic approach to patient assessment to detect the effects of BRMs in an individual. Nurses must be familiar with biotherapy and understand the components of the immune system and their function to make these assessments as well as to educate patients about their treatment program.

8 Blood Component Therapy

PATRICIA F. JASSAK
JOHN GODWIN

Blood component therapy plays an integral role in the comprehensive care of cancer patients. Advances in the use of blood components have affected the overall survival rate of cancer patients by contributing to the success of new cancer treatments associated with prolonged myelosuppression.

The safety of blood products has become a national concern since the recognition in 1982 of the transmission of acquired immune deficiency syndrome (AIDS) by blood transfusion. This concern is especially acute in the cancer patient, who is frequently exposed to large numbers of blood components. The cancer patient is not usually a candidate for autologous blood (self-donated) donation owing to disease and therapy-related bone marrow depression. The risk of AIDS transmission by transfusion can be reduced by ensuring donor selectivity, the use of newer screening methods to detect the AIDS virus, and the development of growth factors to promote autologous cell production and decrease transfusion need.

BASIC PRINCIPLES OF TRANSFUSION

The most common indication for transfusion in the cancer patient is *bone marrow depression,* a general term used to describe a decrease in blood cell production from the marrow. Bone marrow depression is manifested as a decrease

---

See the corresponding chapter in *Cancer Nursing: A Comprehensive Textbook,* by Baird, McCorkle, and Grant, pp. 370–384, for a more detailed discussion of this topic, including a comprehensive list of references.

in one or more blood cell lines (e.g., anemia, thrombocytopenia, or granulocytopenia). The usual cause of bone marrow depression in the cancer patient is the malignancy itself, the therapies the patient is given for cancer, or a nutritional deficiency state.

Knowledge of the patient's type of cancer will enable the medical team to anticipate transfusion needs. Different transfusion requirements can be anticipated among malignancies owing to the manifestations of the disease itself or the specific treatment strategies employed. Leukemic patients are given chemotherapy despite the presence of severe cytopenia. However, when severe cytopenia occurs in patients with solid tumors or other hematologic malignancies, the treatment regimen is usually adjusted by decreasing the dose, extending the length of the recovery period, or doing both. This solution results in less severe marrow depression in solid tumor patients and in a shorter duration of transfusion support for myelosuppression.

SOURCES OF BLOOD COLLECTION

Blood components are available from three different donor sources: homologous, autologous, or directed (designated) donors. Homologous blood is obtained from the general pool of volunteer donors—or, less commonly, paid donors—and is the most common source of blood components for patients. Autologous blood is the recipient's own blood that was donated before its anticipated use. Directed or designated donor blood is obtained when the recipient selects or recruits a specific person for blood donation.

Directed donor programs have been established in response to the AIDS crisis and are mandated by law in some states. Directed donor and homologous units are screened for transmissible diseases and tested for compatibility. When screening tests are positive, the blood units are discarded and the donor is informed confidentially.

RED BLOOD CELL COMPATIBILITY TESTING

The purpose of red blood cell compatibility testing is to prevent the destruction of the transfused cells. When this destruction occurs, it is called a hemolytic transfusion reaction. It is an antigen-antibody reaction.

An antigen is a molecule that is recognized as foreign (nonself) by the immune system. Antigens stimulate B cells of the immune system to produce antibodies and also sensitize monocytes and T cells to react with the antigen. Antibodies are a family of proteins that have in common the ability to bind to antigens. Antigen-antibody binding is one of the major ways that the immune system eliminates foreign substances. Hemolytic transfusion reactions are triggered by antigen-antibody binding.

In 1900, Landsteiner found that human red cells will react with the sera of some persons and not others. He described blood types that were different by virtue of the presence of different red blood cell antigens. He recognized three different blood types, which he called A, B, and O (a fourth group, AB, was later added by Landsteiner's pupils). Red cells contain either an A or B antigen, both, or neither (group O), and serum contains antibodies to antigens not present on the person's red blood cells.

More than 400 different antigens are present on the human red blood cell surface. Families of these antigens with similar antigenic and genetic properties form blood groups. Rh was the name given by Landsteiner and Wiener to the human red blood cell antigen that showed reactivity with sera from animals immunized with red blood cells from the rhesus monkey.

Red blood cell compatibility testing involves a series of pretransfusion tests in the blood bank designed to detect antibodies against blood antigens in the recipient's serum and ensure the acceptance of the donor blood by the recipient. The type and crossmatch order is a request for pretransfusion testing.

TISSUE COMPATIBILITY ANTIGENS (HLA)

The major histocompatibility antigens among humans are termed histocompatibility locus antigens (HLA). They are found on all cells except red blood cells and serve as tissue recognition sites. These antigens can be detected serologically by testing different sera using a patient's lymphocytes. They play an important role when problems with platelet transfusion occur.

Multiple red blood cell or platelet transfusions expose the patient to numerous foreign HLA antigens. In some patients, an immune response occurs and alloantibodies (antibodies to other human antigens) to HLA-A, HLA-B, and HLA-C antigens develop. These antibodies are responsible for the immune destruction of platelets.

BLOOD COMPONENTS AND THEIR ADMINISTRATION

Blood component therapy is the transfusion of a specific part of blood rather than whole blood and offers several advantages. It conserves precious resources and allows the tailoring of treatment for specific problems (e.g., platelets for thrombocytopenia and packed red blood cells for anemia). In addition, it provides an optimal method for patients who require numerous transfusions of a specific blood component. Table 8–1 lists the most commonly used blood components and their characteristics.

Red Blood Cells

Packed red blood cells (PRBCs) are prepared from a unit of whole blood by removing 200 to 250 ml of plasma. Each unit of PRBCs still contains residual leukocytes, platelets,

Table 8-1. BLOOD COMPONENT SUMMARY

Component	Available Forms	Indication	Contents	Volume	Infusion Time	Expected Response
Red blood cells (RBCs)	RBCs	Signs of anemia (Hgb <8 g)*	RBCs; WBCs and platelets are nonfunctional	250–300 ml	2–4 hours	Increase Hgb to 1 g/dl unit
	Filtered PRBCs	Repeated febrile reactions	RBCs, WBCs (<10^8), platelets, plasma	200 ml	2–4 hours	Same
Leukocyte-poor RBCs	Saline-washed PRBCs	Febrile reactions; IgA deficiency with allergic reactions	RBCs, WBCs (<10^8), platelets, minimal plasma	200 ml	2–4 hours	Same
	Frozen, deglycerolized RBCs	Rare blood type	RBCs, no plasma, minimal WBCs, platelets	180 ml	2–4 hours	Same

Platelets	Random donor (RD)	<20,000 platelet count, bleeding	Multiple units, plasma, WBCs, few RBCs	1 unit = 30–50 ml (8 units pooled ~400 ml)	1 unit over 5–10 minutes	Increase platelet count to 5000; mm^3 per unit in 70-kg adult
	Single donor, non-HLA matched	Severe febrile reactions or alloantibodies	Single donor, from apheresis; donor may be family or nonrelated; plasma, WBCs, RBCs	300 ml	30–60 minutes	Equivalent to 8 units RD platelets (~40,000 increase)
	Single donor, HLA matched	Alloantibodies (refractory responder)	Single donor; HLA-A, B, C matched; plasma, WBCs, RBCs	300 ml	30–60 minutes	Equivalent to 8 units RD platelets (~40,000 increase)

Continued

97

Table 8–1. BLOOD COMPONENT SUMMARY *Continued*

Component	Available Forms	Indication	Contents	Volume	Infusion Time	Expected Response
Granulocytes	Single donor granulocyte concentrate	Documented sepsis with PMN* <500; infection worse despite antibiotics	Granulocytes, lymphocytes, platelets, some RBCs, plasma	400 ml	45–60 minutes	Transient (<4 hours) rise in WBC count
Fresh frozen plasma (FFP)	From homologous donor pool and frozen within 6 hours	Coagulation factor deficiency	All coagulation factors, complement	220 ml	30–60 minutes	1 unit increases coagulation factors by 5%–10%
Cryoprecipitate	From FFP cold-insoluble precipitate after thaw at 4–6°C	Deficiency of factor VIII (coagulant or von Willebrand factor), fibrinogen, or factor XIII	Fibrinogen, factor VIII, factor XIII, minimal immunoglobulins	10–15 ml unit	15–30 minutes	Increase factors VIII, XIII, and fibrinogen levels

*Hgb, hemoglobin; PMN, polymorphonuclear leukocytes.

and plasma proteins, but the granulocytes and platelets become nonfunctional because of storage time and conditions. PRBCs contain a portion of the anticoagulant-preservative used when obtaining the whole blood. The most commonly used agent is citrate phosphate dextrose with adenine (CPDA-1). PRBCs are stored at 4° to 6°C for a shelf life of 35 days.

Patients may become sensitized to the white blood cell and platelet antigens still present in the PRBC unit, which often leads to febrile or allergic transfusion reactions. These reactions are more common in patients who have had multiple pregnancies or prior transfusions. Methods to remove unwanted antigens include *filtration,* usually with special in-line white blood cell removal filters, *centrifugation* of the unit in the blood bank with mechanical removal or trapping of white blood cells, *washing* the PRBCs with buffer solutions, and using *frozen* red blood cells (these cells are washed to remove glycerol).

Platelets

One unit of platelets is obtained from each unit of donated whole blood. Each platelet unit has a volume of approximately 50 ml and contains varying amounts of residual leukocytes and red blood cells. Platelet units are stored for 5 days at room temperature (20° to 24°C) with constant gentle agitation. Cold temperatures activate platelets. Multiple units are pooled for each transfusion. For an adult, the average platelet transfusion consists of 6 to 10 units. Platelets are transfused as needed in cases of bleeding and prophylactically to prevent bleeding. Traditionally, the platelet count used for prophylactic transfusion is 20,000/mm³. Platelets are available in three forms: (1) random donor, (2) single donor non-HLA matched, and (3) single donor HLA matched. A single donor platelet transfusion raises the platelet count by approximately 40,000 platelets/mm³. In the absence of normal platelet production, platelet transfusions generally are required every 3 days. Severe exogenous losses, including those that occur in the presence of hemorrhage or fever, will increase platelet transfusion requirements.

Monitoring the posttransfusion platelet count is critical in determining the efficacy of a platelet transfusion. A 1-hour posttransfusion count should be obtained if the random count does not rise appropriately or if there is active blood loss. Evidence by O'Connell et al. indicates that 10-minute posttransfusion counts are as useful as 1-hour posttransfusion counts for evaluating platelet transfusion efficacy.

Granulocytes

The use of granulocytes is controversial. Once initiated, granulocyte transfusions are given daily until bone marrow recovery or resolution of the identified clinical indication occurs. Complications associated with administration of granulocyte concentrates include pulmonary infiltrates, severe febrile reactions, and transmission of viruses, such as cytomegalovirus and hepatitis. In addition, the concomitant administration of granulocytes and amphotericin B has been reported to produce severe adverse pulmonary reactions, although another study failed to confirm this observation. In practice, the administration of amphotericin B and granulocytes should be separated by 4 to 6 hours because either agent alone may cause a severe allergic reaction.

Plasma Products

Plasma component products routinely available are (1) fresh frozen plasma (FFP), and (2) cryoprecipitate (CRYO). These products are used in cancer patients to treat coagulopathies due to secondary disease states, such as disseminated intravascular clotting (DIC) or liver failure.

FFP should be used to replace coagulation factors and not to expand blood volume or to replace fluid. FFP often is indicated for replacement of multiple clotting factor deficiencies. All clotting factors are present in FFP at an approximate concentration of 1 unit of factor/ml of FFP.

Costs of Blood Component Therapy

Blood components vary in cost across the country. Current blood component charges reflect five distinct types of fees. These include (1) a processing fee, (2) a product preparation fee, (3) a type and screen fee, (4) a crossmatch fee, and (5) an administration fee.

HEMAPHERESIS

Technologic advances have allowed the introduction into clinical medicine of sophisticated cell separators. These machines remove whole blood from the donor, separate it into cellular and plasma components by centrifugation, and return the remaining blood to the donor. *Hemapheresis* is the general term used for all procedures for which cell separators are used. Leukapheresis is the selective collection of leukocytes (usually referring to granulocytes).

The most common hemapheresis requested is thrombocytapheresis, which is the removal or collection of platelets. Single donor and HLA-matched platelets are collected from normal donors by this technique (see the earlier section on platelets).

Plasmapheresis is used to selectively remove plasma components in various disease states.

COMPLICATIONS OF TRANSFUSION

The term *transfusion reaction* generally refers to the immediate immune reactions that can occur from blood component therapy. The most frequent acute nonimmune complication of transfusion is congestive heart failure from volume overload. The most common delayed nonimmune reaction is the transmission of infection (Tables 8–2 and 8–3). Iron overload is another delayed reaction that is seen after many red blood cell transfusions (usually more than 100).

Complications Due to Immune Mechanisms

Posttransfusion purpura is a rare, immune-mediated thrombocytopenic complication of red blood cell or plasma product transfusion. A patient with a normal platelet count may receive a red blood cell, platelet, or plasma transfusion for a standard indication and 7 to 10 days later suddenly develop severe thrombocytopenia. The exact mechanism of platelet destruction is not completely understood, but it appears to occur in persons who lack one or more very common platelet-specific antigens.

Graft-versus-host disease (GVHD) is a rare complication of transfusion therapy that has been documented in severely immunocompromised recipients. This complication is a direct result of the transfusion of immunocompetent T lymphocytes, present in whole blood, granulocyte, platelet, and red blood cell fractionated components. Cancer patients at highest risk for developing GVHD from blood component therapy include bone marrow transplant patients and patients with Hodgkin's and non-Hodgkin's lymphoma undergoing combined chemotherapy and radiation.

Irradiating blood components with 15 to 50 Gy (1500 to 5000 rad) abolishes the ability of the T lymphocytes to proliferate without compromising the function of other blood components. The use of irradiated blood components in severely immunocompromised states has been recommended to prevent GVHD.

Infectious Complications

The development of non-A, non-B hepatitis is the most frequent serious risk faced by the recipient of a transfusion. Non-A, non-B hepatitis is responsible for approximately 80% to 90% of the hepatitis seen following transfusion, and the rest represents predominantly hepatitis B.

The next most important infectious complication of transfusion is cytomegalovirus (CMV) infection. This virus is transmitted by viable leukocytes in the blood product. The recipients at highest risk for complications of CMV infection are (1) immunocompromised patients, (2) the fetus in utero with primary CMV maternal infection, and (3) premature infants. Blood components that contain anti-CMV antibodies (CMV-positive units) are more likely to transmit the infection. Bowden et al. reported that CMV-negative bone marrow transplant patients who received only CMV-nega-

Table 8–2. IMMEDIATE IMMUNE TRANSFUSION REACTIONS

Reaction	Mechanism
Anaphylaxis	Antibody to IgA (hereditary or acquired IgA deficiency)
Hemolysis, acute	Red blood cell incompatibility
Fever, nonhemolytic	Antibody to donor leukocyte antigens
Urticaria	Antibody to plasma proteins
Noncardiogenic pulmonary edema	Antibody to recipient leukocytes; complement activation

tive blood products had a significantly decreased incidence of CMV infection compared with those patients who received standard blood products without regard to the presence of CMV.

NURSING IMPLICATIONS

Administration guidelines for nurses to follow to ensure that oncology patients will receive blood components in a safe, efficient manner are identified in Table 8–4.

Standard 170-μm blood filters are required for all blood components and factor concentrates to trap clots. Microaggregate filters have a pore size of 20 to 40 μm. The function of these filters is to remove leukocyte–platelet aggregates that form during blood storage. Leukocyte-poor filters are used when a leukocyte-poor component is clinically indicated (see earlier sections on red blood cells and platelets).

All blood components should be infused within 4 hours after initiation. This decreases the risk of bacterial contamination and ensures component stability. The blood bank can divide the unit into two or more parts, dispensing one part at a time when clinically warranted. Once the component is obtained, it must be used (that is, the infusion begun) within 30 minutes or returned immediately to the blood bank for proper storage.

No medication should be added to blood at any time. Normal saline solution (0.9%) may be added for dilutional purposes, if needed. A large-gauge needle (18 gauge) is recommended for peripheral blood administration. However, many oncology patients may have poor access routes, and a 20-gauge needle may be used.

Thorough and accurate documentation is critical to the transfusion process. Many institutions require frequent monitoring of vital signs (e.g., every 15 minutes for 1 hour, then every 30 minutes until the transfusion is complete), although few clinical data exist to support this practice. Taylor et al. undertook a retrospective chart audit to deter-

Table 8–3. TRANSFUSION REACTIONS

Type	Signs/Symptoms	Onset	Management
Acute hemolytic	Fever, chills, anaphylaxis, decreased blood pressure, nausea/vomiting, flushing, back pain, hematuria, decreased urine output	Usually during the first 15 minutes	1. Stop transfusion 2. Resuscitate 3. Notify blood bank 4. Monitor intake and output 5. Medical management: administration of osmotic diuretics and fluids
Febrile nonhemolytic	Fever, chills, headache, dyspnea, chest pain, decreased blood pressure, nausea/vomiting	Immediately or within 8 hours of transfusion	1. Stop transfusion 2. Notify blood bank 3. Rule out infection 4. Acetaminophen for fever, meperidine for chills, continue transfusion if symptoms not severe
Allergic	Urticaria	During transfusion or within 1–2 hours	1. Decrease transfusion rate 2. Antihistamines 3. Notify blood bank 4. Monitor vital signs
Delayed hemolytic	Decreased hemoglobin level, low-grade fever	7–10 days to weeks	1. Notify blood bank

Table 8–4. GUIDELINES FOR BLOOD
COMPONENT ADMINISTRATION

---

1. Use universal precautions when handling blood components and contaminated equipment
2. Identify the patient
3. Obtain the requested blood specimen
4. Accurately label the specimen
5. Administer premedications, such as acetaminophen or diphenhydramine hydrochloride, if ordered
6. Obtain the ordered blood component from the blood bank
7. PRIOR TO ADMINISTRATION
   - Verify physician order
   - Compare donor identification numbers and ABO-Rh compatibility on transfusion record with information on blood component
   - At the bedside, identify patient with full name
   - Request patient to state his or her full name
   - Compare full name and identity of patient with name and identification on blood component and transfusion record

   DO NOT TRANSFUSE COMPONENT IF INFORMATION DOES NOT EXACTLY MATCH
   - Check expiration date and time on blood component
   - Once it is determined that everything is correct, sign the transfusion record
8. Inspect the blood component for color and consistency, turning component upside down to gently mix its contents
9. Prepare filter, tubing, and 0.9% normal saline flush solution
10. Record patient's baseline vital signs
11. Start transfusion and record date and time of initiation
12. Stay with the patient for the first 5–15 minutes to assess for an acute reaction
13. Record patient's vital signs 15 minutes after initiation of the transfusion and as required by policy
14. Monitor patients frequently during the transfusion
15. At completion, document patient's condition and complete transfusion record
16. Place copy of transfusion record in patient's chart and return copy to blood bank

---

mine when transfusion reactions occurred in relation to vital sign monitoring. They found that fever and chills were the most common reactions reported, with reactions occurring from 30 minutes to 3 hours 35 minutes from the onset of the transfusion.

SUMMARY AND FUTURE TRENDS

Knowledge of modern transfusion principles is essential for oncology nursing practice. Nurses are in an optimal position to provide education to the cancer patient and family regarding transfusion practice. The administration of blood products is a treatment directly provided to the patient and monitored almost exclusively by nurses.

New cancer treatments with biologic agents may prove to be effective and less toxic to the bone marrow, thus reducing transfusion support requirements in the future. Recombinant hormonal agents that stimulate hematopoietic cell production are in early clinical trials. These agents may allow cytotoxic therapy to be given with fewer and shorter intervals of bone marrow suppression. However, treatment methods, such as high-dose chemotherapy with autologous bone marrow transplant, require intensive blood component support. Additionally, the use of such intensive therapies may increase in future clinical practice. An intimate knowledge of the principles of blood transfusion remains essential for the oncology nurse.

9 Bone Marrow Transplantation

ROSEMARY C. FORD

HISTORICAL PERSPECTIVE

The first bone marrow transplants in humans were conducted in the 1950s in patients with end-stage leukemia. These transplants were unsuccessful in that all the patients relapsed. However, the patients did show hematologic recovery. By the late 1960s, several developments had offered encouragement to again try marrow transplant in humans, including advances in tissue typing, improved techniques for pheresis of blood products, and development of more effective and broad-spectrum antibiotics. Clinical trials resumed in the early 1970s, again with patients considered to be in the end stages of their disease. Because of the success of these studies, protocols were initiated for patients earlier in their course of treatment, when their physical condition was better.

Since the early 1970s, the number of long-term transplantation survivors has increased every year. Relapse and long-term survival vary depending on the diagnosis of the patient and the type of transplant.

Marrow transplantation remains a highly experimental procedure. Medical research on transplant units continues to focus on finding optimum conditioning therapies, timing of transplantation in the course of the patient's original

See the corresponding chapter in *Cancer Nursing: A Comprehensive Textbook,* by Baird, McCorkle, and Grant, pp. 385–406, for a more detailed discussion of this topic, including a comprehensive list of references.

disease, and preventing or limiting the major complications, such as infections and graft-versus-host disease (GVHD).

BONE MARROW TRANSPLANT NURSING AS A SPECIALTY

Bone marrow transplantation (BMT) has become established over the last 20 years as a treatment option for patients with aplastic anemia, hematologic malignancies, selected solid tumors, and some genetic disorders.

TYPES OF MARROW TRANSPLANTS

Transplanted marrow can be obtained from several sources, and the source determines the type of transplant the patient receives. In searching for a marrow donor, the human leukocyte antigens (HLA) are identified from blood drawn from the patient and all potential donors. These antigens play a role in the immune response. The HLA-A, HLA-B, and HLA-C loci are identified through a cytotoxic assay using anti-HLA antibodies. The HLA-D locus is identified by a mixed lymphocyte culture of cells from the patient and the potential donors. Reactivity is monitored, and if there is no response, the mixed lymphocyte culture is negative and, therefore, the HLA-D locus is considered matched.

The ABO blood antigens are also identified at this time. A difference in ABO blood groups between patient and donor will not interfere with donor selection, but it does present unique clinical problems. The marrow infusion may have to be depleted of red blood cells (RBCs) to prevent a hemolytic reaction caused by antibodies still circulating from the patient's original marrow.

The most desirable donor in terms of compatibility is an identical twin. Transplants from identical twins are called *syngeneic*. Transplants from persons other than twins are called *allogeneic*. Allogeneic donors may or may not be HLA-MLC matched with the patient. These donors are usually siblings, although other family members can also be used as donors. The odds of a patient matching a sibling are 1 in 4, resulting in only 35% to 40% of patients having a matched sibling. Unrelated but HLA-matched donors have been used successfully for patients without related donors. Mismatched donors also have been used. When the donor and patient differ in only one HLA haplotype, the results are similar to those of patients with matched donors. When differences occur in two or three haplotypes, the incidence of complications is markedly increased.

Allogeneic transplants are the prototype of transplants for hematologic malignancies. The success rates of allogeneic transplants led to trials of autologous transplants in patients without a suitable marrow donor. *Autologous* transplants use the patient's own marrow. When the patient is in remission, marrow is aspirated and frozen. At a later date, usually after the patient has relapsed, the patient undergoes high-dose conditioning in an attempt to destroy all tumor cells. The marrow is then reinfused back into the patient, sometimes after having been treated in vitro with agents to remove any residual tumor cells.

Each type of transplant has advantages and disadvantages. Autologous transplant recipients experience less regimen-related toxicity than allogeneic transplant recipients. Autologous and syngeneic transplants eliminate the complication of GVHD.

THE TRANSPLANTATION PROCESS
Preadmission

The timing of transplantation depends on the patient's diagnosis. Ideally, at the time of diagnosis and before induction therapy is started, it should be determined whether the patient is a candidate for marrow transplantation. Factors that should be considered are the patient's physical, emotional, and psychologic status, the possibility of identifying an acceptable marrow donor, the patient's financial status, including insurance coverage, and the patient's philosophy on entering a research study.

The patient's primary physician usually presents the option of marrow transplantation, with a recommendation as to which center to consider. Once a referral is made to a transplant center, the medical staff at the center determines whether the patient is eligible for entry on a current protocol. When the patient is accepted by the center, the patient and the referring physician are notified, and the patient may be placed on a waiting list for an opening at the center. The length of the wait is determined by many factors, including the acuteness of the patient's condition, the protocol priorities at the center, and the physical status of the patient.

The patient and the donor must both come to the center for about 1 week before admission to confirm the health status of both, the remission status of the patient, and the genetic match of the donor.

A permanent right atrial dual-lumen or, in some cases, triple-lumen catheter is inserted for venous access if the patient does not already have one in place.

Admission to the Marrow Transplant Unit

When the patient has completed the preadmission workup, he or she is admitted to the transplant unit. The inpatient team explains the treatment protocols, responds to concerns, and obtains signatures on research consent forms. The primary nurse should review the teaching begun in the outpatient department and initiate a care plan for this patient. Nurses must individualize patient teaching to match the knowledge base of each patient.

Conditioning Therapy

Conditioning consists of high-dose chemotherapy or total body irradiation (TBI) or both, precisely timed (Fig. 9-1). The purpose is to totally eradicate the patient's original marrow and any residual tumor cells. The common chemotherapeutic agent used is cyclophosphamide, given in megadose. However, dimethylbusulfan, cytosine arabinoside, etoposide, melphalan, and carmustine also are used. Total body irradiation can be given from one or two sources at one session or fractionated over several days.

All patients experience side effects during the days of conditioning, including severe nausea, vomiting, and diarrhea. Owing to the severe gastrointestinal response during high-dose chemotherapy infusion, continuous antiemetic coverage is recommended. The antiemetics can cause profound sedation, and nurses must keep the patients arousable while administering optimal antiemetic relief. High-dose cyclophosphamide can cause cardiotoxicity. Electrocardiograms should be taken before each dose to assess for decreased voltage. Hemorrhagic cystitis can also result from high-dose cyclophosphamide. Bladder irrigation and intravenous hydration should be initiated before and continue 24 hours after administration of this medication.

Total body irradiation usually produces less severe nausea and vomiting than high-dose chemotherapy and so requires less antiemetic usage. The patient may become febrile immediately after TBI. Some patients also develop bilateral parotitis.

The Bone Marrow Donor

On or around the last day of conditioning of the patient, the marrow donor is admitted to the hospital to donate marrow. This is a surgical procedure requiring general or spinal anesthesia. Multiple aspirations from the anterior and posterior iliac crests of the pelvic bone are performed. The volume of marrow is determined by the size of the donor, with a pediatric donor usually yielding a volume of 300 ml and a male adult donor often yielding a volume of more than 1000 ml. The marrow is filtered in the operating room, using a large metal mesh to remove bone particles and fat, and then is placed in blood administration bags.

The marrow donor may require an RBC transfusion after donation because most of the volume of marrow aspiration is whole blood. Often, the marrow donor undergoes pheresis for a unit of blood a week before marrow donation, which is returned during surgery. Donors usually are discharged the day after surgery with oral pain medication, prophylactic antibiotics, and ferrous sulfate supplements.

The donors must be included in the planning of care to the patient–family unit. Some centers require that the donor be in close geographic proximity of the center when the

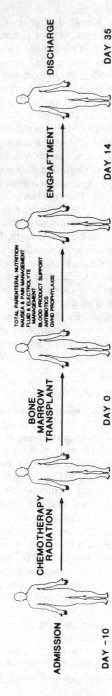

Figure 9–1. Depiction of the process for an allogeneic marrow transplant. In this example, the patient receives conditioning to prepare for the transplant and then receives graft-versus-host disease (GVHD) prophylaxis per protocol.

ADMISSION
DAY –10

CHEMOTHERAPY
RADIATION

BONE
MARROW
TRANSPLANT
DAY 0

TOTAL PARENTERAL NUTRITION
NAUSEA & PAIN MANAGEMENT
FLUID & ELECTROLYTE
MANAGEMENT
BLOOD PRODUCT SUPPORT
ANTIBIOTICS
GVHD PROPHYLAXIS

ENGRAFTMENT
DAY 14

DISCHARGE
DAY 35

patient begins conditioning therapy to ensure the availability of the donor to donate when the patient is ready to receive the marrow. This requirement could call for a 2- or 3-week time commitment. After donating the marrow, the donor may be needed for platelet or white cell donation. This commitment may spread into months if the patient becomes refractory to platelets from other donors.

The psychologic impact of donating marrow must be evaluated for each donor, and appropriate interventions planned. If the patient develops complications after transplant, feelings of guilt may surface in the donor for not having good enough marrow or—in the case of GVHD—of actually causing the problem. A goal should be to help the donor achieve a sense of emotional and intellectual balance before and after the transplant.

The Marrow Transplantation

The actual marrow transplantation is a relatively simple procedure. The marrow is infused into the patient's right atrial catheter, similar to a blood transfusion, except that it is not irradiated or filtered. The rate should be as rapid as possible, determined by the patient's fluid status. Care must be taken to prevent fluid overload because of the colloid load being administered. Side effects are rare. However, chills or a rash occasionally occurs. Rarely, a patient may develop a pulmonary fat embolus or anaphylaxis. These are dealt with as they would be if they resulted from any other cause.

The First 100 Days After Marrow Transplantation

The focus of care in a transplant unit is on optimum support of the patient after the insult of the chemoirradiation and until the marrow graft begins to function. This support requires expert nursing care. Routine nursing tasks, such as taking vital signs, weights, and intake and output, often offer the first clues to the development of a complication and must be performed by a professional staff well educated in the implications of their assessment.

Complications and Side Effects of the Transplantation Process

Acute complications are defined as those occurring during the first 100 days after marrow transplantation. The major complications seen in patients after transplantation are the result of the conditioning regimen (chemoirradiation) used to prepare for transplantation, the lack of a functioning bone marrow, the replacement of the patient's immune system, or iatrogenic (the result of the therapies the patient receives to treat other complications) (Table 9–1). The complications are rarely the result of the patient's original disease. The conditioning is given in supralethal doses, and patients

Table 9–1. CAUSES OF ACUTE AND CHRONIC COMPLICATIONS

Conditioning Regimen (Chemoirradiation Therapies)	Lack of Functioning Marrow	Replacement of Immune System	Iatrogenic Complications
Acute			
Nausea and vomiting	Hemorrhage	Acute GVHD	Renal failure
Diarrhea	Infections		Hypertension
Mucositis	*Cytomegalovirus* pneumonia		Electrolyte imbalance
Alopecia			
Lethargy			
Venoocclusive disease			
Interstitial pneumonia			
Chronic			
Cataracts	Late infections	Chronic GVHD	
Sterility			
Delay or lack of puberty			

GVHD, graft-versus-host disease.

would die if they were not rescued with marrow transplantation.

One complication can cause or exacerbate another, or the treatment of one can cause or exacerbate another. The treatment of one complication may have to be modified or terminated because of the development of another complication, and so the patient is at risk for the development of the complication originally being treated. The clinical onset of many of the complications may be subtle, and the clinical manifestations of different complications can be the same. Nurses must be well educated in assessing patients with complications and in interpreting the results of their assessments.

Graft-versus-host disease

Graft-versus-host disease is unique to marrow transplant patients. In GVHD, the immune system of the donor (specifically the T lymphocytes) recognizes the tissue of the patient as foreign and launches an attack. Three systems of the body are affected by this disease: the skin, the liver, and the gastrointestinal tract. The disease can be manifested in any one or all three systems. Risk factors for developing this disease are age over 30 years, having a donor of the opposite sex, or having a donor who is not a perfect HLA-MLC match. GVHD can be fatal in any of the systems. This disease occurs in one half of all allogeneic transplants, with 16% of these patients dying of GVHD or related complications, such as infection, hemorrhage, or liver disease.

The onset of GVHD coincides with engraftment. Diagnosis is difficult because the symptoms are hard to differentiate from lingering side effects of the conditioning regimen or other complications (Table 9–2).

Much of the medical research conducted on marrow transplant units focuses on protocols to prevent or treat GVHD. The goal of preventive therapies is to remove or inactivate the T lymphocytes. Methotrexate has been administered in low doses to slow the growth of new marrow and, in so doing, slow the production of T lymphocytes. Cyclosporine is an immunosuppressive drug that acts specifically against T lymphocytes and so allows the other cells formed in the bone marrow to grow without interference. Prednisone has also been used for GVHD prophylaxis. Other therapies used to remove T lymphocytes include monoclonal antibodies made specifically against these cells and soybean agglutinin, which is added to the marrow component before infusion.

Infections

Infections caused by bacterial, fungal, or viral pathogens commonly occur alone or in combination in almost every transplant patient. Infections contribute to and often are the major cause of death in transplant patients.

Table 9–2. CLINICAL MANIFESTATIONS AND NURSING IMPLICATIONS OF ACUTE COMPLICATIONS AFTER TRANSPLANTATION

Complication	Clinical Manifestations	Nursing Implications
Mucositis	Initially dry mouth, sore throat, thickening saliva; progressing to copious oral mucus, intense pain, high probability of oral bleeding and infections	• Inspect mouth three times a day, noting color, consistency of mucus, presence of lesions or hemorrhage • Teach patient to perform mouth care with normal saline solution at least every 4 hours • Titrate topical anesthetics and narcotics to patient comfort
Hemorrhage		• Monitor platelet counts • Administer platelets • Avoid invasive procedures when platelet count is less than 50,000 per µl • Avoid medications by intramuscular route
	Epistaxis	• Apply pressure, ice, topicals such as epinephrine, cocaine • In severe cases, the nose may need to be packed • Assess airway for patency • Keep oral airway at bedside • Apply topicals as for epistaxis
	Mouth bleeding often occurs simultaneously with epistaxis	• Encourage frequent mouth care with iced saline solution and cautious use of suction

	Central nervous system bleeding	• Frequent neuroassessment • Lumbar puncture only with platelet count >50,000 • Elevate head of bed
	Gastrointestinal bleeding can be frank or occult	• Guaiac test for all vomitus and stools • Avoid nasogastric tubes, enemas, and rectal medications and temperatures
	Genitourinary	• Assess for blood in urine • Irrigate bladder during administration of cyclophosphamide • Prevent trauma during urinary catheter insertion • Administer medroxyprogesterone acetate to stop menstrual bleeding
Nausea and vomiting	Complaints of nausea Emesis Anorexia	• Assess amount, appearance, color, guaiac positivity, consistency of emesis • Titrate routine antiemetics to patient comfort • Administer total parenteral nutrition until symptoms decrease and appetite returns • Encourage compliance with oral medications
Alopecia		• Support patient in coping with body image change • Suggest hats, scarves, wigs

Continued

115

Table 9–2. CLINICAL MANIFESTATIONS AND NURSING IMPLICATIONS OF ACUTE COMPLICATIONS AFTER TRANSPLANTATION
Continued

Complication	Clinical Manifestations	Nursing Implications
Lethargy		• Encourage patients to ambulate and participate in activities of daily living, schedule times in medication schedule for ambulation, coordinate exercise plan with physical therapists
Venocclusive disease	Sudden weight gain, increase in bilirubin, SGOT, and alkaline phosphatase levels	• Exact assessment of fluid balances and therapy • Check weight twice daily
	Hepatomegaly	• Measure abdominal girth daily
	Ascites	• Postural blood pressure twice daily
	Encephalopathy	• Restrict fluids and sodium intake • Monitor narcotic usage in light of changed liver metabolism • Hemodynamic monitoring if indicated
Renal impairment	Doubling of serum creatinine	• Strict monitoring of intake and output
	Decreased urine output	• Check urine specific gravity every 4 hours
	Decreased quality of urine	• Obtain samples for urine electrolyte and sediment determinations • Monitor patient thirst • Postural blood pressure checks

Graft-versus-host disease	*Initially* Maculopapular rash Nausea and vomiting Green, watery diarrhea Abdominal pain ↑ SGOT *May progress to* Total body skin sloughing Copious watery, guaiac-positive diarrhea Progressive liver failure	• Assess neck veins • Assess for peripheral edema • Monitor patient during dialysis • Daily skin assessment • Daily assessment of stools for quantity, consistency, color • Administer fluids to replace gastrointestinal losses • Protect confused patient
Infections	Fever Increased Erythema at potential site	• Daily hygiene, including bath, dressing, change bed linen • Oral care every 4 hours • Reverse isolation • Good handwashing techniques • Maintain laminar air flow if available • Obtain cultures (blood, urine, throat, stool, catheter site) routinely and immediately on suspicion of development of infection

Continued

117

Table 9–2. CLINICAL MANIFESTATIONS AND NURSING IMPLICATIONS OF ACUTE COMPLICATIONS AFTER TRANSPLANTATION
Continued

Complication	Clinical Manifestations	Nursing Implications
Infections Continued		
Pneumonia	Tachypnea Diffuse infiltrates on chest radiograph	• Administer antimicrobials • Institute measures to lower temperature • Monitor vital signs • Assess breath sounds, quality of respirations, use of accessory respirator, mucositis, skin color, mental status • Support anxious patient and family • Monitor arterial blood gases • Prepare for bronchoalveolar lavage or surgery • Maintain on ventilator

SGOT, serum glutamic oxaloacetic transaminase.

Sites of infection will not resemble those of patients with intact immune systems because there is a lack of white blood cells to make pus and inflammation is usually minimal. Temperature elevation is the main parameter used to detect infection. However, this can be misleading because other factors, such as irradiation, GVHD, and drug or blood product administration, also can elevate temperature. Pancultures should be obtained daily in patients suspected of being infected, although therapy often is started on a best-guess basis before culture results are known.

Risk factors that increase the chance of developing an infection include prolonged granulocytopenia, GVHD, age over 30 years, being in relapse at the time of transplant, and colonization before or early after transplantation.

Treatment of infection includes administration of appropriate antimicrobials, continued surveillance cultures, and close monitoring of patients for development of further complications, such as septic shock. Antimicrobial treatment often is limited by the patient's renal or hepatic function, which may prevent administration of optimal doses. A new therapy currently in initial trials in some transplant centers is the use of granulocyte macrophage colony-stimulating factor (GMCSF). This biologic response modifier has shortened the period of neutropenia in marrow transplant patients, resulting in fewer days of fever and earlier discharge from the hospital.

Interstitial pneumonia: idiopathic or cytomegalovirus

Interstitial pneumonia is manifested as adult respiratory distress syndrome (ARDS), with peak onset being around day 60 after transplantation. This is perhaps the most insidious of the complications, often occurring after patients have been discharged from the inpatient setting. Patients exhibit a rapid onset of symptoms, including a dry cough, dyspnea, nasal flaring, tachypnea, and rales. Diffuse infiltrates are seen on chest radiographs, and marked hypoxia is demonstrated in arterial blood gas analysis. This is the single greatest cause of death in the first 100 days after transplantation.

Pneumonia is diagnosed as *idiopathic* when no infectious organism can be identified. These pneumonias are thought to be caused by the irradiation used during conditioning. Single doses seem to increase the incidence over irradiation doses that are fractionated over several days. Idiopathic pneumonia is responsible for 30% of all pneumonias in these patients. If no infectious organism is found after biopsy, the patient usually is treated with ventilatory support and steroids.

Cytomegalovirus (CMV) is the most frequent cause of pneumonia and carries the highest mortality rate. Risk factors include previous CMV infection, GVHD, age over 30 years, and exposure to the virus through blood products. Prevention of this disease is a major focus of medical research, and new agents, such as ganciclovir and foscarnet, are being tried. The most promising recent finding is that patients who are seronegative before transplantation and receive marrow from a CMV seronegative donor and blood products that have been screened against CMV do not contract CMV infections.

Neurologic complications

Neurologic complications can occur after marrow transplantation as a result of previous chemotherapy and irradiation, conditioning therapy, or infections or as a consequence of therapies to control GVHD, such as cyclosporine. Organ failure in other systems can lead to central nervous system dysfunction. Neurotoxicity can be manifested by seizures, cerebellar ataxia, tremor, depression, expressive asphasia, or quadriparesis.

Graft rejection

Graft rejection, the failure of the new marrow to engraft, has become an increasing problem in recent years. Current studies to increase the available donor pool by using mismatched donors and to decrease the incidence of GVHD by depleting the marrow of T cells before giving it to the patient have increased the incidence of graft rejection.

Psychosocial responses

The decision to undergo a BMT is a major life crisis for the patient and family. In addition to the very real threat of death, patients experience social isolation, bodily discomfort, major body image changes, and a sense of loss of control. These stressors lead to a myriad of emotions, including hope, anger, depression, anxiety, anticipation, guilt, and joy. Pediatric patients often regress, demonstrating behavior of an earlier developmental level.

Nurses have a major role in helping patients cope with the uncertainty and ambiguity of marrow transplantation and in fostering hope. Nurses can plan interventions that give the patient as much control as possible. Fear of the unknown can be decreased through patient education about procedures and potential complications. Nurses can offer strategies, such as relaxation, visualization, and distraction, for coping with pain and nausea. Pediatric patients should have their developmental levels determined before admission and have activities planned that are appropriate for their age and degree of illness.

Long-Term Complications

The causes of long-term complications after transplantation are the same as those for acute complications. Table

Table 9–3. CLINICAL MANIFESTATIONS AND NURSING IMPLICATIONS OF CHRONIC COMPLICATIONS AFTER TRANSPLANTATION

Complication	Clinical Manifestations	Nursing Implications
Graft-versus-Host Disease		
Skin	Rough, scaly skin Malar erythema Generalized rash Hypo- or hyperpigmentation Dyspigmentation Alopecia Joint contractures Scleroderma Loss of sweating	• Use nonabrasive soaps, lotions, sunscreen • Cosmetic support, makeup, wigs • Range of motion activities • Patient–family education • Monitor compliance with treatment protocols
Liver	Jaundice	• Infection precautions until differential diagnosis is made • Monitor liver function test results • Low-fat diet
Oral cavity	Pain, burning, dryness, irritation, soreness, loss of taste Lichenoid changes, atrophy, erythema in oral cavity Candida infection Stomatitis	• Encourage soft, bland diet • Dental hygiene education, soft toothbrush, flossing • Saline rinses • Dental medicine referral or recommendation • Salivary gland stimulants, sugarless mints, artificial saliva

Continued

Table 9-3. CLINICAL MANIFESTATIONS AND NURSING IMPLICATIONS OF CHRONIC COMPLICATIONS AFTER TRANSPLANTATION
Continued

Complication	Clinical Manifestations	Nursing Implications
Graft-versus-Host Disease Continued		
Ocular	Dental caries	
	Xerostomia	
	Grittiness, burning of eyes	• Artificial tears
	Dry eyes	• Schirmer's tear test: if <10 mm of wetting, refer to ophthalmologist
	Sicca syndrome	
Gastrointestinal tract	Anorexia	• Serial checking of weight
	Difficulty eating	• High calorie food supplements
	Painful swallowing	• Recommend nutritional counseling
	Retrosternal pain	
	Weight loss, malabsorption	
	Vomiting	
Vagina	Inflammation	• Water-soluble lubricants
	Stricture formation causing obstruction of menstrual flow	• Recommend sexual counseling
	Adhesions	
	Dry vagina	
	Painful intercourse	
	Marital problems	

Late Infectious Complications

Bacterial, viral, fungal infections	Fever, wheezing, rales, postnasal drip, signs of infection	• Preventive teaching
		• Mask-wearing until 6 months posttransplantation
		• Obtain cultures
		• Administer antimicrobials
		• Patient teaching should include the following
		  (a) Avoid infectious persons (measles, chickenpox, mumps)
		  (b) Avoid school or work until 6 months posttransplantation
		  (c) Avoid hot tubs, public swimming pools until 6–9 months posttransplantation
		  (d) Limit number of sexual partners
		  (e) Avoid live virus vaccines

Varicella-zoster virus infection	Lesions, pain, malaise, tenderness, neurologic manifestation	• Relieve pruritus with calamine lotion • Cool compresses • Prevent secondary infection • Obtain cultures • Administer acyclovir

Continued

Table 9–3. CLINICAL MANIFESTATIONS AND NURSING IMPLICATIONS OF CHRONIC COMPLICATIONS AFTER TRANSPLANTATION
Continued

Complication	Clinical Manifestations	Nursing Implications
Pulmonary Complications		
Interstitial pneumonia *Cytomegalovirus* infection *Pneumocystis carinii* infection	Fever, sepsis, hypotension, lethargy, cough, tachypnea	• Anticipatory preventive teaching • Routine monitoring of vital signs • Chest auscultation and percussion • Monitor pulmonary function test results, arterial blood gases
Restrictive disease	May be asymptomatic or cough	• Anticipatory teaching of pulmonary toilet • Routine monitoring of vital signs • Chest auscultation and percussion • Monitor pulmonary function test results and arterial blood gases
Obstructive disease	Decreased ability to perform daily living activities owing to pulmonary insufficiency	
Cataracts	Poor vision	• Anticipatory teaching of BMT risk factors • Ophthalmologist recommendation

Neurologic Complications

Leukoencephalopathy	Lethargy Somnolence Dementia Seizures Spastic quadriplegia Coma Personality changes	• Early intervention • Multidisciplinary approach with special education program • Routine neurologic assessments

Psychologic Complications

	Depression, weight change Altered body image Survival syndrome Sibling rivalry	• Allow patient–family to verbalize feelings • Identify coping mechanisms, personal strengths • Refer to mental health resources

Impaired Growth in Children

	Subnormal growth and development	• Anticipatory teaching to patients and parents • Annual evaluation of growth pattern • Serial checking of height and weight

Continued

Table 9–3. CLINICAL MANIFESTATIONS AND NURSING IMPLICATIONS OF CHRONIC COMPLICATIONS AFTER TRANSPLANTATION
Continued

Complication	Clinical Manifestations	Nursing Implications
Gonadal Dysfunction		
Female patients	Delayed onset of puberty Premature menopause Sterility	• Careful monitoring of prepubertal girls • Menstrual history • Fertility counseling • Anticipatory teaching and counseling • Sexual counseling
Male patients	Delayed onset of puberty Sterility	• Careful monitoring of prepubertal boys • Fertility counseling • Sperm storage prior to BMT • Anticipatory teaching and counseling • Sexual counseling

Adapted from Buchsel, P. C. (1986). Long-term complications of allogeneic bone marrow transplantation: Nursing implications. *Oncology Nursing Forum*, 13(6), 61–70.

9–3 summarizes chronic complications and the nursing care required.

SUMMARY AND FUTURE TRENDS

As an experimental therapy method, BMT continues to undergo adaptation, incorporating additional therapies and being used in new diagnoses. Currently, much of the medical research is geared toward decreasing the relapse rate by improving the chemoirradiation used in conditioning or by removing tumor cells with monoclonal antibodies, using tissue-specific isotopes or antigens.

In the future, emphasis will be on increasing the marrow donor pool from unrelated mismatched and cadaveric sources and on improving engraftment with hemopoietic growth factors. Major attention will continue to be paid to decreasing the myriad complications following transplantation. The psychologic impact of marrow transplantation needs to be examined at the time of the transplant as well as in long-term survivors.

M. TISH KNOBF

Carcinoma of the breast is the most common cancer and the leading cause of death among American women between the ages of 35 to 54 years. In 1990 in the United States, an estimated 150,000 women will be diagnosed and 44,000 will die from this malignancy. The incidence of breast cancer appears to be increasing worldwide at an average rate of 2% per year. Death rates due to breast cancer over the last decades are relatively unchanged, despite the increasing incidence. The stability of these mortality figures is most easily explained by improvement in the 5-year survival rates. It is unclear whether the prolonged survival is related to early detection and diagnosis, treatment strategies, or both.

EPIDEMIOLOGY AND ETIOLOGY

The incidence of breast cancer varies around the world. Incidence is highest in North America and the countries of northern Europe and lowest in the Asian and African coun-

See the corresponding chapter in *Cancer Nursing: A Comprehensive Textbook,* by Baird, McCorkle, and Grant, pp. 425–451, for a more detailed
discussion of this topic, including a comprehensive list of references.

tries. Incidence rates change substantially for the first- and second-generation descendants of low-risk geographic populations when they migrate to areas in which breast cancer is common. This change strongly suggests that environment and lifestyle are major factors in determining breast cancer risk.

Risk Factors

In the United States, 1 of every 9 women is expected to be diagnosed with breast cancer in the course of her lifetime. Although risk factors have been identified, the exact etiology for the development of breast cancer is unknown.

Screening and Early Detection

The goal of screening in breast cancer is to detect cancers at the earliest stage possible because the extent of tumor at diagnosis is correlated with survival. Women who have small tumors and no spread to the axillary lymph nodes have a very good long-term prognosis compared with those who have large tumors and axillary lymph nodes that test positive.

Physical examination, breast self-examination (BSE), and mammography are three methods of screening proposed by the American Cancer Society. Educational reinforcement is necessary, particularly for mammography, because concern persists among women about radiation exposure from annual examinations. The benefit of identifying tumors that are too small or that cannot be detected by physical examination must be communicated and stressed to the public on an ongoing basis.

PATHOLOGY

Breast carcinomas arise primarily from epithelial cells, with the origin being either ductal or lobular. These carcinomas are invasive or noninvasive. The term *infiltrating* is synonomous with invasive and the term *in situ* with noninvasive. Invasive ductal carcinoma accounts for 70% to 80% of all breast cancers. Lobular carcinomas account for 2% to 3% of all invasive tumors and behave similarly to those of ductal origin.

Historically, the noninvasive carinomas have represented less than 5% of breast cancer that is diagnosed. However, the incidence of the detection of ductal carcinoma in situ has risen dramatically to 15% to 20% with the widespread use of screening mammography.

PROGNOSTIC FACTORS

Axillary lymph node status is the single most important prognostic determinant. The pathologic status of the axillary nodes is the most valuable predictor of recurrence and survival. Women with negative nodes have a 70% to 75%

chance of being disease free at 10 years compared with only 20% to 25% of node-positive patients if no adjuvant therapy is received. The prognosis for node-positive patients worsens as the number of nodes involved increases.

Hormone receptor content is an important prognostic factor as well and is becoming a more critical element in planning treatment. Patients are considered to be estrogen receptor (ER) or progesterone receptor (PR) positive or negative based on the binding capacity. Tumors that are ER positive generally are hormonally responsive, tend to be more well differentiated, have low proliferative activity, are uncommonly associated with visceral metastases, and indicate a better chance of survival as compared with ER-negative tumors.

Progesterone receptor content is a recognized prognostic factor alone, and it adds significantly to the predictive value of ER. Tumors with high ER content are likely to have high PR content, and that combination constitutes a favorable subset of patients. The quantitative values are directly related to response and length of predicted disease-free survival.

A major histologic feature correlated with survival has been tumor grade, a simple grading system that estimates tumor differentiation. The majority of studies have shown that poorly differentiated tumors are associated with a shorter disease-free and overall survival period.

Thymidine-labeling index and DNA flow cytometry are methods that determine the proliferative activity, the percentage of cells in S-phase, and the DNA content (ploidy status) of the tumor. Patients who have a high thymidine-labeling index and aneuploid tumors (those with altered DNA content) have a higher risk for recurrence, early relapse, and shorter survival time when compared with patients who have low S-phase activity and diploid tumors. An important consideration is the number of unfavorable factors for any given patient. The greater the number of poor prognostic features, the worse the prognosis.

STAGING

Staging classifies patients clinically and pathologically according to the extent of disease (Tables 10–1 and 10–2). The staging workup includes a complete history and physical examination, a hematologic and chemical blood profile, and a chest radiograph, mammogram, and baseline bone scan.

Clinical staging guides the individual patient and physician in evaluating treatment options and provides data for comparison of therapies and outcomes in various stages of breast cancer. Because axillary lymph node status is the strongest prognostic factor, pathologic staging, particularly for the patient with locally resectable breast cancer, is required. Pathologic staging is a simple two-stage classifi-

Table 10–1. TNM CLASSIFICATION OF BREAST CANCER

T (tumor)	T_0	No evidence of tumor
	T_{1s}	In situ carcinoma
	T_1	Tumor is 2 cm or less at greatest dimension
	T_2	Tumor is less than 2 cm but not greater than 5 cm at greatest dimension
	T_3	Tumor is greater than 5 cm at greatest dimension
	T_4	Any size tumor with extension to chest wall or skin
N (nodes)	N_0	No palpable homolateral axillary nodes
	N_1	Movable homolateral axillary nodes
	N_2	Homolateral axillary nodes that are considered to contain cancer and are fixed
	N_3	Homolateral supraclavicular or infraclavicular nodes
M (metastasis)	M_0	No evidence of distant metastases
	M_1	Distant metastases

cation: stage I indicates no axillary lymph node involvement, and stage II indicates nodal involvement.

CLINICAL FEATURES AND DIAGNOSIS
Signs and Symptoms

The most common presenting symptom is a lump or thickening in the breast. More than 90% of lumps are discovered by the woman herself, and only 20% to 25% are malignant in nature. Nipple discharge, nipple retraction, scaly skin around the nipple, and skin changes (dimpling, peau d'orange, or inflammation) are observed less frequently and are symptoms that are associated with a more advanced stage of cancer.

Diagnosis

Once a lump has been detected, a physical examination by a physician is recommended. A cyst, a benign tumor, and a malignant tumor are the possibilities for a palpable breast mass. Ultrasonography, a noninvasive diagnostic test without any radiation exposure, can distinguish between a fluid-filled cystic lump and a solid one. In women in the high-risk age group, mammography also should be performed. If a tumor is suspected, a mammogram and a biopsy should be scheduled. Mammography is the superior breast imaging tool, yet false negative results have been reported as high as 30%. Thus, negative findings on a mammogram do not preclude a decision to perform a biopsy on a clinically suspicious mass. Mammographic findings that may indicate

Table 10–2. CLINICAL STAGING FOR BREAST CANCER*

Stage	Tumor	Node	Metastasis
I	T_1	N_0	M_0
II	T_2	N_{0-1}	M_0
IIIA	T_3	N_{0-1}	M_0
IIIB	T_{1-3}	N_2	M_0
IV	T_4	Any N	M_0
	Any T	Any N	M_1

*See Table 10–1 for descriptions of T, N, and M values.

malignancy include asymmetry, clusters of microcalcifications, spicular masses, and masses with a sunburst appearance.

Fine-needle aspiration of solid breast masses to determine malignancy is a recognized diagnostic procedure in a setting in which physicians have extensive experience and in which pathologic expertise is also available. Cytologic diagnosis cannot distinguish noninvasive from invasive carcinoma. Thus, if a positive cytologic result is reported, a tissue biopsy is required. Excisional biopsy is recommended whenever possible, particularly for early-stage breast cancer, in which options for treatment are defined.

Nursing Practice

Emotional support and education regarding the pending procedures are major nursing concerns. For many women, this may represent a first experience with mammography. General guidelines following a breast biopsy include the following: (1) expect mild to moderate discomfort, for which pain relief measures will be prescribed, (2) wear a supportive bra for 24 hours to enhance comfort, (3) avoid strenuous arm activity for the first few days, (4) expect sutures, if present, to be removed in 5 to 7 days, and anticipate that the area will be ecchymotic and tender with gradual dissolution. Indentation at the biopsy site will fill in with fat in a month or two, and significant alterations are rare if incisions follow recommended guidelines according to location of the mass.

Following diagnosis, the nurse continues to provide information and support, expanding the focus to help the patient, spouse, and family process the information to optimize their coping strategies and facilitate decision making.

PRIMARY TREATMENT
Stages I and II, Early-Stage Breast Cancer
Local regional control

The goal of surgery for stages I and II breast cancer is to control local regional disease. Surgical approaches have been modified as new theories of breast cancer have evolved and as radical surgery has failed to alter mortality rates. Breast cancer is a systemic disease, which means that micrometastases could be present at the initial presentation with or without nodal involvement. Consequently, current efforts focus on achieving optimal local regional control and identifying prognostic factors that discriminate patients likely to harbor micrometastases.

The modified radical mastectomy is synonymous with total mastectomy and axillary lymph node dissection. It includes removing the breast and lymph nodes and preserving the pectoralis major muscle with or without preservation of the pectoralis minor muscle.

Breast-preserving surgery combined with radiotherapy is an alternative approach for women who have small tumors (≤4 cm). This approach involves removing the tumor along with some adjacent normal tissue (referred to as lumpectomy), axillary node dissection, and radiotherapy for about 6 weeks. Conservative surgery and irradiation for women with small tumors are equivalent to mastectomy for local control and survival, and they preserve the breast. Considerations for conservative breast surgery and irradiation include the size of the tumor, the existence of more than one foci of tumor, and the extent of microcalcifications on mammographic findings.

Nursing practice

The goal of nursing care is to promote physical and psychologic recovery. It is important to note that physical and psychologic responses are similar in all women regardless of choice of mastectomy or conservative surgery with radiotherapy.

The postoperative period should focus on meeting basic needs, and because hospital stays today rarely exceed 5 days and more often average 2 to 4 days, written information to supplement verbal teaching is strongly recommended. Discharge instructions can facilitate self-care at home and have the potential to decrease anxiety levels (Table 10–3).

Complications of breast surgery

The majority of complications associated with a modified radical mastectomy are related to the axillary lymph node dissection, which is the longest and technically the most difficult part of the surgical procedure.

Seroma is a fluid accumulation in the operative site with an observed incidence of 4.2% to 32%. Treatment of seroma is aspiration, and if fluid accumulation persists after several taps, placement of a Penrose drain and prescription of a course of antibiotics are recommended.

Initiation of early range of motion exercises (postoperative day 1) has been shown to increase the amount and

Table 10-3. PATIENT DISCHARGE INSTRUCTIONS FOLLOWING BREAST CANCER SURGERY

Dressings
Incision

There will be a dry gauze dressing over the incision when you leave the hospital. It is not necessary to change this dressing until you return to see the doctor.

Drain Site

A small dry dressing will be around the site where the drain is placed. Often, there is some leakage of fluid around the drain. Check the gauze dressing for drainage and change if soiled. Some leakage is normal, but if the dressing becomes soaked more than once a day, call your doctor.

Drains

Your nurse has shown you how to empty the reservoir from your drain and how to measure the volume of drainage. You should empty the drain twice a day and record the measurements.

Drains generally are removed when drainage is about 30 ml in 24 hours.

Drains often are removed at the same time as the stitches, generally 7–10 days after surgery.

Bathing

Sponge baths or tub baths, making certain that the area of the drain and incision stay dry, are permitted. You may shower after the stitches and drains are removed.

Hand and Arm Care

You can begin using your arm for normal activities, such as eating or combing your hair. Exercises involving the wrist, hand, and elbow, such as flexing your fingers, circular wrist motions, and touching hand to shoulder, are very good. More strenuous exercises usually can be resumed after the drains have been removed.

Comfort

Some discomfort or mild pain is expected following surgery, but within 4–5 days, most women have no need for medication or require something only at bedtime.

Numbness in the area of the surgery and along the inner side of the arm from the armpit to the elbow occurs in virtually all patients. It is a result of injury to the nerves that provide sensation to the skin in those areas. Women have described such sensations as heaviness, pain, tingling, burning, and pins and needles. These sensations change over the months and usually resolve by 1 year.

Support and Information

Pamphlets on exercises, hand and arm care, and general facts about breast cancer are available from your nurse or volunteer visitor. The American Cancer Society has volunteers who have had surgery similar to yours and are available to visit you.

duration of drainage. Delay of 7 to 10 days for initiation of physical rehabilitative exercises did not alter range of motion function when evaluated at 3 and 6 months, and, therefore, it is recommended that active motion exercises be delayed for at least 1 week.

Sensory changes secondary to trauma to the nerves or transection of the nerves occur in patients with axillary dissection and mastectomy. Subjective complaints include numbness, weakness, increased skin sensitivity, itching, heaviness, pins and needles, and phantom breast sensations, all of which may change in character and persist for up to 1 year.

Lymphedema has been reported in 6.7% to 70% of patients, occurring as early as 2 months after surgery and up to 15 to 20 years later. The major risk factor is removal of the axillary lymph nodes. Lymphedema is defined as the difference between one extremity and its opposite of 1.0 to 1.5 cm. Once lymphedema occurs, management is aimed at prevention of further lymph accumulation. Elevation, mild exercise, massage, salt restriction, avoidance of local heat and trauma, and elastic support are basic interventions. A patient should be measured for an elastic support sleeve when the swelling is at a minimal level and should be reevaluated every 2 to 3 months for a replacement. For moderate to severe lymphedema, an intermittent compression sleeve may be indicated.

Complications of radiotherapy

Fatigue, breast edema, skin reactions, and breast tenderness are symptoms frequently associated with breast irradiation, whereas hyperpigmentation, fibrosis, rib fractures, pneumonitis, arm edema, and myositis are uncommonly observed.

Breast Reconstruction

Removal of the breast is a significant loss, and the impact on body image and adjustment is well documented. The cosmetic benefit for women who receive breast-preserving surgery and irradiation is a more intact body image. Compared with mastectomy patients, irradiated patients have fewer negative feelings about themselves nude, resume sexual relations earlier, and experience less change in body satisfaction.

The nurse should explore with the patient her feelings about the loss, her relationship with her partner, when appropriate, and her adaptation to the prosthesis or reconstructed breast. For women who do not choose immediate reconstruction, a temporary prosthesis should be provided. The American Cancer Society's Reach to Recovery volunteer visitor program can provide a temporary breast form and suggest sources for purchase of a permanent form. A variety of permanent breast forms are available. Evaluation, usage, and satisfaction with the breast form must be integrated into follow-up care.

Breast reconstruction is the alternative to achieve symmetry and preserve body image. Reconstructive surgery creates a breast mound, the most common procedures are implantation of a silicone prosthesis or placement of a tissue expander under the pectoralis muscle. Generally, a 1- to 3-day hospital admission is required for either implant procedure.

Other reconstructive procedures include the latissimus dorsi flap or the transverse rectus abdominis flap, which use autologous tissue and skin. These procedures require more extensive surgery and longer hospitalization and recovery time yet can achieve a more natural symmetry and can provide an option to the patient who is not a candidate for implant reconstruction.

Consideration for reconstructive surgery begins with a physical and psychosocial assessment, a description of the procedure and potential complications, and a discussion about the expectations of cosmetic improvement. Controversy persists about state of disease and timing of the procedure (immediate vs delayed), although opinions appear to be based largely on clinical judgment and personal preference rather than on hard data.

Complications of breast reconstruction include hematoma, infection, delayed wound healing, and capsular contractions (if an implant was used).

Stage III, Locally Advanced Breast Cancer

Ten to thirty percent of breast cancer patients have locally advanced stage III disease, which includes tumors that can be defined as operable ($T_3 N_{0-1} M_0$) or inoperable ($T_4 N_{2-3} M_0$). Stage III disease is associated with a high incidence of local and distant recurrence and a poor 5-year survival rate. Surgery, radiation therapy, and chemotherapy have been used alone and in combination, but the most appropriate therapy or combination of therapies remains controversial. For operable stage III disease, surgery with or without radiation or high-dose radiation alone may be recommended.

Although local control rates have improved with this approach, prognosis is poor because of the incidence of distant metastases. Combination chemotherapy or chemohormonal therapy followed by mastectomy with or without radiation appears to improve the local control rate and may influence disease-free and overall survival rates. Clinical trials with autologous bone marrow transplantation are in progress and may have a role in breast cancer therapy in advanced stages of disease and for patients at high risk for recurrence.

SYSTEMIC TREATMENT OF BREAST CANCER

The purpose of systemic treatment of breast cancer is to prevent distant recurrence, as used in the adjuvant setting, to improve the response and durability of response in locally advanced cancer, and to treat patients who have relapsed with distant metastases. Mortality has been relatively unaffected by surgery or radiation because patients die of disseminated, not local, disease. Beginning in the 1970s and up to the present time, trials focus on particular subsets of patients and factors that influence the efficacy of therapy, such as specific antineoplastic agents, hormones, timing, duration, dose, regimen of choice, long-term effects, cell kinetics, and tumor biology.

Duration of Therapy

In an attempt to decrease both long- and short-term toxicity, shorter courses of 4 to 6 months were compared with the previous 1- to 2-year course of therapy. A review of five major trials from cancer centers and cooperative groups failed to demonstrate any advantage to prolonged therapy, and some data suggest that the shorter courses may be more beneficial.

Regimen of Choice

Combination chemotherapy was shown to be superior to single alkylating agent treatment, and the combination of cyclophosphamide, methotrexate, and fluorouracil (CMF) represents a standard for multidrug adjuvant breast therapy in practice and a reference in the design of many clinical trials. Nodal involvement as a measure of tumor burden is a critical prognostic factor. Premenopausal patients with one to three positive nodes who are treated with adjuvant chemotherapy have a survival advantage, but as the number of positive axillary nodes increases, prognosis is greatly altered despite therapy. Such data have prompted investigators to develop innovative and more aggressive approaches for higher-risk patients, such as the addition of doxorubicin.

Timing

In routine clinical practice, adjuvant therapy is initiated within 4 to 6 weeks after surgery. The optimal time to begin chemotherapy is unknown. It is generally agreed that chemotherapy should be administered early, but whether it is given before, concurrently, or in a sandwich technique with radiation has yet to be defined. Concurrent administration with CMF regimens is feasible with an accepted incidence of increased skin reactions. Concomitant administration of doxorubicin and radiotherapy is not recommended, but doxorubicin-based combinations given before or after primary radiation are safe.

Hormone Therapy

Adjuvant endocrine therapy regained status when the relatively nontoxic antiestrogen tamoxifen became available. A review of nine published studies of tamoxifen vs no treatment or placebo concluded that relapse-free survival is significantly prolonged, as is probably overall survival for postmenopausal women with positive nodes. Response appears proportional to the quantity of the receptor levels. Prescribing for more than 2 years is safe and may provide a continued benefit to patients.

Node-Negative Patients

Although node-negative patients are in the better prognostic group, 25% to 30% eventually will relapse by 10 years and die of their disease. Efforts have focused on identifying subsets of higher-risk patients within the node-negative group who may benefit from adjuvant therapy. Four major study groups have conducted randomized clinical trials of patients with node-negative breast cancer and estrogen receptor-negative tumors. Some patients were given adjuvant chemotherapy and some no therapy. With a median follow-up of 3 to 5 years, all of these trials report a disease-free survival advantage for treated patients. An overall survival advantage has been reported by only one group, but the follow-up time is much too short to make definitive conclusions on the effect of treatment on overall survival.

The National Surgical Adjuvant Breast and Bowel Project conducted randomized clinical trials of 2644 women with node-negative breast cancer and estrogen receptor-positive tumors, some of whom were given tamoxifen and some placebo for 5 years. With a 4-year median follow-up, a significant disease-free survival benefit is noted for the treated group (83%) vs the placebo group (77%). An advantage was observed for both the younger (less than 49 years) and older (more than 50 years) women who received treatment. As with the adjuvant chemotherapy trials, follow-up is still too limited to evaluate the effect on overall survival.

Toxicity

The incidence, frequency, and severity of side effects associated with adjuvant therapy are influenced by the specific drugs, multidrug regimens, combination therapy, hormonal therapy, and duration of treatment. Nausea, vomiting, and hair loss are three side effects feared by patients for whom chemotherapy is recommended. They are, however, not specific for women with breast cancer on adjuvant chemotherapy.

Fatigue

Fatigue is common as part of the disease process, is associated with various cancer therapies, and is correlated with physical and psychological symptoms. Average ratings of distress for fatigue on a 1 to 5 scale for women on adjuvant chemotherapy were in the range of 2.3 to 2.6.

Weight Change

An average weight gain of 4 kg has been observed in patients receiving systemic adjuvant chemotherapy regardless of menopausal status, receptor content, pretreatment weight, duration of therapy, or ingestion of steroids. The total amount of weight gained appears to be slightly greater for women on steroids, for premenopausal patients, and for those on chemotherapy for longer periods of time.

Menopausal Symptoms

The majority of women 40 years or older on adjuvant chemotherapy can be expected to develop some degree of drug-induced ovarian failure that is progressive with drug cycles. Associated menopausal symptoms of hot flashes, sweats, headaches, decreased vaginal lubrication, and dyspareunia have been reported. Information and counseling are critical. Adjuvant endocrine therapy with tamoxifen is associated with hot flashes, vaginal discharge, and irregular menses, particulary in younger women. Menopausal symptoms disrupt routine activities and interfere significantly with sleep. Drug therapy may be indicated to control or minimize symptoms. Diphenhydramine at bedtime may be useful to minimize sleep deprivation, and low-dose clonidine has been reported to reduce the incidence of hot flashes.

Treatment of Metastatic Disease

The greatest risk of relapse in breast cancer occurs within the first 2 to 3 years after diagnosis. Although 90% of those who relapse do so by the fifth year, recurrences have been observed as long as 20 to 25 years later. Bone is the most common site of relapse (40% to 60%), followed by lung (15% to 20%), pleura (10% to 14%), soft tissue (7% to 15%), and liver (5% to 15%). The mainstay of treatment for metastatic disease is hormone and cytotoxic therapy. Indications for surgery and radiotherapy are limited, with the most common being palliative radiotherapy for symptomatic bone metastases.

Endocrine therapy

Hormonal manipulation has been used for decades in the treatment of breast cancer, but not until the discovery of hormone receptors could the selection of patients be refined. Estrogen receptor-negative patients rarely respond; an overall response rate in the range of 30% has been observed, but a higher response rate of 50% to 60% may be achieved with ER-positive patients. Average responses last 12 to 18 months, and response rates are related to the quantity of receptor protein. Clinical experience indicates that postmenopausal patients respond more often than premenopausal patients, bone and soft tissue are the most responsive metastatic sites, and patients who respond to one hormonal therapy will likely respond to another. There are many endocrine correlations with breast cancer, and approaches to inhibit growth are either ablative or additive. The surgical ablative therapies are being replaced gradually by systemic therapy with tamoxifen, aminoglutethimide, and megestrol acetate (Megace). Although side effects are tolerated reasonably well, patients may experience a flare that is defined as transient increased bone pain or hypercalcemia.

Progestins, such as megestrol acetate, have similar response rates in the 30% range and are associated with few side effects except that of weight gain.

Aminoglutethimide is a drug that blocks adrenal steroid synthesis. The adrenal gland is a major source of estrogen in the postmenopausal woman. In essence aminoglutethimide therapy produces a medical adrenalectomy. Because of the complex feedback mechanisms in the endocrine system, a steroid replacement is recommended with aminoglutethimide therapy, usually hydrocortisone 40 mg per day in physiologically divided doses. Side effects of lethargy, visual blurring, maculopapular rash, and dizziness occur in 25% to 50% of the patients during the first 6 weeks of treatment but usually disappear thereafter.

Response to endocrine therapy is associated with a prolonged survival.

Chemotherapy of recurrent disease

Only a few clinical predictors exist for response to chemotherapy. A good performance status, a long disease-free survival, and an absence of liver metastases are favorable factors, whereas pretreatment weight loss, extensive disease, anemia, and prior chemotherapy or radiotherapy are associated with a poorer response rate and prognosis. Combination chemotherapy is superior to single-agent therapy, producing an average response rate of 50%, with a median duration of response ranging from 6 to 12 months. Complete responders are very uncommon and are not associated with a significantly prolonged survival. The average survival time following metastatic disease is 18 to 36 months. The combination of chemotherapy and hormone therapy may increase the response rate, but thus far it has not increased the duration of response or survival.

Many problems are associated with advanced disease and sites of metastases in breast cancer. Hypercalcemia, spinal cord compression, and development of brain metastases are complications of the disease.

MALE BREAST CANCER

Breast cancer in men is uncommon, representing less than 1% of all cancer in males. Its natural history is very similar to that of breast cancer in women, with the major exception being age at onset. The average age of onset for men is 60 to 65 years. Other differences include presentation with a slightly more advanced stage of disease and a greater percentage of hormone receptor-positive tumors. The majority of patients have a firm, painless subareolar mass and a histologic diagnosis of infiltrating ductal carcinoma. Patterns of recurrence and survival as influenced by pathologic stage of axillary lymph nodes are similar to those for women.

Primary treatment is usually modified radical mastectomy, and adjuvant therapy is recommended for pathologic stage II disease. Postoperative radiotherapy may be recommended for improved local disease control. Treatment of recurrent disease is based on hormone receptor status. Orchiectomy and administration of tamoxifen are the first-line treatment choices. Additive second-line endocrine therapy is somewhat more controversial. Data on chemotherapy responsiveness are sparse, and, therefore, it is difficult to make any specific recommendations.

11 Lung Cancer

ADA M. LINDSEY

The incidence of lung cancer is continuing to increase at a rapid rate; approximately 149,000 new cases are diagnosed and 130,000 deaths are reported per year. Lung cancer remains the most common cause of cancer mortality for men, and in the United States, it has now surpassed breast cancer as a cause of death for women in some age groups. The prognosis for lung cancer patients remains poor. Most people have metastatic disease at the time of diagnosis. Thus, the 5-year survival rate is very low, less than 10%.

There are two major classifications of bronchogenic carcinoma: small-cell lung cancer (SCLC) and nonsmall-cell lung cancer (non-SCLC). The non-SCLCs are further classified as squamous cell or epidermoid lung cancer, adenocarcinoma, and large-cell carcinoma. The ratio of incidence of non-SCLC to SCLC is 3 to 1.

Available data suggest that in addition to cigarette smoking, industrial and environmental pollutants are risk factors for lung cancer development. Other carcinogenic substances associated with increased risk include asbestos, ionizing radiation, hydrocarbons, chromium, and nickel. Asbestos exposure in cigarette smokers increases the risk of lung cancer 80 to 90 times.

RISK FACTORS AND INCIDENCE

The primary risk factor in the development of bronchogenic carcinoma is longer total exposure to cigarette smok-

---

See the corresponding chapter in *Cancer Nursing: A Comprehensive Textbook*, by Baird, McCorkle, and Grant, pp. 452–465, for a more detailed discussion of this topic, including a comprehensive list of references.

ing (including number of cigarettes smoked, age when smoking began, duration of smoking, and tar and nicotine content of cigarettes smoked). The role of passive smoking in the development of lung cancer in nonsmokers was studied by pooling data from three large investigations. The risk was greater for older women whose husbands were heavy smokers. The histologic types of cancer that occurred were squamous and small-cell carcinomas.

The rates of lung cancer are higher among those who consume alcohol and those in the lower socioeconomic groups.

Trends in lung cancer incidence and mortality show a continual increase. The incidence is almost double that of two decades ago. Projections indicate the diagnosis of 300,000 new cases in the year 2000. Partial explanations for this increase include an increase in the number of women who smoke, increased exposure to carcinogens in natural and occupational environments, more sophisticated diagnostic techniques, and more accurate classification.

Nurses can assist in the identification of individuals at risk for lung cancer and can encourage them to engage in disease prevention behaviors. The nurse also can educate these individuals and their families about risk factors for development of lung cancer and can provide follow-up consultation and surveillance to ensure that these individuals take advantage of early detection and screening programs.

HISTOLOGIC TYPES
Small-Cell Lung Cancer

Approximately 20% to 25% of lung cancers are histologically classified as small-cell carcinoma. This type of cancer and squamous cell cancer are most frequently linked with cigarette smoking. Approximately 80% of these tumors are located centrally and submucosally. Small-cell cancer is the most aggressive type of lung cancer. It spreads rapidly to submucosal vessels and regional lymph nodes. Small-cell cancer has a cell doubling time of approximately 30 days. Thus at the time of diagnosis, 70%-90% of the patients have extensive metastatic disease. Owing to the frequent occurrence of micrometastases, SCLC is considered to be a systemic disease at diagnosis.

A survival rate of more than 1 year is more likely for those with limited disease. Prognosis and survival remain poor even in the few patients with SCLC who have limited disease and have had surgical resection. The failure of curative resection results from the presence of undetectable, subclinical metastases. Although SCLC cells are quite sensitive to irradiation, failure with radiation therapy also occurs due to the presence of occult metastases. Thus, considering that SCLC usually is disseminated at the time of diagnosis, chemotherapy generally is the first treatment of choice. Although the response to treatment with multiple agents is high initially, the duration of the response is short (6 to 8 months). Because of the frequent central location of the tumor, compression of the bronchial lumen may occur. The occurrence of paraneoplastic syndromes is more frequent with this tumor type. Examples of paraneoplastic syndromes that occur with SCLC include Cushing's syndrome (ectopic production of adrenocorticotropin hormone by malignant lung tissue that stimulates excess production of adrenal gland glucocorticoids) and syndrome of inappropriate antidiuretic hormone secretion (ectopic production of antidiuretic hormone by malignant lung tissue).

Squamous Cell Carcinoma

Squamous cell carcinoma currently represents about 30% to 35% of all lung cancers. The majority of these tumors occur centrally, but they are seen anywhere in the lung. Because of the central location and the tendency for local invasion, bronchial obstruction occurs. There is also a tendency for ulceration and bleeding with squamous cell carcinoma. This type of cancer is much more frequent in males. The cell doubling time is approximately 100 days, and early metastases are less common than is invasion of local structures. This histologic type is more prone to cavitation. Squamous cell carcinoma occurs in areas in which the bronchial epithelium has been chronically damaged.

Patients may experience obstructive atelectasis, pneumonitis, and/or hemoptysis. The tumor may impinge on other thoracic structures, such as the mediastinum, chest wall, ribs, or diaphragm. An inflammatory response and an early positive sputum cytologic evaluation are common findings.

Adenocarcinoma

Adenocarcinoma is the most common type of lung cancer in some geographic areas. Adenocarcinoma represents about 33% of all bronchogenic cancers. These tumors frequently are small and occur peripherally. Adenocarcinoma is seen in areas of previous pulmonary damage with fibrosis, or it may arise from bronchial glands or peripheral mucosa. As a result of its origin, mucin production is frequent. The cell doubling time is approximately 180 days. Adenocarcinoma is detected most often by a routine chest radiograph; at the time of diagnosis, patients frequently are asymptomatic. However, adenocarcinoma has a tendency toward early metastasis, and approximately 40% of patients are considered to have unresectable tumor at the time of diagnosis. Due to the more common peripheral location of this tumor type, an early positive sputum cytologic finding is rare.

Large-Cell Carcinoma

Large-cell carcinomas are extremely undifferentiated forms of other types of lung cancer. Usually, they are large, bulky, peripheral tumors, and they can occur in any part of the lung. They are known to mimic other types of lung cancer. The cell doubling time is approximately 100 days. Early invasion of the mediastinum and central nervous system occurs.

Nonsmall-Cell Lung Cancers

Nonsmall-cell lung cancers represent three (squamous cell, adenocarcinoma, large-cell carcinoma) of the four histologic groups of lung cancer; 70% to 80% of the lung cancers can be classified into these three subgroups. If these tumors are localized, surgery is the treatment of choice. However, in only a small percentage of the cases (10% to 15%) are the tumors considered to be surgically resectable at the time of diagnosis. The 5-year survival rate for those few patients judged to have operable tumors is approximately 30% to 40%. Because most patients with lung cancer have disseminated disease at the time of diagnosis, chemotherapy is used as the major treatment modality.

The remaining lung cancers are classified as relatively uncommon types, such as carcinoid tumors and mucoepidermoid lung cancer.

In addition to histologic classification, tumors may be characterized as endocrine or nonendocrine producing and by the biologic marker or markers expressed. The histologic cell type, degree of differentiation, and paraneoplastic expression are related to prognosis.

CLINICAL MANIFESTATIONS

The presenting clinical manifestations for lung cancer diagnosis are diverse because they may be due to one or more of the following: the primary tumor, metastatic involvement, either local or distant, or systemic, paraneoplastic expression. Some patients who are asymptomatic are diagnosed with lung cancer following a routine chest radiograph. Approximately 15% of those with lung cancer are asymptomatic at diagnosis.

Clinical manifestations caused by local involvement of proximal airways include coughing, hemoptysis, dyspnea, and vague chest pain. Coughing occurs as a symptom of lung cancer in about 40% of patients. However, it may also be due to the chronic bronchitis frequently seen in those with a history of cigarette smoking. A change in an existing cough should be determined. Infection may occur if clearance of mucous secretions from airways is impaired. In lung cancer, a developing cough or a change in cough may be the result of a central airway obstruction or a bronchial mucosal ulceration.

Hemoptysis is the initial symptom of lung cancer. Dyspnea also commonly occurs and is associated with increased coughing and sputum production. Dyspnea may be the result of atelectasis distal to the tumor. Dyspnea is a subjective symptom defined as difficult, uncomfortable breathing. Dyspnea may occur at any point along the disease continuum. Obstructive tumors, pleural effusions, pneumonitis, and cachexia are among the factors contributing to dyspnea.

Lung cancer can occlude airways and invade or compress blood vessels. Wheezing, usually localized unilaterally, is due to airway obstruction from the tumor, but wheezing is an infrequent complaint. Most commonly, lung cancer involves the central airways. Frequently patients have atelectasis.

Weight loss is a clinical feature characteristic of lung cancer, and weight loss for the preceding 6 months is an important factor in determining prognosis. The survival time of patients who have sustained a 5% weight loss is significantly shorter than that of patients who have not experienced a weight loss.

As many as 40% of patients experience chest pain described as being a nonspecific, dull, intermittent ache that is on the same side as the tumor. Chest pain associated with a rib or pleuritic pain is indicative of metastatic disease. Pancoast's tumor, which grows in the apex of the lung, may cause shoulder pain.

Extension of the tumor to the pleural surface of the lung results in a pleural effusion. Usually, the amount of the effusion is large, and unless treatment yields significant tumor regression, the fluid rapidly reaccumulates following removal of the fluid. The majority of lung cancer patients have either regional or distant metastases and will seek health care for symptoms occurring as a result of the metastases.

A potentially life-threatening syndrome occurs with superior vena cava obstruction, and it requires treatment. Patients have upper hemibody edema, appearance of collateral venous circulation on upper body, and increased jugular venous pressure. The syndrome occurs secondary to peritracheal lymphadenopathy and results in compression of the great veins that drain the head and upper trunk. It is seen more often in patients with SCLC. Because of the anatomic location of the superior vena cava, the preponderance is in those with tumors in the right lung. The symptoms include severe headache occurring with cough, blackouts after bending or on rising, dyspnea, and dysphagia. General facial puffiness and periorbital edema may occur. Emergency treatment directed at relieving the edema is required. Diuretics and dexamethasone have been used, but treatment of the tumor by radiation, chemotherapy, or both may be most useful.

Cancer occurring in the lung apex (superior sulcus) may invade the brachial nerve roots; this extension is associated with brachial neuritis. Pancoast described the syndrome associated with tumors involving the superior (apical) sulcus. Patients experience pain, wasting of muscles of the hand, and Horner's syndrome. If the eighth cervical and first thoracic segments of the sympathetic nerve trunk are involved, symptoms indicating Horner's syndrome are observed. These include a small pupil, partial ptosis of the eyelid, enophthalmos, and ipsilateral absence of thermal sweating on the face.

Tumor extension through the pericardium results in pericarditis and abnormalities in cardiac rhythm.

Local spread of lung cancer occurs initially in the hilar glands and usually is present at diagnosis. Metastatic involvement of peritracheal and subcarinal nodes is evident at diagnosis in a third or more of the patients, and spread to supraclavicular lymph nodes and deep cervical chain nodes is observed in about 20% of the patients. Metastatic involvement results in symptomatic disease.

Evidence of systemic disease or the distant effects of lung cancer include lymph node, bone, liver, and central nervous system metastases and paraneoplastic phenomena. Neurologic involvement from intracerebral metastases may be the presenting pathology for lung cancer. Complaints include headache and unsteadiness or difficulty in walking.

Some patients have bone pain, and the ribs, vertebrae, humerus, and femoral bones are those with the most frequent occurrence of metastases. Pathologic fractures may be the presenting symptom. Symptoms of hepatic metastases occur later. Early liver involvement may be observed more commonly in those with SCLC of the bronchus.

Ectopic hormone secretion has been associated with lung cancer. Some patients experience endocrine-related pathologies, such as Cushing's syndrome, that result from increased ectopic secretion of adrenocorticotropic hormone from the lung tumor. Another endocrine-related syndrome seen particularly in patients with SCLC that results from ectopic hormone production by the tumor is the syndrome of inappropriate antidiuretic hormone secretion (SIADH). These patients have high urine osmolality, low serum sodium, and plasma osmolality reflecting a retention of fluid. They may show confusion, lethargy, or other mental disturbances. The presence of SIADH is associated with a poor prognosis. Hypercalcemia may occur as a result of ectopic secretion of parathyroid hormone from squamous cell lung cancer. Hypercalcemia usually occurs in association with a large tumor mass.

An osteitis may occur during the course of lung cancer. The distal parts of the radius, ulna, tibia, and fibula are the most frequently involved bones. Swelling, erythema, and tenderness occur with the symmetric proliferation of subperiosteal tissue of the wrists and ankle joints. This condition is referred to as hypertrophic pulmonary osteoarthropathy. It is seen more frequently with squamous cell carcinoma.

Benedict reported on her study designed to determine the incidence of suffering associated with lung cancer. It is important to recognize the high incidence of suffering experienced by lung cancer patients and the fact that more suffering is associated with the physical aspects of the disease. If the sources of greatest suffering are made explicit, such as from disability, pain, or weakness and fatigue, the nurse can provide suggestions or nursing actions for the patient and family that may alleviate or ameliorate the sources of suffering. The nurse has a major responsibility for assisting the patient with symptom management. Examples include suggesting that the patient limit activity, assisting the patient with essential activity when pain and dyspnea are most severe, providing for nutritional intake when the patient is most comfortable, and providing small amounts of high-calorie, high-protein food frequently when anorexia is present. Provision of oxygen and instruction in breathing techniques may be required. Nursing care is based on the specific clinical manifestations that the patient experiences, and these include a range from local to systemic manifestations.

SCREENING

Early detection through large screening programs has shown only very limited success in reducing mortality. For detection of lung cancer on radiograph, the tumor must be in the range of 1 cm in diameter. This size requires 30 doublings, by which time metastases have occurred. Thus, early detection of lung cancer by chest radiographic screening is unlikely. At 40 doublings, the tumor burden usually results in death.

TUMOR MARKERS

The production of ectopic hormones by some lung cancers has been reported for years. However, no marker has been identified that can be used for screening for lung cancer. A number of tumor markers have been measured in serum specimens from SCLC patients, including adrenocorticotropic hormone, antidiuretic hormone, oxytocin, carcinoembryonic antigen, and calcitonin. Levels of two enzymes, neuron-specific enolase and creatine kinase BB, have been found to be elevated in patients with untreated SCLC.

DIAGNOSIS

Diagnostic techniques include the use of chest radiographs, sputum cytologic evaluations, fiberoptic bronchoscopy and transthoracic needle aspiration biopsy to obtain tissue specimens, and computed tomographic (CT) scans.

The diagnosis of lung cancer must be histologically or cytologically confirmed from tissue or sputum specimens, respectively. Centrally located tumors have a higher percentage of positive sputum cytologic evaluations than do peripherally located tumors. For the most accurate diagnostic results, a series of three or four sputum specimens should be collected and subjected to cytologic examination. Bronchoscopy also is useful in diagnosing centrally located tumors. Tumor tissue can be obtained through the use of bronchial needle aspiration technique. Transthoracic needle biopsies are most useful for diagnosing the more peripherally located tumors and for obtaining pleural and mediastinal tissue. Because pneumothorax is a complication of transthoracic needle biopsies, observation for this problem is critical.

CT is an important adjunct to chest radiographs in the diagnosis of lung cancer. It is particularly useful in evaluating the mediastinal lymph node involvement and the extent of disease. CT and radiographs are used in evaluating the response to therapy. The most sensitive imaging technique for detecting bone metastases is the radionuclide bone scan.

The nurse should describe the specifically ordered diagnostic procedures to the patient and family. This description should include what will occur and what the patient is to do.

STAGING

Staging follows the diagnosis and histologic classification of lung cancer. For non-SCLCs, the TNM (tumor, node, metastasis) classification is used for staging (Table 11-1).

Table 11-1. TNM CLASSIFICATION FOR STAGING NONSMALL-CELL LUNG CANCERS

Stage	Tumor	Node	Metastasis
I	T_1	N_0	M_0
	T_1	N_1	M_0
	T_2	N_0	M_0
II	T_2	N_1	M_0
III	T_3	N_{0-2}	M_{0-1}
	T_{1-3}	N_2	M_{0-1}
	T_{1-3}	N_{0-2}	M_1

Key: T_1 = 3.0 cm or less in diameter without evidence of invasion

T_2 = more than 3.0 cm in diameter or any size with invasion of visceral pleural or associated atelectasis or pneumonitis extending to hilar region

T_3 = any size tumor with direct extension to adjacent structure

N_0 = no demonstrable metastasis

N_1 = metastasis to peribronchial or ipsilateral hilar lymph nodes

N_2 = metastasis to mediastinal lymph nodes

M_0 = no known distant metastasis

M_1 = distant metastasis

For SCLC, the limited or extensive classifications are used more frequently than the TNM system for staging. Limited classification refers to tumors that are confined to the ipsilateral hemithorax; extensive classification refers to tumors that have spread beyond the ipsilateral hemithorax and adjacent lymph nodes. The limited or extensive categories are more useful for SCLC because with the rapid extrathoracic spread of small-cell lung tumors, most would be classified as stage III at diagnosis. The prognosis for those classified as stage I or II also is poor due to the undetected micrometastases. In staging for SCLC, bone marrow aspiration and biopsy may be performed because bone marrow involvement has been observed to occur in as many as 50% of the cases.

TREATMENT

The management of lung cancer depends on the histologic cell type and the extent and pattern of invasion and spread. Generally, the treatment of lung cancer is not very effective. There is no really effective therapy for lung cancer patients with disseminated disease.

Surgery

If the mediastinal nodes are determined to be disease free, surgery is usually the initial procedure. Functional or performance status also is considered in determining treatment. Surgery may be the choice of treatment when there is no evidence of metastatic spread beyond the ipsilateral hemithorax and when other patient characteristics, such as respiratory, cardiac, and cerebral status, are determined to be satisfactory for a favorable surgical outcome.

Surgery is the treatment of choice for patients with stage I or II non-SCLC. For tumor removal, segmental or wedge resections can be used to preserve lung tissue, but lobectomy or pneumonectomy is the more usual approach. The choice of procedure depends on location, size, and extent of tumor spread.

Before surgery, the nurse may have to assist the patient with airway clearance measures to improve ventilatory capacity. Examples of these measures are to teach the patient coughing and deep breathing techniques, to assist with postural drainage, or to provide for inhalation of aerosol solutions. Smoking cessation may be advised before surgery. If infection is present, antibiotic administration will be prescribed. Nursing actions include explanations about the surgical procedure and about what is expected after surgery. Postoperatively, the patient is likely to have mechanical ventilatory assistance for a short time, but positive pressure ventilation is discontinued to prevent or minimize stress to sutured tissues. Following extubation, coughing and deep breathing exercises are necessary. Splinting the incision will help decrease the pain, as will timing the exercises with analgesic administration. Position the individual to facilitate lung expansion. Nursing care depends on the surgical procedure used.

Survival rate decreases as size of tumor increases. Thus, for those with more extensive disease, the evidence of increased survival rate with surgery is more controversial. Surgery may be used in conjunction with adjuvant radiation therapy or in combination with chemotherapy or with chemotherapy alone.

Pulmonary resection may not be possible for those who have coexisting chronic lung disease or compromised pulmonary function.

Radiation Therapy

Radiation therapy is rarely curative for lung cancer, although a small percentage of patients survive 5 years following therapy. Initially, complete regression is seen in about half of those undergoing radiation therapy, but there is a high incidence of local recurrence. The failure of radiation may be due to the presence of radioresistant hypoxic tumor cells. Neutron therapy may be more effective against hypoxic cells. Thus the combination of conventional cobalt-60 radiation and neutrons may improve control of local lung cancer.

Radiation is more successful for those with small, peripheral, non-SCLC tumors with no evidence of metastases. Patients with limited squamous cell carcinoma are those for whom radiation therapy has been the most effective. Primarily, radiation is used for patients with unresectable tumors, for those with regional lymph node involvement, and for those with direct invasion of other thoracic structures. For increased effectiveness of the therapy, the patient should be able to tolerate a 6- to 7-week course of therapy.

Radiation therapy also has been used preoperatively and postoperatively, but the benefit at those times remains controversial. Following tumor resection, radiation therapy may be prescribed for patients who have tumor cells at tissue margins. Radiation may be preferable for those who have resectable tumors but who may not be able to tolerate surgery.

Radiotherapy may be used for palliation of symptoms that result from compression or infiltration of intrathoracic structures by the tumor. It is used also for palliation in chest wall invasion and for relief of bone pain, intractable cough, dyspnea, and hemoptysis. Radiation is used to treat complications, such as bronchial obstruction, superior vena cava syndrome, and rib invasion, and it is used prophylactically for possible central nervous system involvement.

Prophylactic brain irradiation has been used for those with adenocarcinoma of the lung, but there is no evidence of increased duration of survival. Prophylactic cranial irradiation has been shown to decrease the incidence of cerebral metastases and to improve survival, but this improvement has not been statistically significant.

Contraindications for the use of curative irradiation include inadequate respiratory reserve, pleural effusion, distant metastases, large tumor, weight loss greater than 4.5 kg, and a Karnofsky performance status of less than 70.

Complications from radiation therapy increase as the dose increases and as the extent of normal tissue included in the field increases. Pulmonary fibrosis can result from permanent damage to the alveolar endothelium, and the extent of fibrosis is related to the amount of tissue irradiated. One complication that occurs 1 to 3 months after chest irradiation is pneumonitis. The patient experiences dyspnea and a nonproductive cough. Corticosteroids may be used for symptomatic relief, although the efficacy of this treatment is debatable. Because of their effect on respiratory function, pneumonitis and fibrosis can influence the patient's quality of life. If they are severe, respiratory complications may result in death.

Other complications are radiation-induced myelitis that occurs when protection of the spinal cord has been inadequate and pericarditis that results from inclusion of the heart in the irradiated field.

Nurses have a role in explaining the use of radiation therapy and in helping the patient minimize the side effects, such as anorexia, nausea, and fatigue. Because the therapy requires long-term, almost daily treatment, it is important for the nurse to help the patient adhere to the scheduled therapy. The nurse also needs to be alert for clinical manifestations of the complications associated with radiation and to participate in the therapeutic management of the specific complication.

Chemotherapy

The drugs most commonly used alone or in some combination for treatment of non-SCLC are doxorubicin, methotrexate, cyclophosphamide, cisplatin, etoposide (VP-16-213), and vindesine. An increase in survival time after using these agents is not well demonstrated. Most of the drugs in the chemotherapeutic regimen are associated with considerable side effects (morbidity).

Chemotherapy is the main treatment for SCLC. Chemotherapy is less effective for non-SCLCs, except that survival time has been observed to lengthen with the use of cisplatin. SCLC is more sensitive to chemotherapy than are non-SCLCs. However, the response occurs for only a short time, and relapse is frequent. The most effective agents include cyclophosphamide in combination with vincristine and doxorubicin, methotrexate, etoposide or VePesid. Procarbazine, cisplatin, and lomustine (CCNU) are also used.

The major nursing care associated with chemotherapy frequently includes administration of the prescribed agents, assisting the patient in managing the side effects experienced, assessing for signs and symptoms of toxicities specific to the agents used, and monitoring patient responses.

Combination Therapy

Some investigators have shown improved complete response rates and survival using combination radiation therapy of the primary limited small-cell tumor along with chemotherapy. For those non-SCLC patients whose disease is considered inoperable, combined radiation therapy for control of locoregional involvement and chemotherapy for control of distant metastases are used. However, survival rates have not improved greatly, and systemic recurrence remains a problem.

The most common first site of recurrence in patients treated for adenocarcinoma and large-cell undifferentiated carcinoma is extrapulmonary, usually the brain. The most common first site of recurrence for squamous cell carcinoma is local.

Immunotherapy

Lung cancer is an immunosuppressive disease; that is, some lung cancer patients have a depressed immune response, and lymphocytes that have infiltrated the tumor have depressed activity. These immune system defects may contribute to the rapid disease progression. Despite attempts of treatment with immunotherapy, evidence remains controversial.

Although monoclonal antibodies (MoAbs) have been made in response to lung cancer antigens, the antigenic and biologic heterogeneity of SCLC in particular results in the lack of antibody specificity and thus limits the utility of this approach for treatment.

SUMMARY

In those who have no metastatic spread, non-SCLCs are potentially curable by surgery but are relatively resistant to chemotherapy and radiation. For those with SCLC, surgery is relatively ineffective due to the frequent existence of metastatic disease, but the tumor cells are responsive to radiation and chemotherapy.

For some lung cancer patients with extensive disease, supportive care with antibiotics, analgesics, and bronchodilators may be the treatment of choice. For some, quality of life may be increased with symptom management rather than with aggressive anticancer therapy.

12 Genitourinary Cancers

JULENA LIND
ROBERT J. IRWIN, JR.

Cancers of the prostate, kidney, and bladder are common in adults. Testicular cancer, although uncommon, is important to discuss because it is the most common cancer in young men between 25 and 30 years of age.

PROSTATIC CANCER
Definition and Incidence

The prostate is a small, firm organ made up of glands and musculature enclosed in a fibrous capsule through which the urethra passes as it exits the bladder. It is a secondary

---

See the corresponding chapter in *Cancer Nursing: A Comprehensive Textbook*, by Baird, McCorkle, and Grant, pp. 466–484, for a more detailed discussion of this topic, including a comprehensive list of references.

sex organ whose only known function is its contribution to seminal fluid.

Prostate cancer accounts for approximately 20% of all cancers in men and 10% of all cancer deaths.

Epidemiology and Etiology

The peak incidence of prostatic cancer is in men between 60 and 70 years of age. Three major factors are hypothesized to contribute to the causation of prostatic cancer: age, infectious agents, and endocrine factors. Age is the most important variable yet described.

Biology and Natural History

Prostatic cancers are almost always adenocarcinomas, which vary in differentiation and appearance. They are generally staged according to an A, B, C, D system. However, the TNM system also is used.

Also used more frequently today is the Gleason classification. This is a system of histopathologic grading based on the glandular pattern of the tumor at relatively low magnification. Combining clinical staging and histopathologic grading helps predict the biologic potential of prostate cancer.

Local spread to the seminal vesicles and the bladder is common. Prostatic cancer also disseminates hematogenously to the bones and rarely to the lungs and liver. The disease spreads via the lymphatics to the pelvic lymph nodes, then to the periaortic nodes, and occasionally to the supraclavicular nodes.

In the last two decades, the survival rates for prostatic cancer have increased significantly. Five-year survival after prostatectomy for stage A is 88% to 91% and for stage B 73% to 81%. Survival rates for advanced cancer are much less encouraging.

Presenting signs and symptoms

On rectal examination the gland normally feels rubbery. In early cancer, it will feel like a nonraised, firm nodule that may have a sharp edge. Unfortunately, there are no real symptoms in early-stage disease, and small tumors are easily missed. Later, tumors might be detected as a hard lump on rectal examination or as an unexpected finding during histologic examination of transurethral resection specimens.

Urinary disorders, such as frequency, dysuria, and obstruction, are common early symptoms. A frequent symptom of late disease is bone pain related to metastasis.

Differential diagnosis

The urinary tract symptoms of benign prostatic hypertrophy closely resemble cancer. Because only 50% of prostatic nodules are malignant tumors, it is imperative to establish a tissue diagnosis. This is most commonly done by needle aspiration or biopsy. A hardened area felt on rectal examination also could be the result of prostatitis, tuberculosis, fibrous benign prostatic hypertrophy (BPH), or prostatic calculi.

Determination of serum prostatic acid phosphatase by either biochemical or radioimmunologic assay should be included in the prostatic cancer workup. More than 80% of men with stage D disease have an increased serum acid phosphatase level. A bone scan and an excretory urogram (intravenous pyelogram, or IVP) also are usually performed.

Because the sudden discovery of prostatic cancer may take the asymptomatic patient and his family by complete surprise, nursing interventions should focus on education and emotional support. Helping the patient and family to understand the implications of his treatment options—for example, possible impotence or incontinence—is a significant challenge.

Treatment
Surgery

Radical prostatectomy is the surgical removal of the entire prostate, including the true prostatic capsule, the seminal vesicles, and a portion of the bladder neck. It can be done with or without pelvic lymph node dissection. Radical prostatectomy is indicated for stage A and stage B disease, particularly in situations in which the patient is younger, has no metastases, and has a normal acid phosphatase level.

Transurethral resection of the prostate (TURP) also plays a role in treatment. Although it is not used as a curative method, TURP is used to treat obstructive disease in advanced cancer. It may reveal an unsuspected cancer when used as a treatment for BPH.

Complications after radical prostatectomy include impotence, infection, and urinary incontinence. It is thought that postradical prostatectomy impotence is a result of damage to autonomic nerves posterolateral to the prostate, which are required for physiologic erections. The Walsh and Mostwin retropubic prostatectomy (which carefully avoids injury to the pelvic nerves) has shown fewer problems with impotence and incontinence.

Nursing implications involve initially exploring preoperative concerns regarding sexual competence. People in general may hold certain prejudices concerning sexuality in the older adult, which the nurse should avoid. Teaching should be geared to the role of the prostate in sexual activity and alleviating misconceptions that all sexual activity is over.

Immediate postoperative nursing responsibilities include maintaining catheter presence and patency, preventing urinary tract infection, and administering antispasmodics to decrease the discomfort caused by bladder spasms. Interestingly, clot retention after radical prostatectomy is less of a problem than it is after simple prostatectomy.

Radiotherapy

Radiotherapy has been used for curative, adjunctive, and palliative treatment of prostate cancer. Radiotherapy also has been attempted as an adjunct to surgery. Postoperative irradiation for patients with localized disease does not offer any apparent advantage. Prophylactic radiotherapy of the regional lymphatics is often used in patients who are at significant risk of harboring tumor deposits in the regional lymph nodes.

Common side effects of radiotherapy to the prostate are proctitis, diarrhea, and urinary frequency. Potency rates of 60% are possible, although this finding probably applies to younger patients.

Internal radiotherapy via direct implantation also has been used to treat prostate cancer. When the disease is localized to the pelvis, internal radiation can increase the dose directly to the prostate and decrease the exposure to the surrounding tissue. Radioactive iodine (^{125}I) is commonly used. Wound infection, proctitis, and fistula formation are occasional complications described in up to 25% of the patients treated with ^{125}I. However, potency was preserved in 70% to 90% of the patients who were previously potent.

A newer afterloading technique using iridium (^{192}Ir) has been described, with equivocal results. Although early morbidity is low, there is significant later morbidity, including proctitis, ulceration, progressive obstructive symptoms, incontinence, and impotence.

Radiation-induced cystitis usually occurs during the first 2 to 3 weeks of therapy. Education by the nurse would include encouraging the patient to drink at least 2 liters of fluid per day and explaining the benefits of antispasmodics and analgesics in decreasing the discomfort. Nursing care of the patient with afterloading interstitial implants (^{192}Ir) should be done quickly to reduce radiation exposure to nursing personnel. However, seed implants pose minimal risk. Provided that the patient's urine is promptly disposed of, there is no risk to others from ^{125}I radiation because this isotope's decay is by beta emission. Patients are understandably concerned about radiation exposure, and every attempt should be made to provide reassurance for them and their families.

Chemotherapy

Chemotherapy plays a limited role in the treatment of advanced, hormonally unresponsive prostatic cancer. Both single-agent and combination protocols have been attempted.

Hormonal manipulation

Hormonal treatment of adenocarcinoma of the prostate is based on the assumption that prostatic cancer cells are androgen dependent. This treatment is indicated for patients with advanced cancer, but it plays no role in the therapy of patients with localized disease. Dihydrotestosterone is the principal intracellular androgen. Blocking androgen formation or use theoretically will arrest tumor growth.

Hormonal manipulation can take the following forms.
- Administration of estrogen
- Administration of drugs that interfere with androgens
- Orchiectomy
- Adrenalectomy (surgical and medical)
- Hypophysectomy

Diethylstilbestrol (DES) 1 to 3 mg orally is the estrogen usually given. Side effects of DES include thromboembolic disease, congestive heart failure, decreased libido, impotence, and gynecomastia. In some settings, breast irradiation is performed routinely to prevent gynecomastia.

Bilateral orchiectomy decreases plasma testosterone levels, but to virtually unmeasurable levels. Adrenalectomy (either surgical or chemical with aminogluthethamide) blocks adrenal androgens and is used for those persons who orginally responded to hormonal therapy but who have relapsed. Hypophysectomy (surgical removal of the pituitary) ablates both the adrenal and testicular production of androgens, but it is rarely used because of profound endocrine complications.

The most significant nursing implications related to hormonal manipulation include patient teaching regarding the side effects of DES, particularly sodium retention, the potential for cardiac complications, and feminization effects.

Recurrence and palliative treatment

Most prostatic cancers are advanced at the time of diagnosis, and treatment reflects this. Bone metastases to the vertebrae, pelvis, femur, and ribs are very common. Subsequently, pain management is often an issue.

Endocrine manipulation is the usual palliative treatment, although it may be coupled with radiotherapy. Chemotherapy has been attempted, but with only limited success.

Nursing management for patients with recurrent disease focuses on providing for pain relief, teaching the patient how to manage the side effects of hormonal therapy, and offering emotional support.

BLADDER CANCER
Definition and Incidence

Bladder cancer accounts for about 4% to 5% of all cancers in the United States.

Epidemiology and Etiology

Bladder cancer is typically seen in industrialized rather than in underdeveloped countries. The exception to this generalization is countries, such as Egypt, where exposure to the parasite *Schistosoma haematobium* is common.

Hypothesized etiologic factors include cigarette smoking, exposure to the industrial chemicals called arylamines (used in textile and rubber industries), and exposure to *S. haemotobium* (squamous cell cancer of the bladder).

Biology and Natural History

Most bladder cancers in the United States are transitional cell carcinomas arising from the transitional epithelium of the mucosal lining. Although 90% of the cases are localized at the time of diagnosis, as many as 30% to 90% of patients will develop recurrent cancers.

The overall 5-year survival for whites is 76%, and for African Americans, it is 55%.

Presenting signs and symptoms

Gross hematuria is the most common presenting symptom. Other symptoms include irritability of the bladder (dysuria, frequency, or urgency). Symptoms associated with large tumor growth also may be present. For example, tumor pushing on the internal urethral orifice can cause urinary hesitancy and decreased force and caliber of the stream. Obstruction of the ureters can cause flank pain and result in hydronephrosis.

Differential diagnosis

In the evaluation of any patient with gross hematuria, an IVP can help evaluate a suspected bladder tumor by showing the tumor itself or by showing evidence of ureteral obstruction. Cystoscopy provides not only tumor visualization but also an opportunity to perform a biopsy and palpate the tumor. Urine cytology can help in the evaluation of those patients who have hematuria and are suspected of having a malignancy.

Nursing implications at the time of diagnosis include patient and family teaching about what to expect from the diagnostic tests. For example, patients may be anesthetized for cystoscopy. Following the procedure, patients are advised to drink plenty of fluids and to expect some hematuria. As another example, it is useful to know that urine cytology specimens are more reliable if they are not obtained as the first voided specimen of the day. If the specimens are not sent immediately for analysis, the urine should be refrigerated. A further nursing role involves clarifying for the patient and family the test results. If cancer is found, they will need assistance in understanding their treatment options. It must be emphasized here that if cystectomy is indicated, choosing a setting for treatment with access to an enterostomal therapist is extremely important. The patient's future adjustment to treatment and his or her quality of life very well might depend on interactions with an enterostomal therapist.

Treatment
Surgery

Surgical therapy depends on the pathologic stage of the tumor. Frequently, pelvic lymph node dissection is included at the time of cystectomy in an effort to prevent local pelvic recurrence. The urinary diversion associated with radical cystectomy may be an intestinal conduit (such as an ileal conduit) or a continent urinary reservoir. This technique was first described by Kock et al. and was introduced into the United States by Gerber. Most of the reported experience with this procedure is limited to southern California.

Ureterosigmoidostomy, a procedure in which the ureters are implanted into the sigmoid colon and urine is then excreted through the rectum, is rarely done today.

Nursing Implications. Potential problems occurring in the first month after creation of an ileal conduit include wound infections, enteric fistulas, urine leaks, ureteral obstruction, bowel obstruction, and pelvic abscesses. Late complications include stomal stenosis, peristomal hernias, chronic pyelonephritis, ureteroileal obstruction, intestinal obstruction, calculi, and metabolic problems with hyperchloremic acidosis.

Unlike a fecal diversion, the urinary diversion should produce urine from the time of surgery, and a urinary appliance is needed. Ideally, a urinary stoma should protrude 1.25 to 2 cm (0.5 to 0.75 inch) above the skin to allow the urine to drain into the aperture of an appliance.

The color of the stoma should be checked frequently in the early postoperative period. Normal color is deep pink to dark red. A dusky appearance could indicate stoma necrosis.

Because the intestine normally produces mucus, mucus will be present in all urinary diversions that use bowel segments. Excessive mucus can, on occasion, clog the urinary appliance. Increasing fluid intake to 3 liters per day will help.

Skin care and the pouching of the stoma are important nursing considerations. Several excellent sources describe these techniques.

Patient teaching is vital for the person with a new urinary diversion. Concepts that should be emphasized include leakage prevention to protect peristomal skin, comfort and ease in handling the various pieces of equipment, early identification of kidney infections, and resources to call on when at home. Body image issues also should be addressed. Teaching should not begin until the patient's physical discomfort has subsided and the physiologic state has returned more or less to normal. Enterostomal therapists are skilled specialists in technical matters and help the patient and family learn that a normal life is possible with an ileal conduit.

Complications after radical cystectomy with placement of a continent ileal reservoir, such a Kock pouch, include incontinence, difficult catheterization, urinary reflux, obstruction, bacteriuria, electrolyte imbalances, and absorptive deficits.

Immediate postoperative nursing concerns for the patient who has had a Kock pouch include checking the stoma for ischemia and irrigating the Medena tube with normal saline solution to wash out both clots and mucus, which might plug the pouch. Three to four weeks after the operation, when the Medena tube is removed, the nurse will teach the patient to perform self-catheterizations, first every 2 to 3 hours and then every 4 to 6 hours during the day and once at night. With a continent ileal reservoir, there is no need for an external appliance, and intubation of the pouch can duplicate normal bladder function.

A radical cystectomy with urinary diversion affects many aspects of sexual function. The cause of erectile dysfunction after radical cystectomy is similar to that associated with radical prostatectomy for prostatic cancer. However, patients can still achieve orgasm. Because the prostate and seminal vesicles are removed, men experience dry orgasms without emission of semen but still have normal muscle contractions. Women may experience some physiologic problems during intercourse as a result of a shortened vagina. The reader is referred to Chapter 26 for specific information on sexual counseling.

Radiation therapy

Definitive radiotherapy in bladder cancer generally is reserved for patients who are not candidates for surgery. However, outside the United States, invasive bladder cancer frequently is treated primarily by radiotherapy.

Preoperative radiotherapy has been advocated in an effort to reduce pelvic recurrence and decrease the possibility of tumor spread during surgery. A typical protocol using high-dose, short-course radiotherapy is 1600 to 2000 Gy (rad) delivered in fractionated doses over 4 days. A more conventional course would include 4000 to 4500 Gy delivered in 4 to 6 weeks. Although preoperative radiotherapy can be safely combined with surgery, most studies have shown no significant improvement in cure in those patients who received radiation.

Laser surgery to treat invasive bladder cancer has also been attempted.

Complications of radiotherapy include radiation enteritis or colitis and skin reactions. See Chapter 4 for a discussion of nursing care of radiation complications.

Chemotherapy

For superficial, low-grade disease, intravesical chemotherapy (direct instillation of drug into the bladder) has been used to increase the concentration of drug in the area where the tumor cells are located. It may aid in decreasing recurrence by eliminating the residual tumor and stem cells.

Thio-TEPA is the drug most commonly used. However, mitomycin C, bacillus Calmette-Guérin (BCG), and doxorubicin (Adriamycin) also have been used.

Nursing implications include assessment of myelosuppression and handling precautions while the drug(s) are being instilled. See Chapters 22 and 6 for a discussion of myelosuppression and handling precautions.

Recurrence and palliative treatment

Superficial recurrences are managed by repeated transurethral resection and intravesical chemotherapy. Provided that they do not develop invasive disease, patients have a 95% 5-year survival. About 50% of patients with high-stage, high-grade tumor will have relapses after cystectomy. Surgical treatment is seldom used to palliate symptoms in these patients.

Chemotherapy as a treatment for advanced bladder cancer has been investigated and may achieve a complete response in 40% to 50% of the patients, but relapse is inevitable. Single-agent therapy using cisplatin, methotrexate, or vinblastine has been attempted, with partial responses of short duration. Cisplatin has produced the longest responses. Various combination protocols have been tested. Cisplatin, doxorubicin, and cyclophosphamide is one combination protocol that has demonstrated both complete and partial responses in patients with advanced bladder cancer.

The combination programs with higher doses seem to result in higher complete response rates. Unfortunately, they also result in more significant side effects. Nursing management of the side effects of high doses of cisplatin and doxorubicin is challenging. Nausea and vomiting, renal toxicity, ototoxicity, myelosuppression, and the potential for extravasation all must be considered. See Chapters 6 and 20 for a more in-depth discussion of these side effects and their nursing implications.

TESTICULAR CANCER
Definition and Incidence

Testicular cancer is a rare tumor that arises in embryonal tissue. Although rare, it is the most common solid tumor in men between 25 and 35 years of age. Dramatic improvement in the management of this disease has been one of cancer's real success stories. The key to this success was the simultaneous development of effective combination chemotherapy and reliable, noninvasive techniques to assess the extent of disease and its response to treatment.

Epidemiology and Etiology

Although testicular tumors are uncommon, their incidence is increasing among young white men. Cryptorchidism is one of the hypothesized etiologic factors in testicular cancer. Relative risk of testicular cancer in men with an undescended testicle is 3 to 14 times that of normal men.

Exogenous estrogens also have been implicated in the causation of testicular cancer. There is an increased risk in the male offspring of women exposed to DES in the first trimester of pregnancy and of women exposed to the estrogen–progestin combinations that have been used frequently as diagnostic tests to confirm pregnancy.

Biology and Natural History

Most testicular tumors (97%) arise from germ tissue and are called *germinal tumors*. The following is a list of the various types of germinal testicular tumors.

Seminoma (germinoma) (up to 40% of all testes tumors)
    Typical (most common)
    Anaplastic
    Spermocytic
Nonseminomatous germ cell testicular tumors
    (NSGCTT)
    Embryonal
    Teratocarcinoma
    Teratoma
    Choriocarcinoma

Survival from testicular cancer has improved dramatically in the last decade. The overall 5-year survival is 89% in whites and 78% in African Americans.

Presenting signs and symptoms

Two thirds of patients have a history of painless enlargement of the testes. Other symptoms include a dragging sensation in the scrotum and, rarely, a painful mass owing to intratesticular bleeding. Symptoms related to spread of the disease include lumbar pain and abdominal or supraclavicular pain caused by enlarged lymph nodes.

Differential diagnosis

Epididymitis and hydrocele both occasionally mimic the symptoms of testis cancer.

Diagnostic procedures commonly used in testicular cancer include the following.

- Manual palpation of testes and surrounding structures
- Radical inguinal orchiectomy (as biopsy)
- Radiologic techniques
  Chest radiograph (for lung metastases)
  Computed tomographic (CT) scan of chest
    (detects lung metastases)
  Abdominal and pelvic CT scan (detects retro-
    peritoneal nodes)
  Excretory urogram
- Laboratory studies
  Serum α-fetoprotein (AFP)
  Serum human chorionic gonadotropin-β subunit
    (hCG-β)

The laboratory studies determining AFP and hCG-β are used as preoperative tumor markers, and because they reflect the clinical course of the disease, they are very important in the staging of testicular cancer. Elevated serum AFP levels are never seen in men with *pure* seminomas and, therefore, help to indicate the presence of a nonseminomatous testicular tumor. Because liver damage also can produce elevated AFP levels, hepatotoxicity from chemotherapy or radiotherapy should be ruled out.

About 50% to 60% of patients with nonseminomatous testicular tumors will have an elevated hCG-β level, and occasionally patients with pure seminomas will have elevated levels of HCG. HCG is normally produced only in pregnant women.

Nursing implications regarding detection of testicular cancer should include educating the public about testicular self-examination (TSE). A 1986 report stated that a moderate percentage of professional men had knowledge of TSE but that very few practiced it. Of those who knew about TSE, none had learned about it from a nurse.

Patient and family education is the other important nursing function at this time. Young, otherwise healthy young men with testicular cancer need help in understanding their treatment and its sequelae. They especially need help with their sexuality and body image concerns. The psychosocial dynamics may be complex. Independent young adults are often forced to be dependent again on their parents. Nurses can help both the young men and their parents to adjust to the situation.

Treatment for Seminomatous Tumors
Surgery

High radical inguinal orchiectomy, in which the testis, the epididymis, a portion of the vas deferens, and portions of the gonadal lymphatics and blood supply are removed, is routinely done as a diagnostic step.

The remaining testicle will produce enough testosterone to maintain sexual capacity. The orchiectomy has no defined adverse effect on sexual potency or fertility in the otherwise normal patient.

Radiotherapy

Because seminomas are extremely radiosensitive, external beam radiotherapy, directed to the perineum, is used to treat stages A, B1, and B2 disease (stages I, IIA, IIB). If there is retroperitoneal involvement, the mediastinal and supraclavicular nodes also are irradiated.

Complications associated with pelvic irradiation include fatigue, diarrhea, and azoospermia. Radiotherapy, although it does not affect libido or potency, causes infertility in many men. Moderate oligospermia to azoospermia has been reported after a single testicular dose of 8 to 50 cGy.

Nursing implications include teaching the patient and family to manage the side effects of radiotherapy and providing information on sexuality issues.

Chemotherapy

Patients with advanced seminoma [stages B3 and C (IIC, III, and IV)] are candidates for chemotherapy with or without radiotherapy to the pelvis. Most protocols use a combination of cisplatin, vinblastine, and bleomycin, with or without doxorubicin. Because this protocol is very similar to the one used for nonseminomatous testicular tumors, the reader is referred to that section for complications and nursing implications.

Treatment for Nonseminomatous Tumors
Surgery

Although orchiectomy is a standard part of surgical diagnosis, the role of bilateral retroperitoneal lymph node dissection after orchiectomy in treating nonseminomatous germ cell tumors (NSGCTT) remains controversial.

Because many autonomic nerves necessary for ejaculation are located in the retroperitoneal area, infertility may result from this surgery. However, one series reported spontaneous return of normal ejaculatory ability after 3 years in 50% of patients.

Nursing implications after retroperitoneal lymph node dissection include observation for infection and bleeding immediately after the operation and later patient education regarding sexuality.

Radiotherapy

Because nonseminomatous germ cell tumors are relatively radioresistant, radiotherapy is not routinely used in the United States to treat these tumors.

Chemotherapy

The major role of chemotherapy in NSGCTT is in disseminated disease. In August 1974, early studies were begun at Indiana University using a combination of cisplatin, vinblastine, and bleomycin (PVB). The results of this chemotherapy combination on NSGCTT have been remarkable and have revolutionized the treatment of testicular cancer. Einhorn reported a regularly achieved 80% 5-year disease-free survival for patients with disseminated disease.

However, the PVB regimen is highly toxic. Leukopenia, sepsis, nausea and vomiting, and cisplatin-induced nephrotoxicity are common. Raynaud's phenomenon is a long-term side effect associated with vinblastine therapy.

Because the majority of patients with NSGCTT are living longer than 5 years, the focus has turned to evaluation of long-term side effects and survival. One such long-term effect is indicated in the reports over the last 10 years of cases of acute leukemia in men treated for testicular cancer.

Nursing implications for those men treated with chemotherapy are related to the significant side effects of the PVB and the VAB regimens. See Chapter 22 for nursing management of the side effects of cisplatin, bleomycin, vinblastine, dactinomycin, and cyclophosphamide.

Sexuality is an important nursing concern. In one study of men treated for metastatic NSGCTT with a bilateral retroperitoneal lymph node dissection and VAB, only 11% retained ejaculatory ability. The results are better if only unilateral node dissection is done. However, the majority of the patients in the study denied any change in libido.

Recurrence and palliative treatment

Testicular cancer spreads to the retroperitoneal lymph nodes, to the lungs, and rarely to the brain and liver.

As mentioned previously, chemotherapy is used for advanced disease—both seminomatous and nonseminomatous tumors. In tumors that have been refractory to the PVB regimen, combinations of etoposide, cisplatin, or bleomycin or ifosfamide are being evaluated.

Nursing implications for late-stage disease are directed primarily toward relieving the side effects associated with chemotherapy. Emotional support for the patients and families is also very important. This disease affects primarily young men, and the family might include wife, small children, and siblings as well as parents. Concern for all of the members of the family will be an important nursing consideration.

CANCER OF THE KIDNEY
Definition and Incidence

There are two major types of kidney cancer: renal cell and transitional cell cancer of the renal pelvis.

Epidemiology and Etiology

There is a 2:1 male predominance in kidney cancer. This disease is rare in people under 35 years of age.

The rate of renal cell cancer is high in Scandinavia and low in Japan. The North Central part of the United States, especially Minnesota, has the highest kidney cancer incidence in the United States.

Cigarette smoking has been linked to the incidence of renal cell cancer. A hormonal association also appears likely. Diethylstilbestrol and estradiol both have induced kidney tumors in rats. Coffee consumption has been implicated as causing renal cell cancer, but the results have been conflicting and need further clarification. The data also suggest an increased risk of malignancy in patients on chronic hemodialysis.

Presenting signs and symptoms

Gross hematuria is present in more than 40% of patients with renal cell cancer. Pain, described as a dull, aching flank pain, also is a common presenting symptom. Finally, a palpable abdominal mass has been noted. However, it is rare for these three symptoms to appear simultaneously. A wide variety of other vague symptoms also are seen, including fever, weight loss, anemia, and hypercalcemia, which occur infrequently.

Differential diagnosis

The differential diagnosis is a renal mass, most commonly renal cysts and renal tumors. Diagnosis usually is made radiographically because of the variety of presenting symptoms and nonspecific laboratory findings. The advent of renal ultrasound and CT scanning has greatly simplified making the distinction between simple cysts and renal cancer. In many cases, renal angiography is no longer necessary. Tests used in the diagnosis and staging of renal cell cancer include the following: kidneys, ureters, bladder radiograph (KUB), excretory urogram (IVP), nephrotomogram, renal sonogram, renal CT scan, and renal angiogram.

Nursing implications include education about the nature of the diagnostic tests. Allaying misunderstandings about the implications of losing a kidney might also be important.

Treatment
Surgery

Radical nephrectomy is the removal of the kidney and associated tumor, the adrenal gland, the surrounding perinephric fat within Gerota's fascia, and Gerota's fascia itself. This is the treatment of choice for localized renal cell cancer, which also includes tumor extension into the renal vein and vena cava. There is no role for nephrectomy in patients with disseminated disease.

Regional retroperitoneal lymph node dissection often is performed routinely in association with radical nephrectomy.

Nursing implications during the immediate postoperative period include pain management and prevention of postoperative complications. Pain can be quite severe after nephrectomy. As a result of the position on the operating table, the patient experiences not only incisional pain but also muscular strain. Use of moist heat, massage, and pillows to support the back while the patient is lying on his or her side can provide relief. Postoperative nursing interventions include prevention of atelectasis and pneumonia, monitoring renal function of the remaining kidney, anticipating paralytic ileus, monitoring for bleeding, and preventing infection at the incision site.

Radiotherapy

Most renal cell tumors are radioresistant. However, radiotherapy has been used both preoperatively and postoperatively as an adjunct to nephrectomy.

Chemotherapy

There is no effective adjunctive chemotherapy for renal cell carcinoma.

Immunotherapy

Although renal cell cancer has been highly resistant to both chemotherapy and hormonal therapy, preliminary studies suggest that it is particularly susceptible to adoptive immunotherapy with lymphokine-activated killer (LAK) cells plus recombinant interleukin 2 (IL-2). The use of IL-2 alone has been clinically examined in patients with advanced disseminated disease. However, complete and partial responses have been much higher when combined with LAK cells. This treatment, however, is complicated, toxic, and expensive.

Other investigators have examined the use of interferon-α in the treatment of patients with advanced renal cell cancer and have shown that it has modest activity. The side effects reported have been tolerable.

Recurrence and palliative treatment

Renal cell cancer spreads to the medullary portion of the kidney, to the renal vein (sometimes into the vena cava), and to the lungs, bones, brain, and liver. About 30% of patients have metastases at the time of diagnosis.

Palliative nephrectomies are rarely done today. The principal local complications of bleeding, pain, and fever usually can be controlled better by angiographic infarction using a wide variety of materials. The nursing implications for angiographic infarction include watching for hemorrhage.

Chemotherapy has no great impact on metastatic renal cell cancer. Hormonal therapy in the form of progestational agents or therapy has shown responses in rats. Although its mild toxicity makes its use appealing, responses do not significantly improve survival, and this method has largely been abandoned.

As mentioned earlier, therapy employing LAK and IL-2 has been tested in patients with advanced or recurrent disease. Responses thus far have been encouraging.

Nursing implications associated with this experimental therapy include extensive patient education and support and intensive monitoring of the severe side effects, such as hypotension, fever, hepatic dysfunction, thrombocytopenia, and disorientation or somnolence.

13 Gastrointestinal Cancers

GRACEANN EHLKE

CANCER OF THE ESOPHAGUS
Definition and Incidence

Esophageal cancer is more common in men than in women and is most frequently seen in those older than 60 years.

In the United States, the mean survival for patients with esophageal carcinoma is between 3 and 20 months. Five-year survival rate is less than 5%.

Epidemiology and Etiology

Esophageal cancer is common in Japan, the southern shore of the Caspian Sea (Iran), and northern China. Risk factors include alcohol consumption and smoking. Dietary

See the corresponding chapter in *Cancer Nursing: A Comprehensive Textbook*, by Baird, McCorkle, and Grant, pp. 485–501, for a more detailed discussion of this topic, including a comprehensive list of references.

factors include deficiencies in iron or zinc, hot (temperature) beverages, and silica dust (Iranian bread).

Biology and Natural History

The mean survival in esophageal cancer is extremely low. With esophageal cancer, prognosis may depend on location of the tumor. Tumors in the upper esophagus are very difficult to treat with current therapies and have a poorer prognosis than tumors in the lower third.

Presenting Signs and Symptoms

A major indication of cancer of the esophagus is dysphagia for solids and eventually liquids, which is associated with weight loss.

The most serious symptoms are hoarseness and chronic cough. In addition, hemoptysis usually implies that the aorta is involved.

Differential Diagnosis

Diagnosis of some types of esophageal cancer can be made via chest radiograph. For those patients with dysphagia, a barium swallow usually is ordered. This is a procedure for diagnosis of many esophageal tumors.

Esophagoscopy allows a tissue diagnosis. It is accurate 96% of the time. Gallium or cobalt-bleomycin tracers are taken up by squamous cell cancers and have been reliable indicators of tumor in some cases.

Treatment

In an early stage, both radiation and surgery can be used to cure the disease. There are four main purposes of palliative treatment.

1. To open the esophageal lumen. This may be done by surgery, radiation therapy, dilation, prosthesis, laser, or tumor probe.

2. To slow the growth of the tumor. These treatments include surgery, radiation therapy, or chemotherapy.

3. To seal a fistula. This is done with a prosthesis.

4. To provide nutrition. Usually this is done via a gastrostomy or jejunostomy.

Nursing Care

The primary nursing diagnosis for a patient with esophageal cancer is *alteration in nutrition*. This causes difficulty in swallowing, which results from constriction of the esophagus by the tumor.

GASTRIC CARCINOMA
Definition and Incidence

The incidence of gastric cancer has steadily decreased in the last 55 years. The peak age for gastric cancer is 55 to 65 years, and the male/female ratio in 3:2.

Epidemiology and Etiology

The highest incidence of gastric cancer occurs in Japan, followed by Chile.

Gastric cancer has been linked etiologically to heredity, diet, socioeconomic status, and other carcinogens, such as exposure to dust in coal mines and potteries.

Biology and Natural History

Early gastric carcinoma, if treated surgically, carries 5-year survival rates of 85% to 90%. The 5-year survival rate for advanced gastric cancer is 16%.

Presenting Signs and Symptoms

With early gastric cancer, abdominal pain is a frequent symptom as are anorexia, nausea, vomiting, weight loss, fullness, belching, regurgitation, and pain after meals (dyspepsia).

Differential Diagnosis

The best diagnostic tool for gastric carcinoma is endoscopy. Other diagnostic tools that may be used include indirect radiology, gastric juice factors (fetal sialoglycoprotein and lactic dehydrogenase), serum tests (tetracycline test), urine test (Diagnex Blue test), gastric juice (pH, alpha-acid glycoprotein, and carcinoembryonic antigen or CEA), and serologic tests (alpha₁-fetoprotein, CEA, and pepsinogen I).

Treatment
Surgery

The major curative treatment of gastric cancer is surgery. Most often, a subtotal gastrectomy is done.

Radiation

Radiation frequently is used to treat gastric cancer in combination with surgery. The types of radiation employed include preoperative, intraoperative, and postoperative. Radiation is used also in combination with chemotherapy. The combination of chemotherapy and radiation therapy carries a better prognosis than does radiation alone.

Chemotherapy

The most frequently used single agent has been 5-FU. Chemotherapy has been also used as adjuvant therapy. The most positive findings were produced with the 5-FU and methyl-CCNU protocol and with a mitomycin protocol.

Nursing Care

Nutrition is a major problem for the person with gastric cancer. Irritation and ulceration of the gastric mucosa cause abdominal pain. Other gastrointestinal symptoms are nausea or vomiting (or both), abdominal fullness, belching, regurgitation, and dyspepsia.

COLORECTAL CANCER
Epidemiology and Etiology

In the United States, the mortality rate of colorectal cancer is second only to that of lung cancer in the Western world, owing primarily to the diet high in refined carbohydrates. Familial polyposis and ulcerative colitis, diverticulosis, hemorrhoids, adenomatous polyps, villous adenoma, and diet are main contributors to the development of colorectal cancer.

Staging for colorectal cancer includes the Broder, Dukes, and TNM methods of classification.

Asymptomatic patients have the best prognosis. Duration of symptoms is indicative of prognosis also, with patients who have an acute episode of symptoms having the poorest prognosis. Persons under 30 years old have a very poor prognosis (5-year survival rate of 19.5%), and those 70 years old and older have the best 5-year survival rate (67.2%). Prognosis has been linked to CEA levels in the peripheral blood.

Clinical Features and Diagnosis

The most important tests are the digital rectal examination, the Hemoccult test, and sigmoidoscopy. Half of all rectal cancers can be detected by rectal examination alone.

The most common signs of colorectal cancer include rectal bleeding, anemia, and a change in stool. Other possible indications of colorectal cancer include melena, tenesmus, abdominal pain, constipation, and diarrhea.

Treatment
Surgery

Surgery is the primary treatment of colorectal cancer. Surgical approaches include a segmental resection, a radical resection, and a supraradical resection. Patients undergoing radical or supraradical resections do no better than those with segmental resections.

Radiation therapy

The major problem related to irradiation of the bowel is the sensitivity of normal tissues. In many cases, these normal tissues are unable to tolerate the dose of radiation being delivered to the colorectal cancer.

Chemotherapy

Chemotherapy has not been as effective as in other types of cancer. Single agents used in the treatment of the disease are 5-FU, the nitrosoureas, and mitomycin C. By far the most common agent used is 5-FU. Various studies have been done with 5-FU in combination with leucovorin, methotrexate, lavamasol, methyl-CCNU, vincristine, streptozocin, cisplatin, interleukin 2 (IL-2), and lymphokine-activated killer (LAK) cells.

Nursing Care

The various treatments used for colorectal cancer may cause fluid and electrolyte imbalances as well as malabsorption problems owing to changes in levels of enzymes frequently associated with the gastrointestinal system (Table 13–1).

CANCER OF THE PANCREAS

Cancer of the pancreas ranks fifth as a cancer-related death, after lung, breast, colorectal, and prostate cancers. Fewer than 1% live longer than 5 years, and the peak incidence is around age 60 years.

Epidemiology and Etiology

Pancreatic cancer has no known cause. Chronic pancreatitis has been associated with the disease.

Signs and symptoms are jaundice, weight loss, weakness, anorexia, nausea, vomiting, depression, asthenia, and gaseousness.

Jaundice is seen frequently in patients with cancer of the head of the pancreas. Although it is not an early sign, jaundice is usually accompanied by pain, a frequent symptom in pancreatic cancer patients. If the tumor is one in which insulin is produced and excreted, symptoms include fatigue, hypoglycemia, diaphoresis, pallor, and malaise.

Differential Diagnosis

Diagnosis has been made using upper gastrointestinal tests, CT and ultrasonography, arteriography, transhepatic thin-needle cholangiography, and endoscopic retrograde choledochopancreatography (ERCP). Tumor markers include CEA, pancreatic oncofetal antigen (POA), and α-fetoglobulin. Serum immunoreactive elastastase I also has been found to be a sensitive marker.

Treatment
Surgery

Surgery usually consists of either the Whipple procedure or a total pancreatectomy. A regional pancreatectomy involves a total pancreatectomy and extensive lymph node dissection and also removal of the portal vein, transverse mesocolon, and the adjacent soft tissue.

Radiation therapy

Radiation therapy may be used as adjuvant therapy after surgery or for palliative reasons. Radiation combined with chemotherapy produces better survival rates than radiation alone.

Chemotherapy

Single agents most commonly used are 5-fluorouracil, mitomycin C, and streptozocin. Combination chemotherapy

Table 13–1. NURSING CARE PLAN FOR A PATIENT WITH A COLOSTOMY

Assessment	Interventions	Expected Outcomes
Nursing Diagnosis: Alteration in comfort—pain		
Intensity of pain will be influenced by activity of disease process, surgery, or psychologic factors; fear of injuring stoma may cause patient to restrict movements that intensify pain	Report and document nature and site of pain Medicate for pain as needed Reposition and use proper support measures as needed; assure patient that position change will not injure stoma Encourage patient to verbalize Actively listen and provide support Document relief from pain	Verbalizes or displays relief from pain and demonstrates ability to assist in care through use of general comfort measures
Nursing Diagnosis: Potential alteration in nutrition—less than body requirements		
May be undernourished from disease process or illness; some foods are gas- and odor-forming in the digestive process and individual sensitivities to some foods may result in diarrhea or constipation; bulk and residue may need to be restricted depending on bowel activity	Do thorough nutritional assessment; confer with physician and dietitian to correct deficiencies Provide nutrition high in protein and calories to repair tissue and prevent weight loss	

Continued

175

Table 13–1. NURSING CARE PLAN FOR A PATIENT WITH A COLOSTOMY *Continued*

Assessment	Interventions	Expected Outcomes
Nursing Diagnosis: Potential alteration in nutrition—less than body requirements Continued		
	Identify offensive foods and temporarily restrict them from diet; gradually reintroduce one food at a time	Patient is able to plan a diet that meets nutritional needs and limits gastrointestinal disturbances
	Document those foods that are a source of flatus (e.g., carbonated drinks, beer, beans, cabbage family, onions, fish, and highly seasoned foods) or odor (e.g., onions, cabbage family, eggs, fish, and beans)	
	Increase use of yogurt, buttermilk, and cranberry juice	
	Discuss the mechanics of swallowed air as a factor in the formation of flatus and some ways patient can exercise control	
	Avoid cellulose products (e.g., peanuts)	

Exercise caution in the dietary intake of prunes, dates, stewed apricots, strawberries, grapes, bananas, cabbage family, beans, and nuts

Discuss with the physician the patient's nutritional needs and have the dietitian discuss meal planning with the patient and significant others before discharge

Nursing Diagnosis: *Potential fluid volume deficit*

Preoperatively, patient may have been dehydrated from emesis, diarrhea, diaphoresis, and nothing by mouth order

Monitor intake and output carefully, including liquid stool

Monitor blood pressure, pulse, and weight

Monitor hematocrit and electrolyte levels

Intravenous fluid and electrolyte replacement

Instruct patient about need for increased fluid intake during warm weather months

May need to decrease salt intake

Adequate hydration maintained

Continued

Table 13–1. NURSING CARE PLAN FOR A PATIENT WITH A COLOSTOMY *Continued*

Assessment	Interventions	Expected Outcomes
Nursing Diagnosis: Injury: potential for infection		
Myelosuppression may be present owing to disease process; potential fecal contamination at time of surgery; debilitated state may also influence state of myelosuppression	Review signs and symptoms of possible infection Monitor complete blood counts and platelet counts as indicated Avoid medications that may mask signs of infection (e.g., acetaminophen) Provide adequate nutrition, including fluids Monitor any temperature elevations Emphasize good hygiene Promote adequate rest and exercise periods Protect from sources of infection	No evidence of infection
Nursing Diagnosis: Fear—disease with poor control or cure history		
Fear and anxiety may be common problems because life may be threatened and normal coping mechanisms may fail	Review with patient and significant others his or her previous experience with cancer Assist patient and significant others in recog-	Patient and significant others verbalize fears and begin to deal with them effectively; coping mechanisms are iden-

tified and the level of anxiety is reduced

nizing and clarifying fears and to begin developing coping strategies for those fears; may be helpful to coach person by use of examples of coping skills used by others

Nursing Diagnosis: Potential impairment of skin integrity

No sphincter control of stoma, stool, and flatus flow from ostomy; peristomal skin is susceptible to breakdown from bacteria or enzymes in the effluent; consistency of effluent will be affected by the disease process, location of the ostomy, and medications

Measure stoma and order the correct size and make of an odor-proof drainable pouch

Use effective skin barriers, such as Stomahesive (Squibb), karaya gum, Reliaseal (Davol), and similar products

Opening on adhesive backing of pouch should be only ⅛ inch larger than the base of the stoma with adequate adhesiveness left to apply pouch

Provide proper equipment to empty and cleanse ostomy pouch when necessary

This care plan identifies some of the major nursing diagnoses that a patient with a colostomy might have *initially*.

involves 5-FU plus another agent, a nitrosourea or antitumor antibiotic.

HEPATOCELLULAR CARCINOMA

Hepatocellular carcinoma constitutes 2% of all cancers, and it is most common in persons 60 to 70 years old.

Epidemiology and Etiology

Approximately 80% of hepatocellular carcinomas have been attributed to hepatitis B virus. Other etiologic factors include intestinal parasites, hemochromatosis, and aflatoxin from moldy peanuts. Steroids may be a cause of primary liver cancer, particularly oral contraceptives and the androgens.

Biology and Natural History

There are two major types, those involving liver cells (hepatomas) and those involving bile duct cells (cholangiomas). The usual metastatic spread of liver tumors is to the regional lymph nodes, brain, and lungs.

No particular staging system is used for liver tumors. The prognosis for hepatocellular cancer is poor.

Presenting Signs and Symptoms

The presenting signs and symptoms depend on whether or not cirrhosis is present. When cirrhosis is present, the patient's condition deteriorates rapidly, liver failure develops, and death occurs.

For patients without cirrhosis, the initial symptoms may be vague complaints of pain, anorexia, weakness, bloating, and a feeling of abdominal fullness. As the disease progresses, 70% have pain and weight loss. Other signs include an enlarged liver, ascites, and portal hypertension. Jaundice, if present, is mild.

Differential Diagnosis

Liver function tests may indicate elevated levels of bilirubin, alkaline phosphatase, and α_1-fetoprotein. Needle biopsy, radioisotope scans, CT, and ultrasonography are other diagnostic tools.

Treatment

Cure can only be achieved with surgery. The recommended operation is total hepatic lobectomy.

Radiation therapy has not been effective against primary liver tumors, and chemotherapy alone has not had a good response rate. With radiation used in combination with chemotherapy, however, positive results have been obtained.

GALLBLADDER AND BILIARY SYSTEM
Definition and Incidence

The biliary duct system consists of the gallbladder, common bile duct, cystic duct, common hepatic duct, and right and left hepatic ducts. Cancers of the gallbladder and biliary duct system are rare, estimated to affect men slightly more frequently than women, most commonly between the ages of 60 and 70 years.

Epidemiology and Etiology

The cause is related primarily to cholelithiasis, liver fluke infestation and the presence of other parasites, and ulcerative colitis.

Biology and Natural History

The most common gallbladder cancer is adenocarcinoma, found in approximately 85% of all the patients. Other forms include anaplastic and squamous cell carcinomas and adenoacanthomas.

There is no anatomic staging for this cancer.

Prognosis

The prognosis for this cancer is poor.

Presenting Signs and Symptoms

The most common symptom of cancer of the gallbladder is pain and that of the biliary system is jaundice. Other symptoms of cancer of the gallbladder are anorexia, nausea and vomiting, and weight loss. Jaundice usually is indicative of advanced disease. Other symptoms of biliary system cancers may include pruritus and hepatomegaly. It is important to assess for jaundice, usually first noted in the sclera or gums.

Differential Diagnosis

Diagnostic tests include radiography of the gallbladder and liver chemistry tests. An elevated alkaline phosphatase level is indicative of liver involvement.

Common diagnostic tests done for the biliary system cancers include ERCP and liver chemistry tests. In addition to elevations in alkaline phosphatase, the bilirubin level is usually elevated as well.

The 5-year survival rate of people with cancer of the biliary system is approximately 33%. The 5-year survival rate for gallbladder cancers ranges between 2.6% and 6%.

Treatment
Surgery

Complete removal of the gallbladder is the only way to cure gallbladder cancers. This is also the case with the biliary ducts.

Radiation therapy

Radiation therapy has been found to have a good palliative role.

Chemotherapy

Adjuvant chemotherapy has been used infrequently.

SUMMARY

Of all the body systems, the gastrointestinal system continues to have the highest incidence of cancer. Nursing assessments of patients with gastrointestinal complaints could play a major role in decreasing the morbidity and mortality associated with this disease.

14 Gynecologic Cancers

**LUCY K. MARTIN
PATRICIA S. BRALY**

CARCINOMA OF THE UTERINE CERVIX
Incidence

Cancer of the cervix has dropped from second to sixth place in cancers afflicting women in the United States. The number of new cases expected to be diagnosed in 1988 was 12,900, with an expected 7000 deaths. This decrease is due primarily to the availability and use of the Papanicolaou-Traut smear as a screening device.

Etiology

A strong relationship between infection with the human papillomavirus (HPV) types 16 and 18 and cervical intra-epithelial neoplasia (CIN) has been demonstrated.

Biology and Natural History

Cervical cancer is divided into premalignant and invasive forms. Eighty-five to ninety percent of all cervical cancers arise from the squamous epithelium. The junction between the squamous epithelial lining of the ectocervix and the columnar epithelial lining of the endocervix is referred to as the transformation, squamocolumnar junction, or transitional zone. This zone undergoes a process of migration from being located laterally on the ectocervix during adolescence to finally lying high up in the endocervical canal in postmenopausal women. Squamous metaplasia is defined as the encroachment of the squamous epithelium on the area normally occupied by the columnar epithelium.

Squamous cell carcinoma of the cervix is manifested as four typical lesion types. An exophytic lesion, the most common type, is located on the external cervix. This type is friable, polyplike, fungating, and bleeds easily. This lesion arises in the endocervix or ectocervix. A cervix that is rock-hard to palpation usually is a sign of an infiltrating invasive type of lesion in which tumor infiltrates deeply into the cervical stroma. The third type is an ulcerating lesion

---

See the corresponding chapter in *Cancer Nursing: A Comprehensive Textbook*, by Baird, McCorkle, and Grant, pp. 502–535, for a more detailed discussion of this topic, including a comprehensive list of references.

that appears to have eroded a portion of the cervix. A fourth type spreads superficially along the surface of the cervix. Lesions associated with adenocarcinoma of the cervix arise from the mucus-secreting glands of the endocervix and may not become visible for some time. They continue to grow within the cervix, causing it to bulge and become characteristically barrel shaped. These lesions have a high incidence of nodal metastasis and high failure rate for cure, regardless of treatment.

Prognosis

Five-year survival results from treatment with surgery or radiation alone range from 60% to 90%. Poor prognostic factors that have been identified are increased primary tumor size, tumor extension outside of the cervix, and the presence of adenocarcinoma or other aggressive histologic cell types.

As a result of new findings implicating HPV in the etiology of cervical cancer, a new test has been developed that permits examination of the DNA structure of the specimen for the presence of HPV. This new test, called ViraPap, is still under investigation, but it may in the future be performed routinely along with the Papanicolaou smear.

The Papanicolaou Smear

Although the Papanicolaou smear is used only as a screening device, it is essential that it be performed correctly. Papanicolaou smears frequently are performed by nurse practitioners. The results obtained often form the basis for the decision to proceed in a diagnostic workup. For a Papanicolaou smear to be representative, cells must be obtained from the cervical transformation zone. For accuracy, a sample should be scraped with a spatula from the external portio of the cervix and a second sample obtained by swirling a moist cotton swab or brush within the cervical canal. Nursing implications include taking care that the specimen is promptly placed in saline or sprayed with a fixative and not allowed to air dry. Contamination with lubricating jelly may render the specimen useless. The woman should be instructed to avoid douching and intercourse and not to use any vaginal medications before the smear, which should be postponed if menstrual flow is heavy.

Cervical Intraepithelial Neoplasia
Diagnosis

Colposcopy. Colposcopy is the technique of choice for determining the source of abnormal cells seen on the Papanicolaou smear. After application of 3% acetic acid to the transformation zone of the cervix, the examiner visually inspects the entire zone through a colposcope (a low-power microscope). A moistened swab or endocervical speculum is often used to manipulate the exocervical os to increase visualization of the transformation zone in the endocervical canal. The increased ratio of nucleus to cytoplasm in abnormal cells causes the suspected areas to look whiter than the surrounding area, and a biopsy may then be performed. Whitened epithelium, mosaic structure, punctation, and atypical vessels are all examples of abnormal patterns that may be seen, for which a biopsy is indicated. Atypical vessels may indicate the presence of invasive cancer, whereas the other patterns are more typical of CIN.

An endocervical curettage (ECC) should be performed as part of every colposcopic evaluation unless the patient is pregnant. A curette is inserted into the endocervix without cervical dilation. The entire upper half of the endocervical canal is scraped first, followed by the lower half. Patients should be informed that the procedure is moderately painful but not lengthy. During colposcopy, punch biopsies of the external cervix are taken under direct visualization.

Postbiopsy instructions include avoidance of douching, intercourse, and tampons for 2 weeks.

Cone Biopsy. Cold knife conization or a cone biopsy is necessary if the ECC is positive, if invasive cancer has not been ruled out, or if there is a major discrepancy between the Papanicolaou smear and the biopsy results. If the patient wishes to preserve fertility, this technique may be employed as a treatment of CIN as well as a diagnostic technique. During the procedure, a cone of cervical tissue is excised. The apex of the cone contains part of the external os. It is sometimes performed through a colposcope, or the surgeon may be guided by the previous colposcopy diagram.

Conization usually requires general anesthesia, but most patients do not need to be admitted to the hospital unless there is heavy bleeding or other complications. For those patients requiring inpatient observation, routine postoperative monitoring of vital signs and vaginal bleeding from hemorrhage or perforation of the operative site should be carried out. Cervical stenosis, incompetence, and mechanical infertility are rare complications and are related to the amount of endocervix removed.

Management

After satisfactorily establishing the diagnosis of preinvasive disease, several outpatient treatments may be employed. The goal of treatment is to completely obliterate the transformation zone.

Cryosurgery. At present, cryosurgery appears to be the most innocuous and effective treatment option. It is relatively painless, is low cost, can be done on an outpatient basis, and has demonstrated efficacy in eradicating the disease. The gas refrigerant is usually carbon dioxide or nitrous oxide.

The correct size of probe (selected to encompass the entire

abnormality) is coated with lubricating jelly and applied to the cervix until an ice ball 4 to 5 mm in diameter is formed. The cervix is allowed to thaw for 2 to 3 minutes, and the probe is reapplied to form another 4 to 5 mm ice ball. The ice ball should take no more than 2 to 3 minutes to form. Patients should be instructed by the nurse that a watery discharge will be present for approximately 2 weeks, to use pads, and to refrain from intercourse and the use of tampons until the watery discharge has resolved.

Laser Surgery. The newest of the treatments, laser surgery, is another treatment option. Laser stands for *light amplification by stimulated emission of radiation*. The laser is mounted on a colposcope. The beam vaporizes tissue and must reach a depth of 5 to 7 mm to be effective. Physicians and nurses should take precautions to protect the eyes, use nonreflective surfaces, and eliminate inflammatory agents. Smoke and steam that may contain HPV are created with the tissue vaporization. Therefore, masks should be worn, and a suction tube must be attached to the speculum. Patients should be informed that some pain occurs during the procedure, that it will take longer than cryosurgery, and that there may be some bleeding afterward. Pads should be worn and intercourse avoided until spotting and any discharge subside.

Hysterectomy. The patient with CIN who desires no more children and permanent sterilization may choose hysterectomy after examining the other options.

Microinvasive Carcinoma of the Cervix

A microinvasive carcinoma occurs when the tumor penetration into the stroma from the basement membrane is less than 3 mm deep and there is no evidence of lymphatic or vascular involvement.

Management

Simple hysterectomy is the treatment of choice only for cases in which there is solely microinvasion, but as the volume increases and becomes confluent, the condition is treated the same as microcarcinoma or occult cancer (stage IB) because the risk of lymphatic and vascular involvement (and therefore lymph node metastasis) increases.

Carcinoma of the Cervix
Diagnosis and staging

No single symptom occurs that heralds cervical cancer. Contact bleeding, which results from mere touching such as occurs during coitus or a pelvic examination, is the symptom most frequently associated with cervical cancer. The blood is characteristically bright red. The bleeding can vary from a thin, watery, pink discharge to a continuous bloody discharge or frank hemorrhage. Late symptoms include development of pain referred to the leg or flank, which is most often secondary to invasion of the sciatic nerve or pelvic sidewall. Hematuria and renal failure relate to bladder involvement and ureteral obstruction. Rectal bleeding and obstruction attributable to invasion of the rectum are also symptoms of advanced disease. Unilateral or bilateral lower extremity lymphedema indicates lymphatic or venous blockage by tumor extending to the pelvic sidewall. A preterminal condition is often accompanied by uremia, massive hemorrhage, and profound cachexia with inanition.

After thorough history, physical, and pelvic examinations under anesthesia (EUA), bimanual and rectal included, biopsy specimens are obtained and further tests are done to clinically stage the patient's cancer. Radiologic studies include a chest radiograph, intravenous pyelogram (IVP), and barium enema. Rectosigmoidoscopy and cystoscopy often are performed at the time of the EUA. Nursing interventions include providing the patient with the information necessary to understand the workup process and to assist with the physical examination and ensure that the patient's privacy and comfort needs are met.

Management

In most cases, stages IIB and above are treated with radiation therapy. A long-standing controversy has existed as to the optimal treatment for stages I and IIA cervical cancer. Statistics reveal that there is no significant difference in survival rates among patients undergoing surgery alone, surgery plus adjuvant postoperative radiation therapy, and radiation therapy alone for stages I and IIA disease. Advantages of surgery are that ovarian function and vaginal elasticity are preserved and that mortality rate and the occurrence of postoperative ureterovaginal fistula are much less than 1%.

Surgery. Simple, total, or extrafascial hysterectomy (type I) ensures the removal of all cervical tissue but does not require dissection of adjacent structures. It is employed for carcinoma in situ, early stromal invasion, and microinvasive carcinoma of the cervix. The modified radical hysterectomy (type II) is preferred to the more extended versions because of decreased postoperative complications of bladder atony and obstipation. Less paracervical tissue is dissected, and only the upper one third of the vagina is removed. Vital nerve tracts are spared. A pelvic lymphadenectomy also is performed. More deeply invasive (> 5 mm) carcinomas and recurrent cervical cancer after previous irradiation are most often treated with this procedure as long as the cervix is not grossly expanded with tumor. The more commonly seen procedure is the Meigs or Wertheim radical hysterectomy (type III) and pelvic lymphadenectomy. This procedure involves wide excision of parametrial tissue along with the uterosacral ligaments and the upper half of the vagina. Bladder atony and obstipation are more frequent after this procedure.

Complications. Bladder dysfunction appears to be directly related to the extent of surgery. The patient may lose awareness of the need to void and often must perform the Credé maneuver (bending forward while seated) to completely empty the bladder. This appears to be related to damage to the nerve supplying the detrusor muscle to the bladder and, in most cases, resolves over time. Formation of lymphocysts or seromas may occur after lymphadenectomy when there is inadequate internal drainage of the retroperitoneal space. If the lymphocyst is large enough to obstruct the ureteral urine flow or becomes infected, a reoperation may be necessary to drain the sequestered fluid.

Postoperative radiation therapy is used in situations in which the findings at surgery included positive lymph nodes, unclear surgical margins, or a tumor that is large and deeply invasive into the cervix. A delay of no more than 4 to 6 weeks usually is recommended to allow wound healing to occur.

Radiation Therapy. In practice, radical surgery often has been reserved for younger, healthy stage I and stage IIA patients. Radiation therapy is employed for treatment of the rest of the population. The postoperative therapy is administered by either external beam or internal brachytherapy or a combination of both. Whole pelvis irradiation is administered optimally on a linear accelerator megavoltage machine, which will deliver rays to the deeper internal structures with little injury to the skin. Usually 40 or 50 Gy are delivered in a 4- to 6-week period in fractionated doses.

Brachytherapy. Internal radiation therapy, or brachytherapy, usually is accomplished by application of a sealed intracavitary radiation source. In internal radiotherapy, a very concentrated dose is administered in and around the tumor site, and the dosage falls off rapidly so that adjacent structures are not greatly affected.

Radioisotopes, such as cesium-137 or radium-226, are administered by means of a Fletcher-Suit system consisting of a tandem and colpostats (ovoids). An alternative method used for carcinoma of the cervical stump and more advanced or asymmetrical disease is application of an interstitial source, such as iridium-192 via needle implants attached to a vaginal template and obturator.

Usually two applications 2 weeks apart, each lasting 36 to 50 hours, are administered after completion of the course of external radiotherapy. The patient is considered radioactive during the time when the internal sources are in place. In an effort to minimize staff exposure to radiation, the sources are usually afterloaded when the applicators or implants have been properly placed into the patient during general anesthesia and the patient is back in her room. Remote afterloading machines have been developed that withdraw the radioactive sources from the patient and reinsert them when bedside care is completed. Bedside care should be limited to 30 minutes each shift or less if possible.

Complications of Radiation Therapy. Complications are seen both acutely during treatment and with delayed onset and usually are confined to the irradiated area when the patient is managed appropriately (Table 14–1).

Recurrent Carcinoma of the Cervix

Regardless of primary treatment, follow-up is essential for early diagnosis of recurrence. Examinations, including a Papanicolaou smear, should be done every 3 to 4 months. Recurrence most likely will appear within 2 years after completion of treatment. Metastasis is rare.

Management

The goal of most treatment for recurrence is palliation only. Radiation outside the original field may be given for relief of symptoms and comfort for the uncommon occurrence of bone metastasis. Chemotherapy has not proved to be effective for definitive treatment of recurrence. The tumor often recurs within a hard shell of previously irradiated tissue

Table 14–1. VAGINAL CARE DURING AND AFTER PELVIC IRRADIATION

For the first 2 weeks, have partner use condom to decrease irritation to the mucosa from sperm.

Discomfort with intercourse begins at approximately the third week.

Refrain from intercourse when discomfort and mucositis begin.

Begin using vaginal dilator 2 weeks after therapy is finished, daily for 10 minutes.

Use dilator every other day thereafter for the rest of patient's life.

Dilation may be omitted on the day patient has intercourse.

Vaginal dilation

    Make sure dilator is clean.

    Start with the small size dilator.

    Apply water-soluble lubricant or prescribed cream to the dilator.

    Insert dilator between the labia gently and firmly.

    Remove and reinsert three to four times over a period of 10 minutes. Clean well with soap and water.

    Dilation may be done at the same time as a bath, using water as the lubricant if patient is not using a cream that is prescribed.

Douching is not necessary.

and is not accessible via the bloodstream. Historically, squamous cell cancers have not proved to be vulnerable to chemotherapeutic agents, and the majority of all cervical cancers are of this type. Finally, many cytotoxic agents are also nephrotoxic and could not be excreted in a timely manner owing to the prevalence of ureteral obstruction in this patient population. When irradiation has been administered previously, many physicians opt to treat the patient with palliative comfort measures only, after consultation with the patient and family. The patient usually dies from the progression of irreversible uremia.

Pelvic Exenteration

Anterior, posterior, or total pelvic exenteration may be performed.

Nursing care after pelvic exenteration is complex and involves careful observation and coordination of caretakers (Tables 14–2 and 14–3).

Survival

Survival statistics vary according to patient selection criteria. Symptom-free patients with a favorable workup preoperatively survive longer than those who had symptoms or abnormalities on workup. Survival for this group can be more than 50% at 2 years after surgery.

Fistulas

The three most commonly occurring fistulas are of the rectovaginal, enterocutaneous, and vesicovaginal types. Rectovaginal or vesicovaginal fistulas may occur after ir-

Table 14–2. POSTOPERATIVE COMPLICATIONS ASSOCIATED WITH PELVIC EXENTERATION

Early

Pulmonary embolism, pulmonary edema, MI, CVA, hemorrhage

Later (Second Week)

Sepsis because of pelvic abscess or diffuse pelvic cellulitis

Later

SBO because of adherence to denuded surface of pelvic floor or previous irradiation; small bowel fistula related to SBO or irradiation

Long-term

Urinary obstruction of ileal conduit; pyelonephritis because of hydronephrosis

MI, myocardial infarction; CVA, cerebrovascular accident; SBO, small bowel obstruction.

Table 14–3. NURSING CARE PLAN FOR THE PATIENT UNDERGOING PELVIC EXENTERATION

Assessment	Interventions	Expected Outcomes
Nursing Diagnosis: Potential for impaired physical mobility related to presence of lymphedema arising from absence of lymph nodes		
Assess lower extremities (LE) for presence of edema	No intravenous (IV) lines or needlesticks to LEs Prohibit use of knee gatch, pillows under knees Elevate LE in stockinette sling on IV pole or on pillows Consult rehabilitation personnel for pneumatic intermittent compression stocking therapy; obtain order for measurement and construction of Jobst type pressure garment for permanent control; discharge instructions concerning protection of extremity	Patient's LE is free of edema Patient demonstrates no increase in edema
Nursing Diagnosis: Impaired physical mobility related to healing myocutaneous graft donor sites		
Assess LE for full range of motion (ROM)	ROM every shift, passive and active; consult rehabilitation personnel	Patient demonstrates full ROM in bilateral LE

Nursing Diagnosis: *Potential for sexual dysfunction related to neovaginal stricture*

Assess size of neovagina

Assess healing status of neovagina

Obtain compatible size set of vaginal dilators or use syringe covers in gradually increasing sizes; instruct patient in dilation regimen; discuss alternatives to coitus with patient: masturbation, mutual masturbation, oral-genital maneuvers, erotic films; stimulation of erogenous body areas (buttocks, breasts, neck, inner thighs), nudity, and snuggling are other nondemand pleasuring activities

Neovagina will maintain normal anatomic circumference

Nursing Diagnosis: *Potential for infection related to pelvic abscess, cellulitis, or wound dehiscence*

Assess for presence of fever (palpate abdomen for warmth or presence of exudate from suture line, drains, vagina, rectal area, and for pain and tenderness; examine dressings for color and odor)

Wound care as specified: wet to wet, wet to dry dressings every 4 hours; take vital signs every 4 hours

Patient vital signs within normal limits; abdominal area clean and dry radiation therapy in the presence of persistent or recurrent tumor. Refer to Table 14–4 for the nursing care plan for patients with fistulas related to gynecologic malignancies.

ADENOCARCINOMA OF THE UTERINE CORPUS
Incidence

Cancer of the endometrium is the most common of the gynecologic cancers.

Epidemiology and Etiology

Hormonal imbalance is the single most important causative factor. Aberrant pituitary function may be the common factor that links the predisposing conditions. Obesity, nulliparity, late onset of menopause, diabetes mellitus, and hypertension are frequently correlated with endometrial cancer. The presence of the hormone estrogen normally decreases with age. It is thought that the lower concentrations of estrogen may stimulate an increased production of postmenopausal estrogen precursors, primarily androstenedione, in a negative feedback fashion. This prehormone is also produced in increased amounts in the presence of obesity or hepatic disease and when the endometrium has continuous stimulation by unopposed estrogen, creating a state of hyperestrogenism, such as is seen in Stein-Leventhal syndrome.

Exogenous estrogens also may play a role in the development of endometrial cancer. Conjugated estrogens taken to prevent or control the symptoms of menopause, vaginal estrogen creams, or estrogen ingested as additives to meats have been correlated to the development of hyperplasia and cancer.

Biology and Natural History
Endometrial hyperplasia

Endometrial cancer is often discussed in conjunction with a condition known as endometrial hyperplasia, which is generally considered a precursor of endometrial carcinoma, and the relative risk is increased in the presence of the same risk factors discussed for endometrial carcinoma.

Adenocarcinoma of the endometrium

Three main cell types are seen in endometrial tumors. Columnar glandular epithelium is the normal cell type. Adenocarcinoma can be a well-differentiated noninvasive tumor. Twenty percent of adenocarcinomas are adenoacanthomas, a mixed form of adenocarcinoma with benign squamous metaplastic encroachment. The third type is adenosquamous carcinoma, in which both cell types represented are malignant. Adenosquamous and clear cell carcinoma, a rare subvariant type, carry the poorest prognoses. Unlike cervical cancer, cancer of the endometrium is more likely to metastasize.

Table 14–4. NURSING CARE PLAN FOR PATIENTS EXPERIENCING FISTULA(S) RELATED TO GYNECOLOGIC CANCERS

Assessment	Intervention	Expected Outcomes
Nursing Diagnosis: Impaired skin integrity, related to abnormal communication between colon, small intestine, bladder, ureter, or vagina and skin		
Determine output status (high or low)	*Low output:* Apply transparent dressing as prophylactic protection	Patient's skin remains dry
Evaluate characteristics of effluent, skin condition, number of fistulas, and location of orifices	Apply ointments with each dressing change (useful with suction catheter in fistula if unable to use pouch)	Patient reports increased comfort
	Apply skin sealant to perifistular skin to decrease excoriation when frequent tape removal occurs; apply under barriers with adhesives to prevent inadvertent denuding of epidermis	Macerated skin, if present, shows evidence of reepithelialization
	High ouput: Apply skin barriers in presence of caustic drainage	
Nursing Diagnosis: Alteration in bowel elimination, related to incontinence through the enterovaginal fistula		
Evaluate for fecal drainage from vagina	*Low output:* Frequent pad changes and perineal care	Patient reports control of fecal drainage
		Vaginal mucosa remains intact

Apply ointment or skin barrier to perineum

High output: Insert vaginal diaphragm-type device connected to overside drainage bag; remove and clean every shift

- Patient reports no odor
- Patient expresses increased comfort

Nursing Diagnosis: Fluid volume deficit: electrolyte imbalance, related to increased drainage through the fistula

Determine 24-hour volume loss

Observe for symptoms of dehydration and electrolyte balance

Evaluate electrolyte studies

Evaluate fluid intake and output

Observe for odor

Record daily weight and intake and output

Monitor ongoing electrolyte levels

Minimal output: Apply absorbent dressings, secure with stockinette, rolled gauze, or Montgomery straps every 1–4 hours

Apply charcoal-impregnated dressing over fistulas

Low or high output: Apply pouch over skin barrier

Empty pouch when ⅓ full or connect to overside drainage while in bed

Change pouch every 24 hours

Consult enterostomal therapist nurse for assistance with difficult anatomic fistulas

- Patient maintains normal electrolyte status
- Patient maintains normal fluid balance
- Patient expresses feelings of increased control over drainage
- Patient reports increased comfort
- Patient reports no odor
- Patient demonstrates increased mobility

Prognosis

Prognosis appears to be related to the presence or absence of certain factors before primary treatment and possibly the type of pathogenic disease the patient exhibits.

Diagnosis and Staging
Young patients

The profile of the young patient who develops endometrial cancer is one of obesity with a history of anovulation. Spotting and protracted heavy menstrual periods are an indication for further workup for cancer.

Older patients

The normal pattern for cessation of menstruation during menopause is periods that become scantier and farther apart over time. Other patterns of bleeding that occur after menopause are cause for concern. Any bleeding that occurs 12 months after menses have stopped is considered abnormal. Symptoms of advanced disease include generalized abdominal carcinomatosis caused by tumor studding of the entire peritoneal cavity, pain, intestinal obstruction, ascites, and possibly hemorrhage. Histologic confirmation is necessary for diagnosis. Endometrial biopsy or aspiration and endocervical curettage, although uncomfortable, can be performed on an outpatient basis and are associated with little morbidity.

Nursing responsibilities include an explanation of the procedure, including the fact that there is some discomfort. The patient should be advised to take a nonnarcotic analgesic, such as acetaminophen, ibuprofen, or aspirin (if not contraindicated) before the procedure. Pads may be required for the first 24 to 48 hours after the biopsy. With confirmation of endometrial carcinoma, a diagnostic workup and clinical staging should be done.

The grade of the tumor plays a major role in the pathologic aspect of the staging process. The cell type is always classified according to degree of differentiation: grade I, well-differentiated; grade II, moderately differentiated; grade III, poorly differentiated.

Treatment

Radiation usually is given postoperatively for patients with poor prognostic indicators, such as high-grade tumor, deep myometrial invasion, cervical involvement, and disease in the pelvic and paraaortic lymph nodes. For stage II disease, two forms of treatment appear to be effective—surgery (radical hysterectomy and pelvic lymphadenectomy followed by radiation for positive nodes) and external radiation with 40 to 50 Gy with one application of brachytherapy, followed by hysterectomy and bilateral salpingo-oophorectomy 6 weeks later. Occult stage II disease (i.e., stage II with endocervical disease found in the operative specimen) is also managed as stage I, grade 2 and grade 3 disease. In most cases, stages III and IV are treated with surgery, radiation, hormones, and chemotherapy.

Recurrence

Endometrial carcinoma often recurs locally either inside the vaginal vault or above the upper vagina. The recurrences that occur beyond the vagina are difficult to treat successfully with either surgery or radiation. Often, hormonal therapy or chemotherapy becomes the treatment of choice in this situation.

Hormonal therapy

Progestins produce a response in approximately one third of all patients with recurrent carcinoma of the endometrium. Tumors that are well differentiated respond better than do moderately or poorly differentiated lesions. Well-differentiated tumors contain more estrogen and progesterone receptors than those that are poorly differentiated. It is likely that estrogen and progesterone receptor analyses will be done on all biopsied uterine tissue, and depending on the results, progestin therapy will be initiated or the patient will be placed on cytotoxic agents. Progestin therapy is continued unless progression of disease is noted.

Chemotherapy

Overall, neither single agent nor combination chemotherapy has increased survival. With increased use of receptor analysis in the determination of individual patient therapy, response rates may increase.

OVARIAN CANCER
Incidence

Cancer of the ovary ranks fourth in fatalities among cancers of women in the United States. Of great concern is the lack of progress in identifying a cause for this deadly disease.

Epidemiology and Etiology

Most ovarian cancers occur in women between 50 and 59 years of age. Environmental factors play a role in that the highest frequency is found in highly industrialized countries, with the exception of Japan. Lifestyle behaviors, such as ingestion of a diet high in saturated fat, may also be implicated.

Nursing implications include taking as accurate a history as possible when interviewing patients, including exposure to environmental carcinogens or viruses and pertinent lifestyle patterns. Runowicz has described the profile of the high-risk patient as white, nulliparous, and infertile, having a positive family history of ovarian cancer, and living an upper socioeconomic lifestyle.

Biology and Natural History

Ovarian neoplasms arise from cells that were present during the four stages of early embryologic ovarian development. All forms of ovarian cancer spread insidiously along the peritoneum and the surfaces of abdominal organs, encompassing all of the structures of the upper abdomen. The tumor may be of varying consistencies, ranging from a rocky hardness to a rubbery or even a cystlike quality. This phenomenon is caused by a rapid growth of the tumor away from the main sources of blood supply.

Borderline Malignant Epithelial Neoplasms

Borderline malignant epithelial neoplasms account for 15% of all ovarian cancers, are composed of low-grade serous cystadenocarcinomas and mucinous tumors, and have characteristic histologic features.

Prognosis

Long-term survival for ovarian cancer is related to certain prognostic factors. Well-differentiated epithelial tumors of a low grade, small residual tumor volume after surgery (< 2 cm in any one focus), and additional adjuvant treatment after the initial surgery influence survival significantly. Overall survival is 31% after 5 years.

Diagnosis

Ovarian cancer is rarely diagnosed early. Seventy percent of all patients already have metastasis outside the pelvis at diagnosis. These neoplasms grow rapidly and without pain. However, it is a nursing responsibility to encourage any woman older than 40 years of age who complains of persistent low-grade or vague abdominal symptoms of mild indigestion, abdominal discomfort, or urinary abnormalities to seek further evaluation. Late symptoms may include hemorrhage from the necrotizing tumor, sepsis, and profound cachexia. Patients appear gaunt and alert. Often they are hungry but cannot eat without immediately experiencing nausea and vomiting. Gastrointestinal obstruction often occurs, and death usually ensues within 6 months of its onset.

Exploratory laparotomy is the only accurate method for diagnosing ovarian cancer. Even though early diagnosis is important, a careful diagnostic preoperative workup should be completed. Paracentesis is not performed to avoid inadvertent rupture of the tumor and resultant spillage.

Staging

Ovarian cancer is staged surgically.

Treatment
Surgery

Borderline Malignant Epithelial Neoplasms. In most cases, conservative therapy is chosen. If the lesion is unilateral, a unilateral salpingo-oophorectomy with or without contralateral biopsy is acceptable.

A comprehensive staging laparotomy should be done, which includes inspection and biopsy of multiple peritoneal sites, sampling of pelvic and paraaortic lymph nodes, biopsy of the omentum, and possibly endometrial curettage. Nursing management includes instructing the patient of the increased risk of recurrence. The incidence of occult metastasis ranges from 12% to 43% for epithelial neoplasms.

When bilateral involvement is present, more radical treatment is necessary. In such cases, total abdominal hysterectomy and bilateral salpingo-oophorectomy with careful inspection of the entire abdominal cavity are performed. Germ cell tumors, common in young women, are treated with unilateral salpingo-oophorectomy and vigorous chemotherapy, which allows preservation of the remaining gonad and permits possible childbearing at a later date.

Serous, Mucinous, Endometrial, and Clear Cell Types. These cell types are the most common epithelial cancers of the ovary and act similarly in both stage and grade.

The concept of cytoreductive surgery

The aim of cytoreductive surgery is to debulk the poorly vascularized larger portions of the tumor. It is hypothesized that the residual tumor volume responds aggressively by stimulating growth and cell kinetics. This may result in increasing the efficacy and cell kill of the postoperative chemotherapy. The goal of current therapy is to leave no single focus of cancer larger than 2 cm, or less if possible, anywhere in the abdomen.

Radiation therapy

In certain circumstances, radiotherapy is employed as an adjuvant treatment after laparotomy when there is minimal residual disease volume. Techniques used are external irradiation of the total abdomen and pelvis and instillation of intraperitoneal phosphorus-32 (^{32}P).

Intraperitoneal Instillation of ^{32}P. This technique has been used in stage II patients with microscopic residual disease and is advocated by some practitioners for use in stage III patients when second-look procedures reveal persistent microscopic intraabdominal lesions as well. A Tenckoff catheter is inserted, and proper placement and free flow are determined by instillation of fluid and a radiopaque substance.

Chemotherapy

Chemotherapy has proved to be effective as an adjunctive treatment after the initial primary surgery. Ideally, 80% to 90% of the tumor volume has been removed with the cytoreductive surgical effort.

The cell cycle-nonspecific alkylating agents have proved to work most effectively against sluggish tumors. In gynecologic oncology, the following alkylating agents have been used for early-stage disease.

Cyclophosphamide (Cytoxan)
Chlorambucil (Leukeran)
Melphalan (Alkeran)
Triethylenethiophosphoramide (thio-TEPA)

Other single-agent, cycle-specific, nonalkylating agents that have been variably effective for early-stage disease are

Doxorubicin (Adriamycin)
Hexamethylmelamine (HMM)
Methotrexate
Cis-diamminedichloroplatinum (cisplatin)
5-Fluorouracil (5-FU)

Cisplatin has emerged as the most beneficial drug when used as a single agent or in combination with other drugs. DiSaia and Creasman recommend aggressive removal of the tumor and combination multiagent chemotherapy as the optimal approach for improving patient survival in advanced ovarian cancer.

Recurrence

Second-Look Laparotomy. Gynecologic surgeons have employed the second-look operation to assess the control or extent of disease after a course of treatment in selected patients. Second-look operations allow the surgeon (1) to restage a cancer previously staged improperly or that had not been staged at all, (2) to evaluate effectiveness of standard and investigational chemotherapy regimens, and (3) to assess the possibilities of discontinuing further treatment in patients who have received an adequate course of chemotherapy and who appear disease-free clinically.

When recurrence is documented, previously untried second-line chemotherapy combinations are the treatment of choice. The goal is a partial response and control of symptoms, such as malignant effusions. Surgery is reserved occasionally for those patients who had localized disease at the second-look operation, but generally, it is not advised.

Investigational Approaches. Work is being conducted to develop antigens that will alter and intensify the patient's innate antigenic response to ovarian cancer cells. Exploration of the efficacy of diagnostic tumor markers, such as CA125, continues. These would permit earlier diagnosis and determination of recurrence, thus increasing survival.

Intraperitoneal chemotherapy

Administration of chemotherapy via direct instillation into the peritoneum is being investigated at a number of institutions. Pharmacologically, drugs suitable for intraperitoneal instillation must have certain properties. Patients with slight residual disease confined to the abdominal cavity who have had extirpative surgery are considered appropriate candidates. Fluid must be able to be distributed throughout the abdomen for optimal efficacy of this local therapy. Two types of catheter placements are used to achieve this result. A percutaneously inserted Tenckoff catheter, frequently used for home peritoneal dialysis patients, was the first catheter used and still is used in selected circumstances, such as obesity. Implanted ports, such as the Port-a-Cath, have gained favor because no external site care is required between treatments. In both types of catheters, a tip with multiple exit perforations is placed in the peritoneal cavity.

Drugs that have proved to be effective systemically for ovarian cancer have been used in intraperitoneal trials as well. Table 14–5 presents a care plan for the patient undergoing intraperitoneal chemotherapy.

Terminal Management

The goal of end-stage management of this group of patients is maintenance of quality of life. Table 14–6 lists frequent problems associated with very advanced ovarian carcinoma and appropriate medical interventions.

Malignant effusions

Patients with late-stage ovarian cancer often have ascites or pleural effusion or both. Meigs' syndrome is a common manifestation in which the patient has ascites, hydrothorax, and grossly enlarged tumor in the abdomen. It is supposed that lymphatics transversing the diaphragm drain into the pleura. This syndrome resolves after tumor removal.

Management should be limited to paracentesis or thoracentesis to relieve symptoms, such as respiratory compromise or pain. Patients often receive short-term relief of gastrointestinal problems and of nausea and vomiting as well. Nursing implications during these procedures include assisting the patient to attain a comfortable position, using comfort measures, such as pillows, and proper preparation of the aspirated specimen for laboratory or cytologic analysis (Table 14–7).

CANCER OF THE VAGINA
Incidence

Cancer of the vagina is the rarest type of gynecologic cancer. One percent of all genital cancers are of this type.

Table 14–5. NURSING CARE PLAN FOR THE PATIENT UNDERGOING INTRAPERITONEAL CHEMOTHERAPY

Assessment	Interventions	Expected Outcomes
Nursing Diagnosis: Health management deficit: related to intraperitoneal chemotherapy		
Assess current knowledge of patient regarding intraperitoneal chemotherapy	Describe anatomic placement of catheter; show patient a catheter	Patient and significant others will accurately verbalize expectations of this treatment
	Discuss postoperative care and radiologic studies, short- and long-term side effects of chemotherapy; discuss complications: fever, chills, nausea and vomiting, diarrhea, abdominal pain or expansion, shortness of breath	
Nursing Diagnosis: Alteration in fluid volume: excess fluid volume related to retained IP fluid		
Inspect dialysis tubing for kinks	Separate intake and output lines for IP instillations	Intake will not exceed output by >500 ml
Check for clamped tubing in outflow system	Total intake and output every 4 hours	
Check height of tubing	Flush catheter with 10 ml of normal saline solution to lift away fibrin sheath	
Consider if fibrin sheath has formed intraperitoneally	Straighten tubing if kinked and keep tubing lower than insertion site	

Nursing Diagnosis: *Alteration in comfort: pain, related to IP fluid infusion*

Assess all pain parameters

Infuse IP fluids at a slower rate

Reposition to attempt to distribute fluid evenly

Analgesics per orders as necessary

Patient verbalizes comfort; fewer requests for analgesics; able to sleep for longer periods at a time

Nursing Diagnosis: *Potential for infection: peritonitis, related to irritation of cytotoxic drugs*

Assess for abdominal rigidity, distention, rebound tenderness

Auscultate abdomen for decreased bowel sounds

Check IP fluid cultures

Check if febrile

Vital signs every 4 hours; antibiotics as ordered; culture of peritoneal fluids; aseptic technique

Patient shows no signs of infection

Table 14–6. PROBLEMS AND MEDICAL INTERVENTIONS IN ADVANCED OVARIAN CANCER

Problems	Medical Interventions
Fluid and electrolyte imbalance owing to paracentesis or thoracentesis	Replacement of fluids orally and intravenously via vascular access device
Malnutrition, hunger, nausea, vomiting from displacement of intestines by ascites or obstruction	Intravenous alimentation
Intermittent episodes of small and large bowel obstruction owing to carcinomatosis	Surgical bypass, gastrostomy, jejunostomy
Recurrent malignant effusions	Peritoneovenous shunt insertion; paracentesis, thoracentesis, chest tube placement; pleurodesis with tetracycline

Cancer of the vagina occurs most frequently in women older than 70 years of age. A rare type of vaginal cancer, clear cell adenocarcinoma, suddenly appeared in a cluster during the 1960s and continues to appear in diminishing numbers.

Epidemiology and Etiology
Primary cancer of the vagina

It has been hypothesized that irritation of the vagina, such as from trauma, chronic pessary usage for a prolapsed uterus, intercourse, or use of chemical carcinogens, as in sprays and douches, plays a role in the development of squamous cell carcinoma of the vagina, but a relationship has never been established. Current theory considers that cancer in this location may be an extension of a previous cancer of the cervix, vulva, or endometrium.

DES-related cancer of the vagina

Clear cell adenocarcinoma of the vagina is linked to the treatment of women with diethylstilbestrol (DES) during pregnancy, which was used in the 1940s and 1950s to prevent spontaneous abortions.

Biology and Natural History
Squamous cell carcinoma

Premalignant lesions may develop as primary lesions, after radiation therapy, or as a multifocal abnormality. Vaginal intraepithelial neoplasia may occur many years after

Table 14-7. NURSING CARE PLAN FOR THE PATIENT WITH ADVANCED OVARIAN CANCER

Assessment	Interventions	Expected Outcomes
Nursing Diagnosis: Alteration in nutrition, related to extrinsic pressure on gastrointestinal tract or obstruction of gastrointestinal tract by tumor		
Calorie count for 24 hours; assess for weight loss; assess previous food habits	*Intact gastrointestinal tract:* Small frequent meals of patient's choice	Patient's weight will remain stable
	Position from 30 to 90 degrees for maximal stomach expansion	Patient will express increased ability to eat; intestines will be decompressed
	Obstructed gastrointestinal tract	Patient able to ingest food via tube: nasogastric, gastrostomy, or jejunostomy
	Obtain interim order for nasogastric tube; discuss with attending physician the option of gastrostomy or jejunostomy placement; explore options with patient; analgesics as necessary	Decreased requests for narcotic analgesic
Nursing Diagnosis: Alteration in fluid volume: excess, related to malignant effusions of ascites or pleural fluid		
Palpate abdomen for fluid wave or percuss for dullness	Position patient at most comfortable angle between 30 and 90 degrees	Volume of ascites will diminish or stabilize
Auscultate bowel sounds	Prepare patient for paracentesis; assist with paracentesis	
Observe skin turgor	Dress and observe paracentesis site for leakage	
Assess vein filling		

206

Check for edema
Assess for weight gain
Measure abdominal girth

Apply urostomy pouch with drainage bag for continued leakage
Accurate intake and output determinations
Encourage intake of fluids

Nursing Diagnosis: Impaired gas exchange: related to extrinsic pressure of pleural fluid on lungs

Auscultate breath sounds; listen for a pleural friction rub; observe for respiratory distress

Prepare patient for thoracentesis
Assist with thoracentesis; dress thoracentesis site and observe for leakage
Recurrent effusion: Prepare patient for chest tube insertion
Set up chest drainage collection system
Assist with insertion
Dress insertion site with occlusive dressing
Monitor chest drainage output
Prepare patient for pleurodesis (instillation of tetracycline into the pleural space)
Premedicate patient with analgesic
Assist with pleurodesis; rotate patient every 5 minutes to distribute the sclerosing agent

Pleural effusion will diminish in volume or stabilize
Patient will demonstrate adequate respirations

treatment for cervical or vulvar cancer. The lesion most often occurs in the upper third of the vagina. When an invasive lesion is present, it may appear as a round or oblong ulcer with elevated smooth edges, with an excavated crater in the center. If located low in the vagina, the tumor metastasizes to the inguinal and deep pelvic nodes.

Clear cell adenocarcinoma

This type of cancer usually appears on the anterior wall of the upper part of the vagina. It is known to invade the nearby tissue early and metastasize through the lymphatics.

Diagnosis and Staging
Squamous cell carcinoma

The patient usually seeks medical treatment because of a bloody vaginal discharge, which is the most frequent initial symptom. If it is invasive, the lesion is usually visible on examination, and the patient has irregular or postmenopausal bleeding. Urinary frequency or retention is sometimes seen owing to the proximity of the lesion to the neck of the bladder. Diagnosis often is delayed, most probably because of the patient's age, infrequency of pelvic examinations in this age group, and lack of sexual activity.

Clear cell adenocarcinoma

Twenty percent of patients with clear cell adenocarcinoma of the vagina are asymptomatic, and the rest have abnormal bleeding. The cervix can have a hoodlike appearance, surrounded by a collar or with a pseudopolyp protruding from it. The uterus often is hypoplastic and may be the anatomic basis for the infertility problems often experienced by this patient population.

Prognosis
Squamous cell carcinoma

Survival is affected by several factors. The increased volume of tumor in the body, the fact that squamous cell cancers are not very radiosensitive, the high grade of this tumor type, and finally the fact that the vagina is relatively thin and is adjacent to both the rectum and bladder all contribute to the overall poor long-term survival of this group of patients. The 5-year survival rate is between 30% and 35%.

Clear cell adenocarcinoma

The stage at which the cancer is discovered, the prevalent histologic pattern, and the age of the patient are all important prognostic factors that influence survival. It has not been possible to determine long-term follow-up, but the overall 5-year survival rate approaches 80%.

Management
Squamous cell carcinoma

Therapy for carcinoma in situ of the vagina should be individualized according to age, degree of sexual activity, and patient preference. Radiation therapy is the preferred treatment for all stages of vaginal cancer. Radiotherapy is tolerated better in this population of older patients. Three methods of administering radiation are used: external beam to the pelvis, vaginal intracavitary radiation using a tandem and colpostats, or interstitial vaginal implant using an obturator and vaginal template.

Clear cell adenocarcinoma

In contrast to most cancers, follow-up has existed for less than 10 years in these patients. Clear guidelines for the best therapy are nonexistent. This disease tends to metastasize early, although the tumor is not a deeply invasive one.

Recurrence
Squamous cell carcinoma

Nearly 50% of these cancers recur locally within 2 years. Distant metastasis is rare. Chemotherapy is not effective. Resection of inguinal lymph nodes and a combination of internal and external radiotherapy appears to be promising and without the severe morbidity associated with ultraradical surgery in this primarily elderly population.

Clear cell adenocarcinoma

Distant metastasis is more common with this type of vaginal cancer, which tends to make it more difficult to control. Surgery and radiation sometimes have been effective, and efforts to find an effective chemotherapy regimen continue but so far have been without success. Neither single-agent nor combination chemotherapy seems to work. Patients have not responded objectively to treatment with progestational agents.

CANCER OF THE VULVA
Incidence

Vulvar cancer constitutes 3% to 5% of all gynecologic malignancies. The incidence in younger women is rising, and it is the fourth most common gynecologic cancer.

Epidemiology and Etiology

Women in their mid-60s and older are most affected with cancer of the vulva. Historically, obesity, diabetes, hypertension, and arteriosclerosis are correlated with vulvar cancer. Hygiene and age also have been linked with this cancer because it is more common in the poor and the elderly.

There is a strong association between the development of vulvar cancer and the presence of condylomata acuminata (genital warts) caused by HPV or herpes simplex II virus (HSV), but no evidence has appeared to confirm either HPV or HSV as a cause of vulvar cancer.

Biology and Natural History

Vulvar disease occurs in premalignant forms similar to cervical and vaginal disease, and there is a probability that a cancer originating in one area manifests itself at different locations in a skip-lesion fashion.

Invasive vulvar carcinoma

Seventy percent of the lesions of invasive vulvar carcinoma appear on the labia and 13% on the clitoris. A small, hard nodule, which usually arises from a previous area of VIN, begins to ulcerate. Another common presentation is a wartlike, cauliflower-type growth that does not break down. All cell types of invasive vulvar carcinoma spread in the same pattern via the lymphatics.

Diagnosis and Staging

Fifty percent of all patients have had symptoms for 2 to 16 months before seeking treatment or receive medical treatment only. Pruritus is the most common symptom for those with VIN. When it is located on the mucosa, VIN appears red, pink, or macular. If located on the skin, it is pale or whitened. In invasive vulvar cancer, long-standing pruritus, a mass, or lump often is present. The perineum and vulva must be inspected with a bright light. All suspicious-appearing areas, including pigmented regions, are biopsied using a punch technique to obtain 4- to 6-mm cones of tissue. Patients should be instructed to watch for any bleeding and to leave the dressings in place for 24 hours. Instructions should include avoidance of irritating laundry detergent, hygienic sprays, tight clothing, and synthetic underwear, which permit heat and moisture to be trapped in the perineal area. The patient's bathing practices should be reviewed, with education as necessary.

Staging is best done by a combination of surgical and histologic data rather than from a clinical basis, owing to the multiplicity of presentations of this disease.

Prognosis

Prognostic parameters identified for vulvar cancer are the size of the lesion and the grade of the tumor. Invasion of less than 5 mm without lymph or blood vessel involvement is a favorable prognostic factor. The 5-year survival rate approaches 90% for all patients, regardless of stage, when lymph node invasion is negative. The rate drops quite rapidly to 50% to 60% if any lymph nodes are positive at the time of surgery.

Treatment
Premalignant intraepithelial neoplasias and dystrophies

Removal of the involved area of the vulva will arrest the disease at this stage. Surgically, the procedure of choice for extensive or multifocal disease is a skinning vulvectomy and split-thickness skin graft with preservation of the clitoris. The skin graft is usually taken from the buttocks. Bed rest for 6 to 7 days usually is required. Nursing measures to promote adherence of the skin graft to the vulvar area include inspection of the area for suppuration under the graft and maintaining a clean, dry perineum. A transparent dressing may be in place, or application of a heat lamp to the donor site three times a day for 20 minutes may be ordered instead if the site is covered with Xeroform gauze. The donor site is painful when exposed to the air, and coverage with a transparent dressing or Xeroform gauze that remains in place will minimize the discomfort. Patients report the cosmetic result and ability to achieve orgasm to be satisfactory.

Early invasive vulvar carcinoma

The goal is to preserve as much sexual function and to provide the best possible cosmetic result while ensuring cure of the disease. When the primary lesion is less than 1 cm and the depth of invasion is less than 5 mm, the patient is prepared preoperatively for the normally accepted procedural approach of a classic radical vulvectomy and bilateral groin dissection, in the event that positive lymph nodes are encountered. The investigational procedure involves a bilateral exploration of the groin and removal of the *sentinel lymph nodes*—those that would be invaded first by the vulvar cancer. These nodes are examined immediately and analyzed as frozen section specimens. If these nodes are positive, the classic procedure is carried out. If the nodes are negative, the incisions are closed, wound drains are placed, and a wide local excision of the involved vulvar area is performed. Subcutaneous tissue is removed, and margins of 3 cm on all sides of the specimen are established. Either the defect is approximated and closed primarily, or a split-thickness skin graft, usually from the thigh, is sutured into the defect.

Invasive carcinoma of the vulva

The ultraradical procedure—radical vulvectomy and bilateral groin dissection—is the most effective treatment for the advanced stages of vulvar cancer.

Bilateral groin dissections and vulvectomy are made through separate incisions. The perivulvar skin with a 2- to 3-cm margin, labia majora, labia minora, and glans clitoris are all removed. Pelvic exenteration, bilateral groin dissection, and radical vulvectomy are performed in selected advanced cases when the disease is central and not adherent to the pelvic sidewall. The morbidity associated with this type of surgery, especially in the elderly population, is high, and the 5-year survival is only 16%. Boronow has encouraged the use of preoperative pelvic and groin irradiation. Six weeks after irradiation, the patient undergoes a radical vulvectomy with or without a groin dissection. The cure rate is similar, and the patient is spared the assault of a massive surgery.

Recurrence

Patients with pelvic recurrent disease are best treated with wide local excision of the lesion and irradiation to the groin. Within 2 years, 80% of recurrences will appear. More than half of the recurrences are near the site of the original lesion.

GESTATIONAL TROPHOBLASTIC NEOPLASMS
Incidence

Gestational trophoblastic neoplasia (GTN) is the term given to the spectrum of trophoblastic diseases (hydatidiform mole, invasive mole, and choriocarcinoma). It is considered the most curable of all gynecologic malignancies.

Epidemiology and Etiology

Older women have hydatidiform moles more frequently than do younger women.

Biology and Natural History
Hydatidiform mole

An abnormal proliferation occurs in the villi of the placenta within the uterus. The most notable features are hydropic (dropletlike) changes in the stromal layer and absence of blood vessels. The ovary may develop very large thecal luteal cysts. A complete mole will only contain these structures. In contrast, a partial mole will have swollen villi and a less hydropic appearance and may contain an umbilical cord, amniotic membranes, or even a fetus. Both types secrete excessive amounts of human chorionic gonadotropin (HCG).

Diagnosis and Staging
Hydatidiform mole

Cardinal symptoms of the hydatidiform mole are missed periods and vaginal bleeding that ranges from rusty brown spotting to bright red hemorrhage. Often a patient may pass tissue that is grapelike in appearance. Unusual, first-trimester preeclampsia is considered almost singularly diagnostic for hydatidiform mole. The uterus is usually larger than its expected size in half of the patients. Fifteen percent of the patients have large thecal luteal cysts.

Gestational trophoblastic neoplasia

Most patients have abnormal uterine bleeding. If the patient was pregnant recently and GTN appears, it is easier to confirm a diagnosis.

Prognosis

With the discovery of the benefits of chemotherapy in 1956, the mortality rates reversed from 90% to a remission rate of 80% to 90%.

Management
Hydatidiform mole

Evacuation of the uterus is the most effective method of treatment. Suction dilatation and curettage is usually performed, and moderate blood loss is not uncommon. Intravenous oxytocin (Pitocin) is begun partway through the procedure to initiate involution of the uterus. As involution occurs, an instrumental curettage is done, and the specimens are sent for pathologic examination. This procedure often is performed on an outpatient basis. Nursing considerations include very specific instruction to the patient regarding the danger of hemorrhage and the importance of returning for follow-up, avoidance of intercourse until drainage ceases, and contraception information for when intercourse resumes. Simple hysterectomy may be performed if the patient does not wish future pregnancies. Further treatment with chemotherapy is necessary when there is a rise in the HCG level, when the HCG level reaches a plateau and stabilizes, or when metastases are discovered. Regular follow-up is essential.

Gestational trophoblastic neoplasia

Nonmetastatic Trophoblastic Disease (NMTD). Treatment of nonmetastatic trophoblastic disease is 100% successful. Single-agent chemotherapy using high-dose methotrexate with citrovorum rescue is the most effective therapy. If preservation of fertility is not an issue for the patient, early hysterectomy hastens achievement of remission. Hysterectomy is performed as secondary therapy if remission is not achieved with chemotherapy alone.

Good Prognosis Metastatic Gestational Trophoblastic Neoplasia (GPMGTN). Therapy is 100% successful for this category of patients and consists of the same regimen as that for NMTD. Methotrexate, however, is not given in a high-dose regimen. If methotrexate therapy fails, dactinomycin is administered. Multiagent protocols are then attempted for resistant disease.

Poor Prognosis Metastatic Gestational Trophoblastic Neoplasia (PPMGTN). A less favorable but improving outcome occurs with this group of patients. Current therapy consists of methotrexate, dactinomycin, and chlorambucil chemotherapy and concurrent brain or liver irradiation if metastatic disease is documented in these sites. An overall remission rate of 92% has been achieved. All patients who failed to go into remission had a diagnosis of choriocarcinoma rather than invasive mole.

Recurrence

Recurrence develops most often in patients who had advanced initial disease. Remission can be achieved in 100% of patients in both the nonmetastatic and good prognosis categories. Nearly 90% of the patients in the poor prognosis category can achieve remission.

15 Hematopoietic and Immunologic Cancers

COLETTE CARSON
MARY E. CALLAGHAN

See the corresponding chapter in *Cancer Nursing: A Comprehensive Textbook*, by Baird, McCorkle, and Grant, pp. 536–566, for a more detailed discussion of this topic, including a comprehensive list of references.

The hematopoietic and immunologic malignancies are diseases in which there is a proliferation of malignant cells that derive originally from the bone marrow, thymus, and lymphatic tissue. In general, when the bone marrow and peripheral blood are major sites of involvement, the neoplasm is classified as a leukemia. Neoplasms that originate in the lymphatic tissue are collectively referred to as malignant lymphomas.

Hematologic malignances meet immunologic criteria that describe their development as a malignant process. Malignant proliferation of hematopoietic and lymphoid cells usually is marked by monoclonality, that is, cells arising as a single clone, whereas normal tissues are composed of a mixture of cells.

In both leukemia and non-Hodgkin's lymphomas, the proliferating cell often takes the characteristics of a normal cell in a specific phase of maturation. Instead of progressing to the next stage of development, the cell becomes fixed and continues to proliferate in its immature phase. The names of specific leukemia and lymphoma subtypes (e.g., acute myeloid leukemia, small cleaved cell lymphomas) often represent the description of the normal cellular counterpart in a particular maturational phase.

LEUKEMIAS

The common characteristic of all the leukemias is an unregulated proliferation in the bone marrow of a cell of hematopoietic origin. The malignant cell has a growth advantage over normal cells and replaces the normal elements in all areas of hematopoietic bone marrow.

The leukemias are described by the particular cell type of origin and are classified on the basis of their cellular differentiation. The acute leukemias describe disease in which differentiation is very minimal, with early forms of cells or blasts being the cell type. The chronic leukemias describe diseases in which the malignant cells have some degree of differentiation.

Acute Lymphoblastic Leukemia

Acute lymphoblastic leukemia (ALL) is a hematologic malignancy of uncontrolled proliferation and accumulation of immature lymphocytes and their progenitors. Although ALL is the most common childhood malignancy, it accounts for only 20% of adult leukemias.

Etiology

The exact etiology of ALL is unknown, but several factors have been implicated. These factors include radiation, chemicals and drugs, viruses, and genetic abnormalities.

Classification

Two classification systems have been developed that describe the types of ALL. The first is based on the morphologic description of the disease and is called the French-American-British classification system (FAB). The FAB classification recognizes three types of lymphoblasts: L_1, L_2, and L_3. Another classification has been developed that is being used with some success.

This approach to the classification of ALL is based on immune properties of the leukemia cells. The subtypes include the common T-, B-, or null-cell ALL.

Data from studies evaluating prognosis in the immunologic classification seem to indicate that adults with T-cell ALL have the best prognosis, those with common ALL have an intermediate prognosis, and those with null-cell ALL have a slightly inferior prognosis. Patients with B-cell ALL have the least favorable prognosis.

Other factors are reported to influence negatively the remission rates. These include male sex, initial presentation with central nervous system leukemia, high white blood count on presentation, older age, and presence of a mediastinal mass. These factors have been reported to influence a poorer prognosis but do not always confirm a poor prognosis.

Clinical features

The classic clinical features of fatigue, fever, bruising, and pallor are manifestations of failure of normal bone marrow. Most patients have these symptoms less than 3 months. Common laboratory findings include leukocytosis with immature blasts or cells, anemia, thrombocytopenia, and bone marrow packed with poorly differentiated lymphoid blast cells. The peripheral leukocyte count can range from 1000 to 400,000/mm³. Although more commonly seen in patients with chronic myelogenous leukemia (CML) blast crisis and acute myelogenous leukemia (AML), intravascular clumping of leukemia cells may occur in patients with blast counts in excess of 100,000/mm³.

Other clinical features associated with ALL are lymph node enlargement, hepatic or splenic enlargement, meningeal leukemia, bone or joint pain, and genitourinary manifestations, including hematuria, cystitis, pyelonephritis, priapism, renal failure, hyperuricemia, uric acid nephropathy, and testicular involvement. These symptoms are related to leukemic infiltration of extramedullary lymphatic tissue.

Infections are common in patients with the disease and as a cause of death. ALL causes marked impairment in the host defense system. There is a marked reduction in the number of phagocytic leukocytes and an impairment in ability to mobilize against infection. Patients with ALL show a decreased response to mutagen, have reduced delayed hypersensitivity reactions, and often have low levels of immunoglobulins at diagnosis. Diagnosis is based on morphologic and cytochemical analysis of bone marrow.

Treatment

The treatment of ALL generally is divided into two phases termed *induction therapy* and *postremission therapy*. The purpose of induction chemotherapy is to eradicate all detectable leukemic cells, induce a remission, and restore normal bone marrow function. Postremission therapy usually consists of central nervous system prophylaxis, consolidation-intensification chemotherapy, and maintenance chemotherapy. The goal of postremission therapy is to eradicate undetectable leukemic cells and thereby prevent a relapse.

At present, most induction regimens include vincristine, prednisone, daunorubicin, and L-asparaginase. Consolidation-intensification chemotherapy is considered useful, but specific drugs and duration of therapy have not been determined. As in maintenance therapy, which is important in the treatment of childhood ALL, the drugs and duration of therapy are yet to be determined in adult ALL.

In general, current chemotherapy regimens using an anthracycline, usually daunomycin, can achieve 70% to 80% remission rates. With optimal postremission therapy, 3- to 5-year actuarial leukemia-free survival has been achieved in 20% to 35% of unselected patients.

Central nervous system prophylaxis

In childhood ALL, the role of central nervous system prophylaxis in prolonging survival is well documented. In adult ALL, the usefulness of central nervous system prophylaxis in prolonging survival has been difficult to document. In general, most treatment regimens in adult ALL include intrathecal methotrexate with or without central nervous system irradiation.

Relapsed and resistant leukemia

Hoelzer and Gale have reviewed the experimental drugs used in patients who have relapsed and resistant ALL. The most active regimens appear to be moderate- to high-dose methotrexate with L-asparaginase or folinic acid rescue, the combination of teniposide and cytarabine, and high-dose cytarabine in combination with amsacrine or an anthracycline.

Bone marrow transplantation

Champlin and Gale have reviewed the data evaluating bone marrow transplantation (BMT) in adult ALL. In patients with advanced disease, the 2- to 4-year survival rate is 10% to 20%. Patients in first or second remission have a 2- to 4-year survival rate of 30% to 50%. These statistics are using allogeneic transplants and vary in different studies.

Autologous BMT in adult ALL has been performed. Disease-free survival of approximately 20% in 2 years is reported in individuals with ALL in second or third remission. The value of autologous transplantation in ALL remains an area for further critical investigation.

Nursing care

The mainstay in the treatment of ALL is effective elimination of leukemic cells in the bone marrow by chemotherapeutic agents. The resultant pancytopenia is a nursing challenge.

Acute Myelogenous Leukemia

Acute myelogenous leukemia (AML) or acute nonlymphocytic leukemia (ANLL) is a group of diseases in which an abnormal hematologic stem cell gives rise to a monoclonal population of myeloid cells whose ability to differentiate beyond early forms is impaired. These abnormal cells have a growth advantage, and therefore blasts and other early forms eventually replace the normal hematopoietic marrow cells.

Etiology

The exact etiology of AML is unknown, but several factors have been implicated. These factors include radiation, chemicals and drugs, viruses, and genetic abnormalities.

Classification

The FAB classification is a widely accepted classification system for AML. This system is based on the morphologic description of the malignant cell line involved.

Clinical features

The clinical presentation of patients with AML usually reflects the degree of replacement of normal bone marrow by leukemic cells. Zigelboim et al. estimated that 20% of patients experience symptoms of anemia, pallor, weakness, and fatigue.

Bleeding is another important manifestation of this disease. Twenty to fifty percent of patients with AML will have moderately severe thrombocytopenia at the time of diagnosis. Patients with acute promyelocytic leukemia (M_3) can have additional coagulation abnormalities. These abnormalities present unique challenges in the induction phase of a patient with acute promyelocytic leukemia.

Patients with AML commonly have infections. Bacterial infections are most common, but fungal, viral, and protozoal infections can occur.

Patients also have physical complaints that reflect the

infiltration of normal tissues with leukemic cells. Bone or joint pain can reflect infiltration of the bone marrow. Hepatomegaly, splenomegaly, and lymph node enlargement have been reported in 10% to 60% of patients. Renal abnormalities may occur as a result of direct infiltration, gout from increased uric acid, and gastrointestinal symptoms, including distention, satiety, and obstipation, as a result of organ infiltration.

The most common skin lesions are petechiae related to thrombocytopenia. Leukemic skin infiltrates are uncommon but can be found in patients with monocytic and myelomonocytic leukemia, relapsed or resistant leukemia, and high white blood cell counts. In addition to skin infiltrates, patients with monocytic leukemia can have hypertrophied gums, oral ulcers, palpable spleen, anorectal ulcerations, and central nervous system involvement.

Central nervous system involvement in AML is uncommon but is primarily seen in patients with monocytic (M_2) and myelomonocytic leukemia.

AML is diagnosed by bone marrow aspiration and evidence from biopsy specimens.

Prognostic variables have been investigated in an attempt to identify patients who will respond favorably to therapy. In general, older age, previous cancer, previous therapy, and chromosomal abnormalities are variables that are associated with an unfavorable prognosis. A favorable prognosis is associated with patients in the younger age group, with the presence of Auer rods, and with a shorter time between treatment and complete remission.

Treatment

The goal of induction therapy in AML is to achieve hematologic remission. Hematologic remission is defined as the reduction of leukemia cells to undetectable levels, restoration of bone marrow function, including normalization of hemoglobin, granulocytes, and platelets, resolution of hepatosplenomegaly, and return to a normal performance status.

Various drug regimens have been used in the treatment of AML. It is not unusual for patients to undergo two induction courses to obtain a remission. The drugs used at the second induction may be the same ones used during the first induction, or the regimen may be different. Once remission has been achieved, the goal becomes one of preventing relapse. If no further therapy is given, recurrence of leukemia occurs in a majority of patients. It is believed that recurrence is related to the presence of residual leukemic cells that are undetectable by current methods. The approach to preventing relapse is to administer chemotherapy to the patient in remission.

Various protocols have been employed in the chemotherapy of postremission AML. Gale and Foon reviewed these protocols, stating that most contained two to six additional cycles of cytosine arabinoside (ara-C) and 6-thioguanine with or without daunomycin. They found that occasionally other drugs were used alone or in combination. These drugs included 5-azacytidine, amsacrine, methotrexate, prednisone, vincristine, cyclophosphamide (Cytoxan), doxorubicin (Adriamycin), and carmustine. More recently, high-dose cytosine arabinoside (HDARAC) has been used in postremission therapy.

Another chemotherapy regimen being investigated is high-dose cytoxan (50 mg/kg) and VP-16 (3600 mg/m²) without bone marrow transplant for high-risk and relapse leukemias. This regimen has produced about 30% remission rates in patients who have relapsed after initial therapy. Studies are continuing to determine the role of this therapy for leukemia. Most centers do not use maintenance therapy in the treatment of AML.

Most patients relapse within 1 to 2 years. Remission can be achieved in 25% to 50% of patients with resistant or recurrent leukemia. Although remission in resistant or relapsed leukemia may occur, the duration of remission is short.

Before the advent of chemotherapy, the median survival for patients with AML was 3 months. With current drug regimens, remission occurs in 60% to 80% of patients. The median duration of remission has been reported to be 9 to 16 months, with some reports of 20% to 40% of patients in remission for 2 years or more. Despite these advances, AML remains a fatal disease for the majority of patients.

Bone marrow transplantation

BMT has been used in the treament of AML. Several centers using allogeneic transplants report continuous disease-free survival of 45% to 57% at 2 to 5 years after transplantation. These figures have led some investigators to recommend that allogeneic BMT be the treatment of choice for patients under the age of 50 who have a suitable donor. This issue remains controversial, however. Studies continue to ascertain the role of BMT in patients in first remission.

Autologous BMT is being investigated at various centers. Results are preliminary, and further studies need to be carried out (see Chapter 9).

Nursing care

Nursing care of patients with AML can be very challenging. Bone marrow hypoplasia and pancytopenia will occur. Nursing care is critical during the recovery period of bone marrow after chemotherapy.

The newer regimens using high-dose chemotherapy offer

newer challenges for oncology nurses. With total white blood cell counts below 500 and platelet counts below 20,000, life-threatening infection and bleeding are common problems. Knowledge of the administration and side effects of chemotherapy agents, as well as the administration of blood components is important for nursing intervention.

Chronic Lymphocytic Leukemia

Chronic lymphocytic leukemia (CLL) is a hematologic malignancy characterized by proliferation and accumulation of relatively mature looking but immunologically ineffective lymphocytes. It is the most common leukemia in Western countries, accounting for about 30% of all leukemia cases. It is extremely rare in the Orient.

CLL generally occurs in older individuals (median age is 60), although occasionally it can develop in young adults and even children. It occurs twice as often in males as in females.

Etiology

The exact etiology of CLL is unknown, but various factors seem to be important. CLL has been the most common type of leukemia associated with familial leukemia.

In CLL, the malignant transformation occurs most frequently in the B lymphocyte, with a small proportion occurring in T lymphocytes.

In general, patients' first symptoms of the disease are fatigue and reduced exercise tolerance, enlargement of superficial lymph nodes, or splenomegaly. In many patients, the signs and symptoms have occurred gradually so that a specific date of onset is unknown. In about a quarter of the patients, the diagnosis is discovered by accident, in a routine examination, during which enlarged lymph nodes, splenomegaly, or abnormal blood counts are found.

Classification

Two types of staging systems have been used to describe CLL. The Rai system categorizes paients into 5 stages on the basis of the lymphocyte count and the presence or absence of lymphadenopathy, splenomegaly, hepatomegaly, anemia, and thrombocytopenia.

The Binet system categorizes patients into 3 groups. The prognosis for patients with stage A disease equals that of the general population, for patients with stage B disease, median survival is approximately 7 years, and for patients with stage C disease, median survival is less than 2 years.

Natural history

During the early phase of CLL, no treatment is given. Patients are usually asymptomatic, but as time goes on, fatigue and reduced exercise tolerance may worsen. Lymph nodes gradually increase in size, with new lymph nodes becoming involved. The spleen enlarges, and hepatomegaly may develop. Lymph tissue may grow in unusual areas, such as the scalp, orbit, subconjunctiva, pharynx, pleura, lung parenchyma, walls of the gastrointestinal tract, liver, prostate, and gonads. Obstructive jaundice can occur from periportal infiltration, and, very rarely, congestive heart failure can occur as a result of myocardial infiltration.

As the CLL becomes more aggressive and advanced, patients may experience severe fatigue, recurrent or persistent infection with fevers, pallor, edema, or thrombophlebitis from nodal obstruction, and increasing back tenderness and pain.

The absolute lymphocytic count in CLL ranges from 10 to $150 \times 10^3/\mu l$, but counts up to $1000 \times 10^3/\mu l$ can occur in patients who are untreated. The abnormal lymphocytes in CLL are smaller than the lymphoblasts and myeloblasts of acute leukemia. Therefore, the incidence of thrombotic and embolic complications is small.

As the tumor burden of lymphoid tissue increases, the proportion of normal marrow precursors decreases until eventually only lymphocytes remain in the marrow. It is not unusual for the differential white blood cell count of these patients to contain 90% to 100% lymphocytes, with only a few of the other types of white blood cells in the peripheral blood. As replacement of the marrow with lymphocytes occurs, granulocytopenia, thrombocytopenia, and anemia occur and can be mild to severe. Most patients will die from the complications related to pancytopenia.

Treatment

The treatment of CLL varies, depending on the stage of disease. In general, when patients experience organomegaly or cytopenias, treatment is initiated. Several treatment modalities have been used in the treatment of CLL.

Chemotherapy. The chemotherapy used in the treatment of CLL is either a single-agent or a multiagent regimen. The initial treatment for patients who require intervention is usually chlorambucil or cyclophosphamide with or without prednisone.

Chlorambucil is the most common drug. A response rate of 60% is common using chlorambucil, with 10% to 20% complete remission reported.

Cyclophosphamide is reported to be as effective as chlorambucil. It often is administered to patients who are unresponsive to chlorambucil.

Corticosteroids are used to control the increase in leukocytic count and to treat the immune-mediated hemolytic anemia and thrombocytopenia.

In patients with advanced disease, combination chemotherapy with cyclophosphamide (Cytoxan), vincristine, and prednisone (CVP) has been used, as has cyclophosphamide, hydroxydaunorubicin (Adriamycin), vincristine (Oncovin), and prednisone (CHOP).

New drug therapies are being investigated in the treatment of CLL. Pentostatin (2'-deoxycoformycin) has shown activity in controlling lymphoid malignancies, including CLL. Initial studies using this drug identified considerable toxicities, although current studies testing pentostatin at low-dose levels indicate toxicities have been reduced.

Another drug that has shown antilymphocytic activity is 2-chlorodeoxyadenosine (2-CDA). In one study, 78% of patients had a reduction of circulating lymphocytes, with 55% of patients demonstrating objective clinical responses. Investigations with this drug continue.

Fludarabine is another drug under investigation. Complete responses have occurred in 13% of patients in a study. Further investigations are continuing to establish the schedule for dosing and the length of response to treatment.

In summary, patients who develop organomegaly or cytopenia are treated initially with single-agent chemotherapy. As the disease progresses, multiagent chemotherapy is used to control the disease.

Biologic Response Modifiers. The role of monoclonal antibodies is being investigated in the treatment of CLL. An approach using monoclonal antibodies is the development of anti-idiotype monoclonal antibodies. These antibodies are tailor-made specifically for an individual patient's tumor cells.

Interferon, another BRM, has been studied in patients with CLL. Although reported responses from the initial trials have been low in numbers, interferon's activity in combination with alkylating agents and as maintenance therapy continues to be investigated in patients with CLL.

Splenectomy. The benefits of splenectomy in patients with CLL have been debated over the years. Today, splenectomy is used in selected patients with hemolytic anemia, thrombocytopenia, pancytopenia, and painful splenomegaly.

Radiotherapy. The primary role of radiation therapy in CLL is one of palliation and symptom control. Radiation therapy generally is used to treat enlarged lymph nodes, painful bony lesions, or massive splenomegaly that is resistant to chemotherapy.

Leukapheresis. When the number of circulating white blood cells is great enough to produce vascular thrombosis or embolism in patients who are unresponsive to chemotherapy, removal of the lymphocytes by pheresis has been used.

Systemic Complications of CLL. Complications usually occur as the disease advances and becomes refractory to therapy.

Nursing care

Nursing care of patients with CLL begins with the initial diagnosis. Patient and family education about the disease and its treatment is an important area in which nurses can intervene. As the disease progresses, education related to the treatment and the side effects of treatment must be undertaken with patients and families.

Bone marrow replacement with ineffective lymphocytes results in neutropenia, thrombocytopenia, and anemia. Chapter XX provides nursing interventions for these problems.

Infiltration of bone and other organs with lymphocytes will cause the patient pain. Chapter XX discusses comfort measures nurses can provide.

Hemolytic anemia associated with CLL requires the nurse to have expertise in blood component therapy. Patient education and support are important because some patients may require weekly transfusions. Other complications associated with CLL—hyperviscosity syndrome, hyperuricemia, and hypercalcemia—although uncommon, are challenging to the nursing and medical team.

Patients with CLL can live long lives. As the disease progresses, quality of life issues become important.

Chronic Myelogenous Leukemia

Chronic myelogenous leukemia (CML) accounts for approximately 20% to 30% of the adult leukemias. It is a relatively rare disease in children. The peak incidence of CML has been in the fourth decade of life but has been found to be shifting to a later age. This leukemia occurs more frequently in men than in women.

Etiology

Exposure to radiation has been implicated in the development of CML. Approximately 1 person in 15 or 20 who develops the disease has had unusual exposure to any form of radiation or chemical. Any chemical capable of damaging hematopoietic stem cells is potentially leukogenic, although identification of causative agents can be difficult. The chemical that has clearly been identified as one that increases the incidence of myelogenous leukemia in humans is benzene associated with heavy occupational exposure.

In most cases, the etiology of CML is unknown.

Biologic manifestations

CML is a hematologic malignancy that results from the development of an abnormal hematopoietic stem cell that gives rise to offspring that have the Philadelphia chromosome. With the development of cytogenetic studies and the enzyme marker glucose-6-phosphate dehydrogenase (G-6-PD), it has been established that CML is a clonal disorder resulting from the malignant transformation of a pluripotent hematopoietic stem cell.

The chromosome abnormality, found in 90% to 95% of patients, is thought to be a key element in the steps of the malignant transformation.

The transformed malignant stem cell in CML shows a marked increase in proliferation of marrow granulocytic and occasionally megakaryocytic progenitor and precursor cells. The marrow cells with increased proliferation seem to have a growth advantage and to overproduce in the marrow itself, replacing normal myeloid cells and expanding into the peripheral blood. Thus, large numbers of immature and mature granulocytic cells accumulate in the blood. With further expansion into the peripheral blood, the malignant cells proliferate in the spleen, replacing the normal lymphoid elements of that organ, and accumulate in the sinusoids of the liver. This extramedullary proliferation results in enlargement of both the spleen and the liver.

Diagnosis

The diagnosis of CML is based on sustained granulocytosis, which is usually associated with splenomegaly, a low leukocyte alkaline phosphatase (LAP) score, and the presence of the Ph¹ chromosome. Chemical abnormalities associated with CML include hyperuricemia, low LAP score, increase in vitamin B_{12} levels, increase in lactate dehydrogenase, and increase in K^+.

Clinical phases

CML is characterized by three phases: chronic, accelerated, and acute. During the chronic phase, there is an overproduction of relatively normal granulocytes that respond to treatment. At diagnosis, patients will experience malaise, fatigue, lack of exercise tolerance, and weight loss. As the disease progresses, aching in the bones that contain red blood cell marrow, tenderness in the lower half of the sternum, and discomfort and fullness in the upper abdomen that indicate hepatosplenomegaly are present.

The symptoms usually subside with treatment, and patients may be asymptomatic during these periods from 1 to 4 years. After this period, the signs and symptoms gradually become worse and less responsive to treatment.

The accelerated phase is characterized by progressive symptoms and resistance to chemotherapy. Systemic symptoms (fever, night sweats, weight loss), increasing hepatosplenomegaly, lymphadenopathy, and extramedullary leukemia are common manifestations. The blood counts that were so responsive to therapy during the chronic phase now become unresponsive.

The acute phase is highlighted by a significant increase in the blast count and further progression of anemia, thrombocytopenia, or myelofibrosis. Extramedullary leukemia with tumors or diffuse infiltration involving skin, mucous membranes, lymph nodes, orbit, pleurisy, synovia, extradural tissues, peripheral nerves, and meninges occurs in approximately 40% of patients. Most patients will develop the acute or blast crisis phase, in which the disease now resembles acute leukemia. Approximately 5% to 10% of patients move from a chronic phase, in which the disease seems to be controlled, to a sudden acute or blast crisis phase.

During this phase, the manifestations of CML resemble those of acute leukemia. The cells no longer differentiate to mature granulocytes, and maturation arrest occurs at the blast or promyelocyte stage of maturation. The blast crisis generally occurs in one of two forms: myeloid and lymphoid. Approximately 70% of patients will develop a myeloblastic acute leukemia, and the remaining 30% will develop a lymphoblastic leukemia. To determine the appropriate treatment, it is important to determine whether the blast crisis is of lymphoid or myeloid origin.

Treatment

The purpose of treating CML is to control the white blood cell count and to relieve symptoms. The growth of malignant cells is controlled by chemotherapeutic agents, the two most common being busulfan and hydroxyurea. During the busulfan treatment, peripheral blood counts must be monitored to prevent life-threatening pancytopenia. After prolonged use of busulfan, pulmonary fibrosis, skin pigmentation, hypogonadism, or a muscle-wasting syndrome with features of Addison's disease may develop.

Hydroxyurea, which must be given daily, is another commonly used drug that effectively suppresses myelopoiesis.

The chemotherapy drugs control the growth of the malignant cells but do not eradicate the disease. Patients who achieve normal white blood cell counts continue to have Ph[1] chromosome-positive cells in their bone marrow. Chemotherapy relieves the symptoms of the disease, but no single agent has been shown to delay the development of a blast crisis or to prolong survival.

Splenectomy has been suggested as a potential treatment of CML. In general, splenectomy has not proved to be beneficial in prolonging the chronic phase or the patient's survival.

Combination chemotherapy has been attempted in patients with CML. It has resulted in significant toxicity and has provided no convincing evidence that the duration of the chronic phase is prolonged or that the probability of survival is improved.

Interferon is beginning to be evaluated for the treatment of CML. In initial studies, interferon has been effective in controlling granulocytosis and thrombocytosis in CML.

The prognosis for patients in the acute phase is poor. Once patients have entered the acute phase, survival without treatment may be limited to 2 to 6 months

Patients who experience the acute lymphocytic leukemia-type crisis are treated with ALL standard therapy: vincristine and prednisone. At least half of these patients will respond to this therapy with complete remission that can last from 2 to 18 months, using aggressive induction or cyclical reinduction therapy.

Patients who experience the acute myelogenous leukemia-type crisis do not respond to vincristine and prednisone, nor do they respond to the type of therapy used for acute myelogenous leukemia. Only 20% to 30% achieve a remission with this intensive chemotherapy, and their remissions are brief.

Bone marrow transplantation

In the past several years, BMT has been used to treat CML. Approximately 65% of patients in the chronic phase who received syngeneic transplants and 20% who were treated in blast crisis have achieved complete remission. Allogeneic transplantation has yielded a complete remission rate of 63% in the chronic phase and 12% in the acute phase. Younger patients tolerate this procedure better than do older patients. Most centers do not perform transplant operations on patients older than 50 years. Investigation into the role of BMT as a treatment measure in CML continues.

Nursing care

During the chronic phase, educating the patient and family about the disease and the initial chemotherapy is important. As the disease progresses and as patients develop more symptoms, nursing care will address alteration in protective mechanisms, nutritional status, and comfort and other areas, depending on the manifestations of disease progression.

Hairy Cell Leukemia

Hairy cell leukemia is described as a lymphoproliferative disease similar to CLL. It is seen usually in patients older than 30 years of age; the ratio of males to females is 5:1. It represents 2% of all leukemias.

Etiology

The etiology of hairy cell leukemia is unknown.

Clinical features

Hairy cell leukemia is considered primarily a B-lymphocyte disorder. The term *hairy* describes the projections on the abnormal lymphocyte that are characteristic of the disease.

Patients may be asymptomatic, but they usually have symptoms caused by splenomegaly, pancytopenia, or infection.

Splenectomy treatment

When patients become symptomatic, treatment for hairy cell leukemia is initiated. Splenectomy is usually the first treatment. The cytopenias related to the splenic sequestration are improved by splenectomy, although not completely in most cases. Splenectomy is usually beneficial to all patients, but approximately half will require further therapy at a later date.

Chemotherapy

Hairy cell leukemia progresses in two different forms. One, in which the bone marrow is replaced by hair cells, causes pancytopenia. In the other, the disease appears with an increasing white blood cell count and resembles a leukemia. Usually, chemotherapy is required for both forms of disease.

Interferon has shown high response rates in large numbers of patients. The length of response to the interferons is being investigated. Approximately 80% of patients treated with interferon-α achieve beneficial clinical responses, but there are few complete responders (<10%).

Radiation therapy

Radiation therapy provides symptomatic relief of bone pain. Radiation therapy to local areas of involvement can provide symptomatic relief of pain and radiographic changes of lytic bone lesions.

Nursing care

Some patients with hairy cell leukemia have a very indolent course, with little nursing intervention required. Others require nursing care similar to that performed for CLL, depending on symptoms.

LYMPHOMAS

The lymphomas consist of two major subtypes: Hodgkin's disease and non-Hodgkin's lymphomas. In 1932, Thomas Hodgkin first described a disease that was characterized by progressive enlargement of the lymph nodes. Many years later, Hodgkin's disease became distinct from other lymphomas when the giant Reed-Sternberg cell was recognized in some lymphomas and not in others. This differentiation resulted in the classification of Hodgkin's disease, which is characterized by the presence of Reed-Sternberg cells, and non-Hodgkin's lymphomas, which are characterized by an absence of Reed-Sternberg cells.

Hodgkin's Disease

The treatment for Hodgkin's disease and the survival rate have improved dramatically in the past two decades. Once a fatal disease, the current 5-year survival rate is estimated to be between 80% and 90%, and the 10-year survival rate is an estimated 60% to 70%.

Hodgkin's disease may develop at any age, from early childhood to advanced old age. A bimodal curve of age incidence is found, with a peak in the United States in the mid to late 20s and a second peak after the age of 50 years. The young adult group is composed equally of men and women, and the predominant disease is the nodular sclerosis subtype. Among older patients, men exceed women. Survival and disease-free survival decrease as age increases.

Etiology

The etiology of Hodgkin's disease is unknown. Several peculiar characteristics of Hodgkin's disease have implicated viral, possibly genetic, and environmental factors.

It appears that Hodgkin's disease arises as a single focal area, beginning in lymph nodes in more than 90% of patients. In the early stages, the disease remains confined to lymph nodes for a variable period, making diagnosis sometimes difficult until multiple nodes are involved. Disease usually spreads to adjacent lymph nodes. This orderly pattern of contiguous spread is most evident in nodular sclerosing Hodgkin's disease. There are exceptions.

The most important fact influencing both staging and treatment is that Hodgkin's disease is a unifocal disease that usually spreads in a contiguous manner.

Histopathologic classification

Hodgkin's disease differs histologically from other lymphomas. In Hodgkin's disease, the diagnostic cell—the Reed-Sternberg cell—rarely predominates on a biopsy section and sometimes is difficult to find.

According to the Rye classification, which was developed in the 1960s and is widely used, Hodgkin's disease is divided into four categories. The histopathologic identification reflects the host's resistance and subsequently the prognosis, which proceeds from favorable to less favorable. The four categories are lymphocyte predominance, nodular sclerosis, mixed cellularity, and lymphocyte depletion.

As prognostic indicators, the histologic subtypes are dependent on other important variables, which include volume and site of disease, extent of disease spread, and presence of systemic symptoms (known as staging), age, and sex.

Clinical presentation

One characteristic symptom of Hodgkin's disease generally is progressive, painless, rubbery lymph node enlargement, usually localized in the neck region in 60% to 80% of cases. Most patients are asymptomatic, but 40% of patients may have associated B symptoms (systemic symptoms) of fever, night sweats, and unexplained weight loss. Occasionally, a patient is diagnosed after a mediastinal mass is discovered on a routine chest radiograph or after a persistant cough provokes a visit to a physician. When disease originates in the retroperitoneal area, it may be accompanied by prolonged fever. Rarely, a patient may have complaints indicative of an extranodal lesion, for example, gastrointestinal bleeding or pain due to obstruction.

Diagnosis and staging

The initial evaluation of Hodgkin's disease requires an adequate surgical specimen for the histologic diagnosis. A detailed clinical history is required that establishes the presence or absence of systemic symptoms, including fever, night sweats, and weight loss. A complete physical examination includes an examination of all lymph node chains, including Waldeyer's ring, and a determination of abdominal involvement, such as that of the liver and spleen.

Extent of Disease. The extent or stage of disease strongly influences the choice of treatment and must be determined carefully in each patient. This process is referred to as staging. *Clinical staging* usually refers to all procedures except a staging laparotomy. *Pathologic staging* refers to findings indicated from a staging laparotomy.

After the initial staging workup is completed, the extent of the disease is staged by a widely used system called the Ann Arbor Staging Classification of Hodgkin's disease. The Ann Arbor system divides Hodgkin's disease into four stages based on the extent of disease involvement. Stages range from a single node or region of involvement (stage I) to a diffuse disseminated involvement (stage IV). In the first three stages, extranodal involvement is delineated using the subscript E, meaning direct extension rather than that of hematologic dissemination, as in stage IV. Additionally, all stages are given the letter A to indicate the absence of systemic symptoms or the letter B to indicate the presence of systemic symptoms. Patients with B symptoms have unexplained fever, night sweats, or weight loss of more than 10% of body weight in the preceding 6 months. The presence of B symptoms indicates a less favorable prognosis.

Laparotomy. A number of investigators are questioning the routine application of staging laparotomies in Hodgkin's disease. There is no question that the use of laparotomies in research treatment centers has provided important information on the origin and spread of Hodgkin's disease. The controversy rests on the issues of whether—and if so, when—to perform surgical staging laparotomies.

Staging laparotomies are usually restricted to patients in

whom radiotherapy alone will be used for treatment. Patients with a clinical stage of IIIB or IV Hodgkin's disease require chemotherapy and, therefore, would not be candidates for a staging laparotomy. Similarly, patients with a clinical stage of IB, IIB, or IIA with mediastinal involvement generally require chemotherapy and radiotherapy (combined modality) and would not be candidates for laparotomy. Therefore, candidates eligible for staging laparotomy given no medical contraindications are patients with clinical stages of IA, IIA without mediastinal involvement, and IIIA Hodgkin's disease. Because the clinical staging process is not always absolute, some claim advantages to doing staging laparotomies on all patients who are not clearly in stage IV. Nevertheless, the routine use of staging laparotomies should be considered only at institutions that conduct clinical trials in which the results of therapy can be related to sites and volume of disease.

Disadvantages of doing a staging laparotomy include the risk of significant morbidity (0.7%) and mortality (0.7%) that is associated with the surgical procedure.

Prognosis

Many factors influence the prognosis of Hodgkin's disease in an individual patient. Although current treament has resulted in a dramatic increase in survival, some patients still respond poorly. Many factors contribute to a favorable or a less favorable prognosis.

Treatment

The goal of management of Hodgkin's disease is cure. The success of the treatment for Hodgkin's disease has improved dramatically over the past 20 years. Several factors have contributed to this success. They include

- The orderly process by which the disease spreads and the ability to stage the disease clinically and pathologically.
- Modern megavoltage techniques in radiation therapy, which allow beam direction to specific sites but shield normal tissue to prevent unnecessary damage. Consequently, tumoricidal doses of radiation can be administered, thus eradicating disease.
- Combination chemotherapy, e.g., mechlorethamine (Mustargen), vincristine (Oncovin), procarbazine, and prednisone (MOPP), doxorubicin (Adriamycin), bleomycin, vinblastine, and dacarbazine (ABVD), which is curative in many patients with disseminated disease.

The basic goal of radiation therapy is the eradication of all tumor in a specific tissue volume or in all sites of disease. Hodgkin's disease is very radiosensitive, and it has been documented that eradication of tumor is proportional to the dose of radiation administered.

Patients with stage IA or IIA disease can obtain a complete response following either involved field or subtotal nodal irradiation.

Patients with stage IB or IIB disease have a higher rate of relapse after radiation therapy than patients with stage IA or IIA disease. Therefore, treatment of early-stage disease with B symptoms is often combination chemotherapy.

Patients with stage IIIA disease present a more controversial therapeutic group. There are several approaches to treatment for these patients. Some institutions recommend radiation therapy, followed by salvage treatment with chemotherapy on relapse. Total nodal irradiation as a primary treatment has been associated with a 5-year relapse-free survival.

In patients with advanced disease, defined as stage IIIA with five or more nodules in the spleen, stage IIIB, or stage IVA or IVB, combination chemotherapy is clearly the treatment of choice. Various regimens have been evaluated over the years, with cures using chemotherapy alone ranging from 25% to 60% in advanced disease. The first successful combination of drugs—the well-known and widely used MOPP regimen—was developed by DeVita and colleagues in 1964 at the National Cancer Institute (NCI).

Over the years, several other chemotherapy or combined modality programs have been compared with the success of MOPP. The approach is to use a different noncross-resistant regimen. These combinations support the Goldie-Goldman hypothesis that the earlier the tumor is exposed to all potential therapeutic methods, the better is the chance of avoiding refractoriness to treatment, which is the greatest obstacle to cure.

The best and most studied is the ABVD combination of drugs doxorubicin, bleomycin, vinblastine, and dacarbazine, developed by Bonadonna and colleagues in Milan. ABVD has the advantage of efficacy without showing evidence of the sterility and secondary malignancies found in patients receiving MOPP.

The success of chemotherapy, like that of radiation therapy, is dependent on the dosage and timing of the drug. Reduction of the dose or dose rate by as little as 20% in animal models can totally abolish the curative effect of combination chemotherapy. Because of some of the severe side effects from the most successful regimens (MOPP, ABVD), patients may request dose and schedule changes to avoid disruption in their lifestyles. It is extremely important for the oncology nurse to explain to the patient that such alterations will decrease the effectiveness of treatment and ultimately may lead to the loss of life.

Side effects

The most commonly used chemotherapy regimens, MOPP and ABVD, cause nausea and vomiting. Anticipatory nausea and vomiting are not unusual and should be prevented. Early recognition and avoidance of anticipatory nausea and vomiting are the most effective nursing interventions. Regular nausea and vomiting require skilled nursing prevention and intervention and are discussed in Chapter X. Other side effects, such as hair loss, are related to administration of individual drugs and are discussed in Chapter 22.

Fatigue and lack of energy during treatment and at 1 year after treatment had been reported in several studies of patients with Hodgkin's disease. Patients receiving radiation to the chest experience sore throats, difficulty swallowing, nausea, and vomiting. The nutritional status of the patient may be compromised owing to difficulties in eating and lack of appetite. Radiation to the abdominal and pelvic areas can cause the patient discomfort from diarrhea, which then leads to fluid and electrolyte loss. Good skin care is essential because a common side effect in radiation therapy is skin desquamation. Measures for nursing intervention are addressed in Chapter 20.

Complications of treatment

Hypothyroidism. Late complications of high-dose irradiation include chronic hypothyroidism. Hypothyroidism is most common in patients receiving radiation to the cervical nodes and can be expected to occur in 60% to 70% of patients. A thyroid-stimulating hormone (TSH) level should be followed periodically after treatment to evaluate for thyroid hormone replacement.

Sterility. MOPP chemotherapy is known to cause sterility. Several studies have indicated that fertility may still be possible for some young patients treated for Hodgkin's disease (teens to early 20s). Little suppression of fertility occurs in young women; suppression is greater in men receiving MOPP.

Women receiving MOPP chemotherapy have associated ovarian failure after six cycles of MOPP. Alternating MOPP and ABVD reduces the number of MOPP cycles and, therefore, the risk of sterility.

Second Malignancy. Among chemotherapy drugs commonly used for Hodgkin's disease, nitrogen mustard, chlorambucil, procarbazine, and lomustine (CCNU) are the ones most associated with therapy-related leukemias. In addition, patients treated with chemotherapy and radiation therapy (combined modality) are at greater risk for late-onset acute leukemia and non-Hodgkin's lymphoma.

Non-Hodgkin's Lymphomas

Non-Hodgkin's lymphomas are a heterogeneous group of malignant neoplasms that originate in the lymphoid compartment of the immune system. It has long been recognized that they possess a wide and often bewildering spectrum of clinical and biologic behavior from indolent to very aggressive.

Non-Hodgkin's lymphomas can be defined as malignancies of the lymphatic tissue, with the exception of Hodgkin's disease, acute and chronic lymphoid leukemias, multiple myeloma, Waldenström's macroglobulinemia, and hairy cell leukemia.

In the United States, non-Hodgkin's lymphomas occur three times as often as Hodgkin's disease. The American Cancer Society estimates that approximately 32,000 new cases and 17,300 deaths will occur in 1989. The incidence of lymphoma is increasing yearly, especially in patients with autoimmune deficiencies (e.g., AIDS). The peak age incidence is higher than that for Hodgkin's disease, with about 25% of cases occurring between the ages of 50 and 59 years and the greatest risk occurring between the ages of 60 and 69 years, with males predominating.

Etiology

The cause of non-Hodgkin's lymphoma remains unknown, although several theories have been postulated. A number of lymphomas have been associated with chromosome translocations and rearrangement of proto-oncogenes (e.g., bcl-2, c-myc). In addition, certain viruses and the competence of the immune system play a role in some lymphomas.

Current data suggest an etiologic role for HTLV-1 in some adult T-cell lymphomas. Burkitt's lymphoma, which is confined almost exclusively to Africa, is associated with the presence of the Epstein-Barr virus, a lymphotropic herpesvirus. The precise role of this virus is unknown.

Compared with the general population, individuals with congenital and acquired immunodeficiencies (e.g., AIDS) and those receiving immunosuppressive treatment are at increased risk for developing non-Hodgkin's lymphoma.

As mentioned, chromosomal abnormalities also have been linked with both immunodeficiency and lymphoma. Genetic abnormalities of chromosome 14 are recognized in many follicular lymphomas and in Burkitt's lymphoma.

Pathophysiology

Lymphomas, for the most part, are the malignant counterpart of the maturing lymphocyte. Therefore, different lymphomas are related to different maturational phases of the lymphocyte. In non-Hodgkin's lymphoma, an abnormal proliferation of neoplastic cells occurs that resembles a phase or site of maturation. Instead of progressing to the next phase, the cells remain fixed at one phase of development and continue to proliferate. These neoplastic cells also may take on functional characteristics and activities of their normal counterparts.

Lymphocytes consist of two functional classes of cells in the immune system: the T lymphocyte, which is involved in regulation of antibody synthesis and cellular immune processes, and the B lymphocyte, which contributes to the humoral immune response that requires antigen sensitization for maturation to occur. A third class of lymphocytes, the natural killer (NK) cells, occurs early in the T-cell lineage and does not require prior sensitization by antigen.

The majority of lymphomas, approximately 70%, are B-cell lymphomas. Lymphoid malignancies of T-cell origin are less common, consisting of approximately 20% to 30% of lymphomas.

Cellular Origin. The cells of the immune system have different locations in the peripheral lymph nodes. Because lymphoma cells often retain certain characteristics of their cell of origin, it is often possible to relate tumors to their function and anatomic properties. Normal lymph nodes include B cells, T cells, and histiocytes. Approximately 10% of lymphomas are of unknown origin, and less than 1% are from true histiocytes.

Classification of non-Hodgkin's lymphomas

The many different categorization systems for non-Hodgkin's lymphomas have led to controversy and confusion and have made interpretation of treatment difficult for many practitioners. The Working Formulation of non-Hodgkin's Lymphoma for Clinical Usage was developed from a National Cancer Institute international cooperative study. In the working formulation, tumors are divided into low-, intermediate-, and high-grade lymphomas, depending on the activity of the specific lymphoma. Lymphomas listed under each category are defined by histologic, anatomic, and immunomorphic characteristics.

Most clinical protocols divide lymphomas into two broad categories: (1) indolent, or low grade, and (2) aggressive, or intermediate and high grade. Patients with low-grade non-Hodgkin's lymphoma usually have a relatively long survival with or without aggressive treatment. Tumors can be controlled with chemotherapy, but they are rarely cured. High-grade tumors may result in death for the patient within 1 or 2 years, but paradoxically, with aggressive treatment, certain subsets of patients can be cured.

Clinical presentation

The clinical presentation of patients with non-Hodgkin's lymphoma is similar to that of Hodgkin's disease and various other disorders involving the lymph system. Because palpable nodes often are found on normal individuals, differential diagnosis is dependent on size, shape, feel, and location of lymph nodes.

The most frequent clinical presentation in Hodgkin's disease and non-Hodgkin's lymphoma is painless superficial lymphadenopathy. A history of waxing and waning lymph-adenopathy over a period of months is not unusual. Except for an awareness of lymph node enlargement, patients with lymphadenopathy are generally asymptomatic.

Systemic symptoms (fever, weight loss, night sweats) may be present but are seen more frequently in Hodgkin's disease and do not have as strong an association with poor prognosis as they do in Hodgkin's disease. Non-Hodgkin's lymphoma is commonly more extensive, most often stage III or stage IV disease at diagnosis. Non-Hodgkin's lymphoma frequently involves lymphoid sites, such as epitroch-lear nodes and Waldeyer's tonsillar ring. Localized disease is uncommon. Extranodal disease, bone marrow infiltration, and bulky disease are often characteristic features. Truly localized disease is rare, appearing in approximately 10% of patients with non-Hodgkin's lymphoma.

Manifestations of specific lymphomas

Low-Grade Lymphoma. Lymphomas that exhibit a nod-ular type of histologic pattern display a more indolent be-havior pattern than those possessing a diffuse histologic pattern and, therefore, a more aggressive nature. Low-grade lymphomas, according to the working formulation, consist of small lymphocytic lymphomas and follicular lymphomas, both small cleaved cell and mixed small cleaved cell. Nearly all low-grade lymphomas are neoplasms of mature B-cell origin. The terms *good risk, indolent, favorable,* and *low-grade* as categorizing lymphomas often are used synony-mously, although even in these subgroups there is a degree of clinical heterogeneity. These lymphomas are character-ized by considerably longer survival, but various treatment approaches have failed to yield permanent cures.

Most often, patients with low-grade lymphomas have widespread disease. Because of the indolent nature of the disease, patients remain asymptomatic, and, therefore, the disease remains unnoticed. By the time the patient is di-agnosed, the low-grade lymphomas show wide dissemina-tion of disease to lymph nodes, bone marrow, and occa-sionally the liver. Mediastinal lymph node involvement is less common than in Hodgkin's disease, but abdominal lymphadenopathy may be evident and is far more common in non-Hodgkin's lymphoma than in Hodgkin's disease.

Spontaneous regression of disease has been observed in various subtypes of lymphoma.

Histologic conversion over time from a low grade to a higher, more aggressive grade also is evident in low-grade lymphomas. Progression is from nodular to diffuse and from small to large cell. The most common progression is from nodular, poorly differentiated lymphoma or follicular small cleaved cell lymphomas (working formulation) to more ag-gressive lymphoma.

Although the picture regarding low-grade lymphomas initially appears optimistic, the disease usually is fatal. Clinical morbidity and life-threatening problems are related to increasing tumor bulk. Eventually, symptoms include fever, night sweats, weight loss, and infection. Bone marrow involvement and renal and hepatic dysfunction are manifested in widespread disease.

Aggressive Non-Hodgkin's Lymphomas. Patients with aggressive lymphomas exhibit a large-cell or mixed histologic pattern. Before the improvement of combination chemotherapy, complete remissions for patients with intermediate and high-grade lymphomas were rare, with median survival for those with diffuse histologic findings being rarely more than a year. These findings were attributed to the fact that most patients presented with advanced-stage disease and a rapidly growing tumor. Typically, aggressive lymphomas exhibit high-fraction tumor growth with rapid doubling times. Paradoxically, these aggressive lymphomas respond better to chemotherapy and, therefore, have a greater potential for cure than do most low-grade, indolent lymphomas. Salvage therapy after relapse results in few and short-term remissions, although many combinations of drugs, radiation therapy, and BRMs have allowed a greater potential for cure.

Diagnosis and staging

Once a histopathologic diagnosis is established by lymph node biopsy, further clinical evaluation is needed to determine the sites and extent of disease involvement. This process, referred to as *staging*, is necessary to plan effective treatment methods and to establish parameters to follow the patient's response to therapy. It is also helpful in predicting the clinical course and prognosis of the specific lymphoma.

For the majority of patients, accurate assessment of extent of disease and subsequent treatment can be made based on the results of the previously mentioned tests. A staging laparotomy is not used in non-Hodgkin's lymphoma because, in contrast to Hodgkin's disease, the majority of non-Hodgkin's lymphoma patients have disease below the diaphragm and do not require further staging workup. Therefore, laparotomy, if used, is reserved for the few patients with clinical stage I_E and II_E disease in whom evidence of abdominal involvement would change the course of treatment from radiation therapy to combination chemotherapy.

The Ann Arbor staging classification for Hodgkin's disease is used also for staging non-Hodgkin's lymphoma but has some deficiencies when applied in non-Hodgkin's lymphomas. This staging system does not account for such facts as histologic findings, bulk of disease, and site of disease, such as extranodal involvement, all of which are important prognostic indicators in non-Hodgkin's lymphoma.

Treatment

The treatment of malignant non-Hodgkin's lymphoma is a rapidly evolving area with the continuous introduction of new drugs, drug regimens, and other therapeutic methods, such as autologous BMT, monoclonal antibodies, and BRMs. Radiation alone is a limited option that is used for early-stage disease. Chemotherapy or combined modality therapy represents the most common treatment because most patients have late-stage disease. Chemotherapy regimens have evolved over the past several years, with different combinations of noncross-resistant drugs being used for optimum benefit. Because the goal is cure, especially with the aggressive lymphomas, regimens are often vigorous and cause side effects.

Indolent Lymphomas—Low Grade. Various treatment approaches have failed to demonstrate durable remissions in low-grade lymphomas, although these lymphomas are characterized by a relatively long survival. Indolent lymphomas have demonstrated a high sensitivity to a wide range of chemotherapeutic agents (with complete remissions ranging from 60% to 70%), but the duration of remissions is short (between 17 and 24 months). Unfortunately, at 4 years, 80% of patients initially treated have relapsed. At 5 years, the survival rate is greater than 70% but at 10 years it is less than 30%.

Treatment of patients with low-grade lymphomas is controversial. Although early treatment has demonstrated longer remissions, long-term survival appears to be equal. At present, there are no convincing data to suggest that early, more aggressive treatments have any survival benefit, although clinical trials are ongoing.

Aggressive Lymphomas. The aggressive lymphomas are all considered to be intermediate or high-grade lymphomas as defined by the working formulation, except for lymphoblastic lymphoma and Burkitt's lymphoma. The probability of remaining free of disease after 10 years is better for patients with diffuse aggressive lymphomas than for those with indolent lymphomas. In the last decade, a major change in the prognosis of aggressive lymphomas has evolved with the advancement of chemotherapeutic regimens. The best-known regimens include COP-BLAM-III, MACOP-B, and Pro-MACE-CytaBOM. Some regimens add midcycle chemotherapy. Chemotherapy is interspersed between the main cycle because disease regresses quickly, but often it regrows before the next cycle of chemotherapy begins. These regimens have produced complete remission in approximately 80% of patients with aggressive large-cell lymphomas. These results are especially significant because the response rate includes patients with previously described poor prognostic factors, such as bulky abdominal disease. It is important to treat the patient with as full a dose as possible because the most important factor affecting outcome is dose intensity.

Patient selection for these regimens is important for disease characteristics and patient tolerance. Age appears to be a limiting factor, with drug toxicity being more formidable in patients older than 50 years of age.

Side effects

Studies have suggested a strong relationship between the side effects of disease and treatment and the patient's psychologic morbidity.

The intensity of treatment regimens for aggressive lymphomas results in potential side effects and toxicities. Side effects have included substantial hematologic and mucosal difficulty, such as infection and mucositis. Hair loss should be anticipated with treatment using regimens including doxorubicin and cyclophosphamide. Patient preparation involving wig selection and potential body image concerns requires nursing intervention (see Chapter 25).

Major toxicities resulting from chemotherapy include pulmonary, related to bleomycin, and severe neuropathy, either gastrointestinal or peripheral, as a result of vincristine therapy.

Oncologic emergencies

Patients with progressive lymphoma are at risk for several oncologic emergencies, such as superior vena cava syndrome in patients with mediastinal masses, spinal cord compression from tumor growth, and tumor lysis syndrome as a result of the rapid breakdown of cells from aggressive chemotherapy. Patients with central nervous system involvement are at risk for intracranial pressure. Oncologic emergencies are discussed extensively in Chapter 31.

Cutaneous T-Cell Lymphoma—Mycosis Fungoides

Mycosis fungoides is a rare cutaneous lymphoma of the T lymphocyte. In the United States, this malignant skin disease affects only 400 to 600 patients per year, who range from 45 to 69 years of age at diagnosis. First described by French physician Alibert in 1806, the name *mycosis fungoides* resulted from the mushroomlike appearance of the tumors. Although indolent in nature, with a median survival of 8 to 10 years, systemic spread to peripheral blood, lymph nodes, and other organs is common. The prognosis is highly dependent on the stage of disease, which is determined by the type of skin lesions and peripheral blood, lymph node, and visceral involvement.

Three clinical stages have been identified: (1) premyotic or erythematous, (2) plaque, and (3) tumor. The first stage is characterized by a general itching and superficial skin eruptions of varying sizes. At this early stage, the disease can be confused easily with other skin disorders, such as psoriasis and dermatitis. The lesions may wax and wane and spontaneously disappear and reappear. These lesions usually appear approximately 6 years before most patients are diagnosed. Usually, the relentless itching and fear of contagion lead the patient to seek diagnosis. The premyotic stage may last from several months to 10 years.

The plaque stage of mycosis fungoides is an aggravated symptom and causes great discomfort. This stage is characterized by an irregular thickening of the skin, with raised and irregularly shaped plaques, which may be accompanied by palpable lymph nodes. Lesions are no longer transitory and may lead to painful fissures of the palms and soles. Scalp involvement may result in alopecia. Itching may become an annoying symptom, especially if it was present in the premyotic phase.

The tumor stage is characterized by mass lesions, which can appear in previously normal skin, in plaques, or in previous mycotic lesions. They may appear anywhere but are found most often in the face and body folds, such as the axillae, groin, cubital folds, neck, and breasts. The most frequent cause of death with cutaneous T-cell lymphoma is infection followed by progressive dissemination.

Treatment for mycosis fungoides includes topical as well as systemic chemotherapy, radiation therapy, BRMs, and supportive care. Patients respond better with early treatment, but at present there is no cure.

Innovative nursing care is required for the patient with mycosis fungoides, which includes skin care, infection control, and nutritional support. Comfort measures are necessary for pruritus and pain relief (see Chapters 3 and 4). The psychosocial impact of this disease, including the insult to body image and self-esteem, presents multifaceted challenges for nursing intervention.

Problems Associated with Survivorship

The successful treatment of the lymphomas has resulted in cure for many patients and progressively longer lives for others. Studies of patients with Hodgkin's disease and non-Hodgkin's lymphoma have identified several physiologic and psychologic difficulties of long-term survival.

Lack of energy or tiredness is a common complaint, often accompanied by depression. Loss of libido and problems with infertility have been documented in patients with Hodgkin's disease. Impairment or disturbance of short-term memory may be a short-term or long-term effect. Anxiety and fear of relapse and further treatment are also problems but appear to decrease as the patient lives longer free of disease.

Those returning to work often experience job discrimination or difficulties at work and problems obtaining insurance. Marital difficulties and an increase in divorce among survivors of Hodgkin's disease have been attributed to role changes, stress of treatment, and anger at the well spouse. Educating the patient about potential psychosocial difficulties during treatment and recovery is a suggested intervention to decrease the impact of these difficulties once they occur.

Future Treatments

Current studies are using various and new types of BRMs in the treatment of low-grade lymphomas. Biologics are used alone or in combination with other biologics, chemotherapy, radioactive molecules, or toxins (see Chapter 7). Other areas of research include the consequences of higher doses of chemotherapy, with or without whole body irradiation, followed by autologous bone marrow transplantation. Encouraging preliminary results of this research as a salvage program for patients who have had relapses after treatment have been identified.

16 Head and Neck Cancers

JEAN L. REESE

Cancerous processes in the paranasal sinuses, nasal and oral cavities, salivary glands, pharynx, and larynx can affect speech, appearance, eating, and breathing. The person with head and neck cancer often bears concomitant health problems associated with aging, malnutrition, smoking, and alcohol abuse.

TRENDS

Head and neck cancer is increasing among women, the elderly, and African Americans. More than 50% of all cancers occur in persons over 65 years old. This percentage

See the corresponding chapter in *Cancer Nursing: A Comprehensive Textbook*, by Baird, McCorkle, and Grant, pp. 567–583, for a more detailed discussion of this topic, including a comprehensive list of references.

holds, with slight variation in different sites, for the elderly who have cancers of the head and neck. In addition, the 56% 5-year survival rate for the over-61 age group compared unfavorably with the 79% survival rate among patients aged 40 years or less.

Both incidence and death rates have been increasing more rapidly among African Americans than among whites. Factors thought to be related are poor nutrition, earlier tobacco and alcohol consumption, and other environmental or personal factors. Another concern is the use of smokeless tobacco by teenagers, in whom oral mucosal changes are evident.

ORAL CAVITY AND PHARYNX
Definition

Oral cavity cancer occurs in the lips, oral tongue, floor of the mouth, buccal mucosa, upper and lower gingiva, retromolar trigone, and hard palate.

The pharynx, composed of the nasopharynx, oropharynx, and hypopharynx, extends from the base of the skull superiorly to the level of the esophagus inferiorly. The soft palate forms the floor and anterior wall of the nasopharynx. The eustachian tube orifice and the adenoids are located in the nasopharynx. The extensive submucosal capillary lymphatic plexus present in the nasopharynx leads to frequent metastasis from this region to the neck. The oropharynx includes the base of the tongue, the tonsillar areas, the soft palate, and the posterior pharyngeal wall. The base of the tongue is bounded by the circumvallate papillae anteriorly, by the epiglottis posteriorly, and by the glossopharygeal sulcus laterally. The hypopharynx extends from the level of the hyoid bone to the lower border of the cricoid cartilage, where the esophagus begins. The pharyngeal walls, pyriform sinus, and postcricoid area make up the hypopharynx.

Incidence, Mortality, and Survival Rates
Cancer of the mouth and pharynx

More than 90% of all oral and pharyngeal cancers occur in people over 45 years old. An exception arises with nasopharyngeal carcinomas, of which 15% to 20% appear in persons under 30 years old.

Survival rates vary depending on the site of cancer in the mouth, with the malignant gradient increasing as the site of the cancer moves posteriorly in the oral cavity. Thus, cancer of the lip has the best survival rate when compared with other oral structures.

Cancer of the tongue

An estimated 6000 new cancer cases in the United States arise annually from the tongue. The lateral border of the middle third of the tongue is the most common site for cancers. About 75% of the cancers occur in the mobile portion of the tongue, and the rest originate in the posterior third of the tongue.

Floor of the mouth carcinomas

Floor of the mouth carcinomas are nearly as common as those occurring in the tongue. Metastasis to the cervical lymph nodes occurs in 35% to 70% of the cases but develops later in the disease process than does metastasis from cancer of the tongue.

Carcinoma of the palate

Carcinoma of the palate frequently occurs in men in their 60s. The tumors are usually ulcerated, are surrounded by leukoplakia, and have indistinct borders.

Signs and Symptoms
Oral cavity carcinomas

A painless mass present for varying periods of time, persistent ulceration, difficulty wearing dentures, local or referred pain to the jaw or ear, and blood-tinged sputum are common complaints with oral cavity carcinomas. Later complaints include dysphagia, difficulty chewing, or changes in articulation. Some lesions may be discovered during a dental examination. In other cases, patients first note a mass in the neck.

Mashberg and Samit emphasize that mucosal erythroplasia rather than leukoplakia is the earliest visual sign of oral and pharyngeal carcinomas. In addition, if mucosal redness or inflammation persists for more than 14 days in the high-risk areas (floor of the mouth, ventrolateral tongue, and soft palate) without obvious cause, the area should be biopsied.

Nasopharyngeal cancers

Presenting symptoms are vague and variable. A painless enlarged neck node is a common first indicator of tumor presence. Nasal discharge (sometimes bloody), nasal stuffiness, and hypernasal speech are other indicators. Spread of the tumor can produce unilateral conductive hearing loss, atypical facial pain, and paresthesias, diplopia, trismus, nasal regurgitation, tongue paralysis, and shoulder weakness.

Oropharyngeal cancers

Cancers of the oropharynx tend to be highly metastatic, aggressive, and undifferentiated. The majority of these cancers are beyond the T_1 designation when first seen. Tumors of the base of the tongue frequently occur without ulceration. Tumors often are visually apparent or palpable at presentation. Other manifestations include local pain and dysphagia.

Hypopharyngeal cancers

The common presenting symptoms include a sore throat and neck mass. Localized pain with swallowing and referred pain to the ear also are typical. Weight loss and dysphagia occur with enlargement of the tumor.

Risk Factors

Tobacco is strongly associated with oral and pharyngeal cancers. Chewing pan, a mixture of betel leaf (a climbing pepper), areca (or betel) nut, lime (calcium hydroxide), and catechu, is common in India, where oral carcinomas abound. The effect of tobacco is multiplied by the ingestion of alcohol.

Other identified risk factors include poor nutrition and poor oral hygiene. Currently, the evidence suggests that chronic oral irritation has little influence on the development of squamous cancers. The three intraoral areas that most frequently show squamous cell carcinoma are the floor of the mouth, the ventrolateral tongue, and the soft palate complex.

Boot and shoe manufacturers and repairers have exhibited an increased incidence of buccal cavity cancer owing to exposure to noxious substances in their work. In addition, cotton, wool, and asphalt workers have had a higher than expected incidence for mouth and pharyngeal cancers. Sun exposure has long been associated with the development of lower lip cancer in outdoor workers.

Leukoplakia, a relatively common mucosal disorder, becomes malignant in about 5% to 6% of the cases.

Asian Chinese have a high rate of nasopharyngeal carcinomas.

The relationship of the Epstein-Barr virus (EBV) to nasopharyngeal carcinoma is well established. Genetic predisposition, environmental factors, and exposure to EBV are variables associated with increased risk of nasopharyngeal carcinomas.

Diagnosis

Locating the site of the tumor is of great importance for exact staging. Needle and simple open biopsies are common methods of determining tissue histology. The use of toluidine blue to differentiate the margins of squamous cell carcinoma is helpful with leukoplakia or erythroplasia. Routine radiographs of the area serve initially to localize a suspected lesion, and chest radiographs rule out lung metastasis. Computed tomography (CT) shows soft-tissue densities as well as bony structures, muscles, fascial planes, opacification, and enlarged lymph nodes.

Medical Treatment
Surgery and radiation

The choice between radiation or surgery as the initial treatment hinges on many factors. Tumor location and volume, patterns of spread, and the impact of treatment on function, rehabilitation, and cosmesis are a few of the considerations. With lip lesions, irradiation or local excision is used. Neck dissection is performed for metastatic disease, not for prophylaxis. Cancers of the lower gingiva that are less than 3 cm require wide local excision with radiation. Initial surgical treatment produces better results than does radiation. Tumors over 3 cm are treated with radical excision, radical neck dissection, and postoperative radiation.

Survival rates for T_1 and early T_2 lesions of the mouth floor are similar whether treated with radiation or surgical excision. Invasive tumors, regardless of size, require wide excision with reconstruction using tongue or nasolabial skin flaps. Deltopectoral or pectoralis major myocutaneous flaps are used for more extensive surgical removal of a tumor, and ipsilateral radical neck dissection is highly recommended. If the tumor is close to the midline, the suprahyoid lymph nodes are removed. If positive nodes are present contralaterally, a modified neck dissection is in order.

Tumors of the hard palate require wide resection involving partial or total maxillectomy. Plans for use of an obturator with an upper denture are completed before surgery. Radical neck dissection is not performed unless lymph nodes are involved. High-grade malignant salivary tumors, epidermoid carcinoma, and cylindroma require radiation.

Nasopharyngeal tumors are treated by radiation because surgical removal is nearly impossible and bilateral metastases develop early. However, some extensive surgical procedures are being initiated with an infratemporal fossa or transparotid approach.

Tumors of the anterior two thirds of the tongue that are 2 cm or less can be treated equally well with radiation or partial glossectomy. Although combined external beam and interstitial radiation have been successful, partial glossectomy demands less treatment time and causes minimal speech and swallowing problems. Larger lesions necessitate total or subtotal glossectomy, regional lymphadenectomy, and radiation.

Base of the tongue lesions have access to a rich lymphatic bed that penetrates the pharyngeal wall. Poor prognosis is associated with squamous cell carcinomas in this area. Surgical management includes glossectomy, or partial or total laryngectomy. Because soft palate tumors do not metastasize early, surgical resection or radiation is recommended at stage I. If metastasis does develop, radical neck dissection is performed. Small tonsillar tumors can be resected through an intraoral approach, followed by radiation. Again, large tumors warrant wide resection, including the pharyngeal wall, radical neck dissection, and radiation.

Tumors of the hypopharynx, because of their late discovery, usually require a laryngopharyngectomy with a radical neck dissection.

Chemotherapy

Chemotherapy has been used skeptically in the treatment of head and neck cancers. Drug trials have been largely unimpressive, failing to control such variables as dose schedules, response criteria, and eligibility criteria.

NASAL CAVITY AND PARANASAL SINUSES
Definition

The nasal cavity connects laterally with the maxillary sinuses and superiorly with the frontal, ethmoid, and sphenoid sinuses. The nasal passageway acts as a sieve, warmer, and humidifier for the inhaled air. The paranasal sinuses supply additional mucus to the nasal cavity.

Incidence, Mortality, and Survival Rates

The annual adjusted incidence rates of sinonasal cancers (SNC) is 0.8 for men and 0.5 for women per 100,000 in the United States.

Several studies have found up to 80% of sinus cancers originating in the maxilla. Squamous cell carcinoma is the most frequent neoplasm (80% to 90%) in both the nose and sinus. Adenocarcinoma (7% to 15%), transitional cell carcinoma, and sarcoma follow in decreasing order.

Five-year relative survival rates for localized lesions are about double those of regional spread. Local recurrence is the most common cause of failure, with 30% to 40% of recurrences developing in the nasal cavity and ethmoidal-sphenoid complex. The maxillary sinus has about a 60% local recurrence rate, with metastasis taking place 20% to 25% of the time. Because advanced lesions resist current treatment modalities, 60% to 75% of the patients with sinonasal carcinomas die within 5 years. Treatment with radiation alone for unresectable lesions results in a 12% to 19% 5-year survival rate. Malignant tumors of the paranasal sinuses involve the orbit and sinus wall in 60% of the cases, of which 45% will require exenteration.

Risk Factors

Numerous environmental substances have been implicated, including nickel, chromium, wood dust, boot and shoe dust, wool dust, mustard gas, isopropyl oil, nitrosamines, aromatic hydrocarbons, and radium. Because of the low incidence rate of sinonasal cancers in the general population, even a small increase in a group exposed to these substances is sufficient to constitute increased risk.

Diagnosis

Knowing the extent of the tumor is paramount for determining treatment. This determination is based on a history and on direct and indirect examination of nasal cavity and nasopharynx. CT scans and tomograms aid detection of bony and soft-tissue changes.

Medical Treatment
Surgery and radiation

Radiation or surgical removal or both are employed, depending on the extent of the tumor. Surgical intervention with radiation has produced better results than radiation alone. Survival rates have ranged from 29% to 48% for combined therapies, compared with 10% to 34% for radiation alone.

Surgical procedures may leave the patient with a severe facial deformity requiring specially made prosthetic devices to cover cavities and aid swallowing and articulation. The sequelae, depending on the surgical approach and anatomic position of the tumor, may include loss of smell, loss of vision, numbness of the face, temporary facial paralysis, and facial deformities.

SALIVARY GLANDS
Definition

The salivary glands are divided into the major glands, comprising the parotid, submandibular, and sublingual glands, and the minor salivary glands, found in the mucous membrane throughout the upper aerodigestive tract.

The auriculotemporal nerve, arising from the mandibular branch of the trigeminal, supplies parasympathetic secretomotor innervation to the parotid. After parotidectomy, redness and sweating may occur over the distribution of this nerve after eating. This phenomenon, known as Frey's syndrome, results from faulty regeneration of the secretory nerve fibers to the sweat glands in the skin.

Incidence, Mortality, and Survival Rates

Malignant tumors of the major salivary glands are rare, the incidence rate being 0.8 to 1.0 per 100,000 for the years 1983 and 1984.

The parotid gland is involved in approximately 90% of salivary gland neoplasms. About 80% of these are benign, and 20% are malignant. Tumors of the submandibular gland are rare, representing about 10% of all salivary gland neoplasms. However, up to 50% of submandibular tumors are malignant. Sublingual neoplasms are very rare, but close to 80% are malignant. Tumors of the minor salivary glands also develop rarely, but about 60% are malignant.

Risk Factors

Occurrence of salivary gland tumors is associated with prior radiation exposure in the head and neck region.

Diagnosis

Parotid tumors present a diagnostic problem because of their notorious heterogeneity. Needle aspiration biopsy is viewed favorably as a diagnostic method. Open biopsy is used to make a diagnosis when other methods have failed and to plan palliative radiation or chemotherapy.

Medical Treatment
Surgery and radiation

A parotid tumor less than 4 cm in size can be removed by a subtotal parotidectomy that preserves the facial nerve. Conversely, large stage III tumors require a radical parotidectomy with facial nerve sacrifice. Facial nerve repair with an autogenous nerve graft is accomplished at the time of surgery, and regional flaps are used to cover extensive resection.

LARYNX
Definition

The larynx extends from the superior tip of the epiglottis to the inferior margin of the cricoid cartilage. The larynx is divided into three regions—supraglottic, glottic, and subglottic. The absence of midline divisions in the supraglottis and subglottis allows tumors in these areas to spread circumferentially. In addition, anatomic structures that separate the supraglottis from the glottis and the subglottis from the glottis prevent extraglottic tumors from immediate extension into the glottis. Consequently, hoarseness develops later in the course of the disease, making early detection less frequent.

Incidence, Mortality, and Survival Rates

The 1987 annual adjusted incidence rate for cancer of the larynx among whites in the United States is 9.0 for men and 1.5 for women per 100,000. The supraglottic, glottic, and subglottic regions of the larynx have a ratio of tumor occurrence of 40:59:1, respectively, in the United States.

The most frequent abnormalities (90%) arise from the squamous cell. Other cell types are verrucous carcinoma, carcinosarcoma, adenocarcinoma, lymphoma, and sarcoma.

Risk Factors

Laryngeal cancer, as with most other head and neck cancers, is closely associated with smoking and alcohol consumption. Increased incidence of laryngeal cancer occurs among persons who work with asbestos and wood. Communities in which paper, chemicals, or petroleum are manufactured show a higher incidence of laryngeal cancer. Decreased amounts of vitamins A and C in the diet have been associated with increased risks of laryngeal cancer.

Diagnosis

The diagnostic workup includes viewing the larynx with a mirror (indirect laryngoscopy), a flexible fiberoptic endoscope, or a laryngoscope—or all three. Radiographic studies, xerography, and CT add other dimensions to the diagnostic process.

Medical Treatment
Surgery and radiation

Stage T_1 vocal fold lesions are treated equally well by radiation or by local excision. The T_2 glottic lesion may be treated with either a hemilaryngectomy or radiation, although the surgical approach tends to have better survival rates. Total laryngectomy is recommended for most stage T_3 glottic lesions. Neck dissections are also advocated with stages T_3, N_0, or N_1. Positive nodes indicate adjuvant radiation therapy. Stage T_4 lesions require total laryngectomy with radical neck dissection and postoperative radiation. The majority of supraglottic lesions can be treated adequately with a horizontal supraglottic partial laryngectomy. Although early stage T_1 supraglottic lesions can be treated with radiation, if radiotherapy fails, a total laryngectomy must be performed. Postoperation complications include fistula formation and wound infections.

A supraglottic laryngectomy, while preserving the voice, invites aspiration. A total laryngectomy, on the other hand, avoids the problem of aspiration but requires a major adjustment in communication. Persons can learn to communicate by means of esophageal speech, artificial larynges, or voice buttons placed in a primary tracheoesophageal fistula.

NURSING MANAGEMENT
Prevention

The high correlation of smoking and alcohol consumption with head and neck cancer demands unrelenting education of the public and individual discouragement of usage by health professionals.

The newly diagnosed patients tend to be more receptive to changing their personal habits because of perceived vulnerability and knowing the results of that habit. Teaching patients oral self-examination skills empowers them to improve their health status. Knowledge of the symptoms arising from cancerous lesions alerts patients to changes that otherwise may be discounted.

Detection

Inspection of the oral cavity is of particular significance because asymptomatic cancerous lesions remain undetected.

Mashberg and Samit describe these lesions as characterized by "innocuous-appearing red inflammatory or erythroplastic mucosal changes, . . . [the] lesions are less than 2 cm in diameter; are predominantly red, with or without a white component; and are smooth, granular, or minimally elevated."

Patient Preparation for Treatment

Treatment methods include surgery, radiation, and chemotherapy. Surgical intervention for head and neck tumors ranges from minor to extremely complex. Preparation and continuing support of the patient to meet this challenge on a day-to-day basis falls to the nurse.

Preoperative care

Areas to probe are usual daily activities, eating habits, living arrangements, and availability of the support of significant others. Explanations about incisions, tubes, alterations in airway, swallowing, or speech, and changes in appearance must be given in terms and in ways the patient can understand.

Postoperative care

Airway Management. Airway management for patients with surgery of the oral cavity or pharynx entails keeping the temporary tracheostomy patent. Instillation of sterile saline solution in small amounts (2 to 5 ml) stimulates coughing and allows easier expulsion of thick mucus. Suctioning with sterile equipment may be done as often as every hour depending on the amount of mucus produced. Humidification, by ultrasonic nebulization or oxygen mist, provides an essential element in liquefying secretions in the early postoperative period.

Usually, plastic disposable cuffed tracheostomy tubes are used to prevent aspiration of oral secretions until the patient gains control of swallowing. Release the cuff around the tracheostomy tube every shift to remove secretions that have collected above the cuff. The amount of tension the cuff exerts on the tracheal wall can be controlled by checking the amount of pressure in the cuff's bladder using a sphygmomanometer, 10 ml syringe, and stopcock.

The inner cannula can be removed, without risking the loss of the airway if it suddenly becomes plugged. Disposable vs reusable inner cannulas have been shown to save time in the cleansing procedure, with no difference in the infection rate. After the need for a cuffed tracheostomy tube passes, it is replaced by a metal tracheostomy tube.

Corking of the tracheostomy tube allows evaluation of the patient's ability to breathe through the upper aerodigestive tract before removing the tube. The tracheostomy incision closes without suturing by applying an airtight pressure dressing over it. The patient is instructed to press fingers over the dressing when coughing to prevent air flow from separating the incision.

If a total laryngectomy is performed, a plastic stent may be placed in the tracheal stoma to reduce contraction of the stomal opening.

Complications, such as fistula formation, may require reinsertion of a cuffed plastic tracheostomy tube. The cuffed tracheostomy tube prevents secretions from draining into the lungs and also provides a seal for mechanical hyperinflation of the lungs.

Regional Flap Management. The success of reconstructive surgery of the head and neck using a flap rests on the viability of that flap. Because the myocutaneous flap crosses the neck to its destination, all constricting items around the neck are avoided, such as gown ties, humidification mask cords, and tracheostomy ties. Plastic cuffed tracheostomy tubes may be held in place with sutures rather than ties the first few days after the operation. Humidification delivery by T-piece rather than mask obviates the use of an elastic band encircling the neck. Changes in the temperature and color of a flap need to be reported immediately to the surgeon. The blood flow in free flaps may be monitored with Doppler ultrasound. Loss of the Doppler signal indicates the need for immediate wound evaluation and possible exploration.

Neck dissection requires either pressure dressing or drain placement. The dermis must adhere to the underlying structures to reestablish its blood supply. Functioning drains help prevent the occurrence of hematomas or seromas. Drains are attached to collecting devices and are removed when the daily output becomes scant. In addition to measuring the drain output, the nurse observes the color of the drainage. If it becomes milky rather than reddish, chyle is leaking owing to accidental severance of a lymphatic duct during surgery.

Neck dissection incisions often leak serous fluid, which is removed with hydrogen peroxide, followed by normal saline solution and sometimes ointment application. Zinc oxide ointment may be applied on the skin below the tracheostomy stoma for protection from secretions.

Communication. The patient with a tracheostomy is without a voice. The patient's call light or some other communication device must always be within reach. Labeling the public address apparatus with the room numbers of patients who cannot speak reminds nurses to tell the patient by public address that they will respond immediately. Paper and pen, flash cards, and pictorial boards are ways in which the patient can let the nursing staff know what is needed. After removal of the tracheostomy tube, the patient may have difficulty with articulation as a result of the oral cavity or pharyngeal surgery. Listening and verifying the communication are essential nurse behaviors to gain the confidence of the patient.

For the patient who has had a total laryngectomy, the loss of voice is permanent. For those persons who have had hemilaryngectomies or supraglottic laryngectomies, the removal of the tracheostomy tube allows return of the voice, albeit somewhat altered from its original timbre. Loss of the voice results in an inability to sing, whistle, make quick verbal retorts, laugh, or change voice inflections. The voice conveys much more than words; it holds emotions—joy, pain, anger, fear, delight. This revelation of self to the world is gone for the laryngectomee. Replacements, such as with esophageal speech, the voice button, or the artificial larynges, give the laryngectomee a means to communicate, but they lack the expressiveness of the normal voice. Yet it is not unusual for an individual with a laryngectomy to overcome this handicap and continue a lifestyle with style.

Camouflaging the stoma may be important to some laryngectomees. Bibs, ascots, lace collars, or shirts with a tie provide cover for appearance in public and prevent inhalation of small particles. The laryngectomee must unlearn some reflexes: covering the mouth when coughing, blowing on liquids to cool them, and blowing the nose. Other restrictions include prohibition of swimming or fishing from a boat. As the integration of this change occurs within the self, the patient may develop depression, especially if alternative forms of communication are difficult and if talking was a major way of meeting emotional needs.

Preoperatively, patients often suffer from deficient intake owing to alcoholism or dysphagia. Postoperatively, a patient may have insufficient intake because of swallowing difficulties and aspiration. This is particularly true of patients who have had surgery that interferes with the changing positions of the upper aerodigestive tract structures that control swallowing. Drooling, pocketing of food in the lateral sulcus, and losing food into the pharynx while chewing are examples of swallowing problems. Procedures that are used to help with swallowing include postural changes and alterations in food consistencies, exercises to strengthen muscles and increase jaw range of motion, and exercises with specific instructions to change the coordination of the swallow.

Psychosocial Aspects. Persons who have cancer of the head and neck often have a history of alcoholism and, with it, lack of close personal relationships, unstable work histories, and dysfunctional family interactions. Characteristics of dependence, inability to change habits, and poor adaptive coping skills make adjustment to the disfigurement and dysfunction from the treatment methods especially difficult. Other factors that impede adjustment are isolation, fear of rejection, negative changes in family interaction, and the patient's dependence on physical appearance for self-concept.

The alterations in appearance and function of speech, swallowing, or breathing require self-image adjustments and learning of self-care tasks.

If the family interaction is dysfunctional, a spouse or significant other can hinder the progress of the patient in accepting physical changes and taking care of physical needs. Trying to alter long-standing interaction patterns during the short hospitalization period is unrealistic. Giving information about what to expect, both physically and psychologically, listening to concerns and giving direction, and including significant others in home care planning will—it is hoped—provide some stability for the patient and family.

Not all patients who have major head and neck surgery are alcoholics or have dependency needs. Many travel through the grieving process without unusual aberrations and retain their self-esteem despite physical changes. The team approach, with nurses coordinating the work of social workers, pastors, dietitians, speech therapists, physical therapists, and surgeons for physical and psychosocial support of the patient, increases the probability of a better life adjustment to the treatment outcomes.

17 Soft-Tissue and Bone Sarcomas

AMY SMITH-BRASSARD

SOFT-TISSUE SARCOMAS
Definition and Incidence

By definition, soft tissue is the extraskeletal supportive structures arising from the mesoderm. These connective tissues include muscles, tendons, fat, and synovial and fibrous tissues.

Soft-tissue sarcomas are tumors arising from these connective tissue structures. Sarcomas can occur most anywhere in the body but are most commonly found in the extremities.

According to the 1990 Cancer Facts and Figures, an estimated 5700 new cases of soft-tissue sarcomas would have been diagnosed in 1990, with approximately 3100 deaths. The incidence of soft-tissue sarcomas is higher in children under 15 years, ranking behind leukemias, lymphomas, and tumors of the central and sympathetic nervous systems.

Epidemiology

No definable causes or trends have been noted in the incidence of soft-tissue sarcomas. A genetic predisposition has not been found, although isolated cases of soft-tissue sarcomas among siblings have been documented. Cases of genetic disorders have been linked to the development of sarcomas, but these are rare. However, within the past decade, medical researchers have reported a much higher incidence of Kaposi's sarcoma in association with AIDS. Pre-

---

See the corresponding chapter in *Cancer Nursing: A Comprehensive Textbook,* by Baird, McCorkle, and Grant, pp. 597–607, for a more detailed discussion of this topic, including a comprehensive list of references.

viously, Kaposi's syndrome was seen mainly in elderly men of Jewish or Mediterranean origin. The disease in AIDS patients is a more aggressive form involving the viscera and lymphatic system.

Reports have linked soft-tissue sarcomas and environmental exposure to phenoxyacetic acids and chlorophenols. There have been case reports of patients developing soft-tissue sarcomas years after radiation therapy for a malignant tumor, such as breast cancer or Hodgkin's disease.

Biology of Sarcomas

Because connective tissue is found throughout the body, soft-tissue sarcomas can occur nearly anywhere.

Soft-tissue sarcomas usually first appear as asymptomatic soft-tissue masses. These tumors often grow insidiously, so that early detection is difficult. Soft-tissue sarcomas take the path of least resistance in their growth, pushing surrounding tissues before them. They compress surrounding tissue, and so the tumors can grow quite large before clinical symptoms develop. This tumor forms a pseudocapsule yet contains invasive extensions of malignant tissue. Local signs of tumor besides the presence of a mass include peripheral neuralgia, paralysis, or ischemia if the tumor is impinging on nerve or vascular supply. The tumors may also obstruct bowel, ureters, or mediastinal structures.

Anatomic staging uses the TNM classification plus an A or B to denote tumors that are less than or greater than 5 cm. Nodal involvement occurs rarely. With the exception of rhabdomyosarcomas and synoviosarcomas, soft-tissue sarcomas rarely infiltrate surrounding lymph nodes but instead tend to metastasize via the hematogenous route.

It is this hematogenous dissemination and local invasion into surrounding tissues that generally dictate a poor prognosis. Another prognostic factor is location, for example, trunk vs extremity. The primary site influences resectability and ability to cure the tumor. In the extremity, proximal lesions are believed to be less curable than distal lesions. Age and sex seem to have little influence on prognosis with the exception of fibrosarcomas, which tend to do better in children. An estimated 80% of all lesions recur in about 2 years after surgical resection. More than 50% of cases recur as pulmonary lesions. Local recurrence is the next most common site. Aggressive pulmonary resection for isolated lesions is recommended. Without resection, the median survival after pulmonary mestastases have developed is 6 to 12 months.

Diagnosis of Soft-Tissue Sarcomas

As with any suspected malignancy, the medical workup should include history, physical examination, soft-tissue radiograph of the affected part, CT scan or magnetic resonance imaging (MRI) of the region, plus radiographs and CT scans of the lung.

The histologic grade of the tumor is the most important factor in prognosis and in treatment decisions. An incisional biopsy is usually done to diagnose a soft-tissue mass. Incisional biopsies on an extremity should be placed longitudinally so to not interfere with muscle group excisions during a major curative surgical procedure.

Occasionally, an arteriogram may be obtained to visualize the vascular supply of the tumor. A bone scan may delineate bone invasion or, more likely, periosteal reaction to nearby tumor growth and increased blood supply. During any surgical biopsy, extra caution is necessary to prevent development of hematomas. These can result in further spread of the tumor.

Because soft-tissue sarcomas rarely invade lymph nodes, a lymphangiogram has little diagnostic value.

Treatment

The oncology nurse plays a pivotal role in the support and teaching of patients as the treatment plan evolves. The major goal is to eradicate the tumor with minimal loss of function.

The first step in optimal control of the disease is surgical excision with a microscopic tumor-free margin.

The excision of a soft-tissue sarcoma should be done by a wide en bloc resection. This should include previous biopsy sites and a wide expanse of muscles, tendons, fascia, neurovascular structures, and lymph nodes. The entire specimen should be removed at one time without violating any tumor. Preferably a margin of 2 to 3 cm is left.

En bloc resections of truncal sarcomas depend on the skill and ingenuity of the surgeon. In an extremity, however, if a wide resection is not possible, the alternative is amputation in selected cases. Indications for amputation include the following.

- The mass cannot be encompassed by wide excision.
- An operation would leave a useless extremity with compromised vascular or neurologic supply
- The mass is a recurrence from a previously excised tumor.
- The tumor is difficult to palliate owing to pain, odor, and so forth.

In a large retrospective study at Memorial Hospital from 1949 to 1968, investigators found that amputations did lower recurrence rates at the stump site. However, 5- and 10-year survival rates were lower than those for patients receiving en bloc resections.

Radiation is used to treat the microscopic extensions of tumor. This can spare the patient extensive surgery. Using radiation in an adjunctive and more limited fashion avoids the late sequelae of high-dose radiotherapy.

Before surgery, 5000 to 6000 cGy are given in the hope that reduction in tumor bulk will occur. An advantage of preoperative radiation therapy is that it reduces the risk of intraoperative contamination of vascular space by viable tumor cells. Another advantage is that patients who would have needed an amputation if surgery had been done initially may now be eligible for limb preservation procedures. Surgery should take place 2 to 3 weeks after radiation. Postoperative radiation is used to sterilize an area that has known residual microscopic tumor or is at risk for developing recurrent disease. Because most soft-tissue sarcomas occur in an extremity, the desire to salvage the limb is paramount for the patient.

Despite the success of achieving local control with surgery and radiation therapy, the 5-year survival rate of patients with soft tissue sarcoma is only 40% to 60% overall. The multimodality approach has improved 5-year survivals in patients with high-grade soft-tissue sarcomas of an extremity to 70% to 80%. The main cause of death is disseminated disease.

In the 1970s, trials with doxorubicin alone and with doxorubicin in combination with cyclophosphamide, dacarbazine (DTIC), and vincristine showed an increase in survival. The study by Rosenberg et al. demonstrated an increased survival in those patients receiving chemotherapy as opposed to the group not receiving systemic therapy (57% vs 83%). This increase in survival, however, has been seen only in patients with soft-tissue sarcoma of an extremity. In a randomized trial of patients with head, neck, and trunk sarcomas, the 3-year disease-free survival was 77% with chemotherapy, compared with 49% without chemotherapy. However, there was no difference in overall survival.

It appears that adjuvant chemotherapy with a combination of drugs including doxorubicin increases disease-free and overall survival in patients with high-grade sarcomas of an extremity. The role of adjuvant chemotherapy in sarcomas elsewhere in the body is doubtful at the present time. Doxorubicin is considered the drug of choice whether used alone or in combination. The Southwest Oncology Group has randomized patients to one of three study arms: doxorubicin plus DTIC; doxorubicin, DTIC, and cyclophosphamide; or doxorubicin, DTIC, and dactinomycin. The median survivals in each group were 37, 45, and 50 weeks, respectively. Chemotherapy in advanced soft-tissue sarcoma offers hope for partial response and a prolongation of survival, but this result is short lived.

BONE SARCOMAS
Definition and Incidence

Primary malignant tumors of bone are rare, constituting about 0.5% of all cancers. The incidence of bone tumors is highest during adolescence, when it reaches a rate of 3 per 100,000. Osteogenic sarcoma is considered the most common primary malignant bone tumor. However, multiple myeloma, a nonosseous cancer of the bone marrow, is actually the most prevalent type of bone tumor. Chondrosarcoma is the most common malignant cartilage tumor. Most bone cancers are actually metastases from a separate primary carcinoma.

Most bone tumors involve the appendicular skeleton, usually the knee joint.

Etiology

This disease occurs 1.5 to 2 times more often in males. Owing to the high incidence in children and adolescents, it is speculated that areas of rapid growth may be more susceptible to developing a neoplasm. Metabolic stimulation from Paget's disease has been linked to the development of osteosarcomas. Radiation has also been a culprit in the development of osteogenic sarcomas, chondrosarcomas, and fibrosarcomas.

Biology of Bone Sarcomas

Bone sarcomas have their own specific characteristics. The tumors are composed of spindle cells that grow centrifugally and form a pseudocapsule. Around the tumor is a zone of reactive tissue, which usually contains inflammatory cells. Tumors often interdigitate with surrounding tissue through this reactive zone. An important yet ominous characteristic of bone sarcomas is the ability to break through the pseudocapsule and form satellite lesions. High-grade sarcomas have the ability to develop skip metastases, which are tumor nodules within the same bone but not in continuity. These are believed to be caused by embolization of tumor cells within the marrow sinusoids. Skip metastases are usually indicators of poor prognosis.

Bone sarcomas spread along the path of least resistance. Their growth is characterized by compression of normal tissue, resorption of bone by reactive osteoclasts, and direct destruction of tissue.

Low-grade malignant tumors remain relatively localized, with occasional nodules being found within the reactive zone. These lesions can be treated successfully by surgery alone if a margin of normal bone is allowed. Malignant, high-grade bone sarcomas have a normal history of rapid growth and metastasis. Bone tumors disseminate through the blood, usually to the pulmonary bed. High-grade tumors warrant the use of systemic therapy.

Diagnosis

Radiographic evaluation, patient history of pain, and tissue biopsy are integral to the diagnosis of a bone sarcoma. Patint history often includes complaints of pain and sometimes of swelling. Occasionally, a mass is felt as an extension of the primary tumor. Routine radiographs are the most informative method of depicting the type of bone destruction and the margin between tumor and normal bone. Radiographic findings will include periosteal reaction and both lytic and blastic features.

Tomography is helpful in delineating tumor margins, internal mineralization, and pathologic fractures. CT is more helpful in assessing lesions of the central skeleton than those of the extremities. In the preoperative staging, CT scans of the chest are very important in depicting metastatic lesions of the lung.

The isotope bone scan is helpful in detecting additional lesions, but owing to its nonspecificity, this technique is not particularly helpful in defining characteristics of the lesions.

A high alkaline phosphatase level is indicative of bone destruction and can be of diagnostic value. Aggressive bone tumors also may cause an increase in serum calcium level and urinary calcium excretion.

An accurate diagnosis requires an open biopsy to obtain sufficient tissue. As with soft-tissue sarcomas, the biopsy site should be chosen that will not interfere with a definitive surgical procedure. Likewise, a biopsy site needs to be planned so that the region can be removed en bloc with the tumor resection. Often, a biopsy and definitive resection will be done at the same time. This requires a frozen section and a pathologist who is experienced in diagnosing malignant bone tumors.

Specific Histologic Types

Owing to the rarity of these tumors, only chondrosarcomas and osteogenic sarcomas are discussed here.

Chondrosarcoma is a malignant tumor composed of cells that produce hyaline cartilage. The tumor has a long, slow evolution, and some variants are so similar to their benign counterparts that diagnosis is difficult. Thus, mismanagement can occur. Ordinary chondrosarcoma occurs most often in middle-aged or older adults. The diaphysis of the femur is the most common site. Patients with a low-grade tumor have a longer disease-free and overall survival than those with higher-grade lesions. Five-year survival is approximately 50%.

Osteosarcoma accounts for about 20% of all bone sarcomas. Although osteogenic sarcoma tends to occur in adolescents and young adults, Paget's disease is a known precursor of osteosarcoma, accounting for a secondary peak incidence in the fifth and sixth decades of life. It affects men more often than women, and about 50% of tumors occur in the distal part of the femur. Most patients with osteosarcomas have a long history of pain and swelling, occasionally revealing a palpable mass. Osteosarcoma is usually a destructive lesion with indistinct borders. It generally extends into the cortex and even into adjacent soft tissue. Osteosarcomas metastasize to the periphery of the lung, as opposed to deep within lung tissue. Metastasis tends to occur within the first 2 years after diagnosis.

Treatment

A multimodality approach of surgery, radiotherapy, and chemotherapy is most often used in the treatment of bone sarcomas. Limb-sparing surgery is a procedure that removes a soft-tissue or bone sarcoma while preserving the extremity's function and cosmetic appearance. Treatment is dictated by the grade and staging of the tumor. Low-grade lesions can be treated more conservatively, whereas a high-grade tumor requires more aggressive therapy. Simple excision or curettage is used in benign or low-grade tumors as long as adequate excision of the tumor is achieved. If the tumor is not thoroughly removed, recurrence is likely. An en bloc resection is possible if wide enough margins can be achieved yet still leave useful function of the limb. According to Sim, the criterion for conservative surgery is that the tumor be largely interosseous and involve a short segment of bone. Any extraosseous extension should be small.

If at the time of surgery it is known that the margin is not clear or the wound is contaminated with tumor cells, it is best to carry out amputation. An amputation should leave a margin of 8 to 10 cm of healthy tissue. In large, extensive lesions, an adequate margin may mean disarticulation to include possible skip metastases.

Despite radical surgery, either by excision or amputation, only 25% to 30% of patients survived 2 years. Similarly, despite local control, 80% of patients died from pulmonary metastases. Micrometastases were believed to have been present, probably at diagnosis, and needed to be treated systemically. In the 1970s, both doxorubicin and high-dose methotrexate were found to be effective agents in extending survivals after amputation. Technologic advances at this time enhanced limb-sparing procedures because bone replacement could be done with cadaver allografts or internally fixed metallic prostheses. Metal endoprostheses, usually of titanium, are used most often.

At the NIH Consensus Conference on Limb-Sparing Treatment of Adult Soft Tissue and Osteosarcomas, the conclusion was reached that disease-free survival and overall survival were comparable for selected patients treated with limb-sparing vs amputation. Limb-sparing surgery is the treatment of choice when local tumor can be completely resected. Limb-sparing procedures are not warranted for lesions in which it is impossible to achieve adequate margins or lesions that involve major vessels or nerves.

Some evidence suggests that adjuvant chemotherapy is beneficial in long-term survival in osteosarcoma. Chemotherapy is advocated for advanced disease. Jaffe et al. achieved disease-free survival in 50% of the patients using a vincristine and high-dose methotrexate regimen.

Cortes et al. reported using doxorubicin (30 mg/m^2 for 3 days every 4 to 6 weeks), with resulting long-term survivals of up to 5 years. Ettinger et al. obtained results by alternating doxorubicin (30 mg/m^2 for 3 days) with cisplatin (110 mg/m^2 every 3 weeks).

Rosen et al. obtained excellent long-term survivals with neoadjuvant chemotherapy of high-dose methotrexate, doxorubicin, bleomycin, cyclophosphamide, and dactinomycin given 4 to 16 weeks before surgery. Neoadjuvant therapy avoids delay in treatment by causing necrosis and usually makes less aggressive surgical procedures possible.

Surgical resection of accessible pulmonary metastases is recommended when warranted by the patient's condition.

Bone sarcomas vary in their sensitivity or resistance to radiotherapy. Osteogenic sarcomas and chondrosarcomas are considered radioresistant, and how they respond to radiation depends on the degree of cell differentiation. The role of radiation in osteosarcomas is not clearly defined except to enhance tumor necrosis either before or after surgery. In a few research settings, hyperthermia has been tried in the treatment of locally advanced and bulky sarcomas that have been unresponsive to other treatment methods.

Because osteosarcoma is most common in adolescents, patients have body image and peer group identification as major developmental tasks. The adolescent must be included in treatment plans and decisions. The nurse plays a major role in helping the patient understand the treatments. The numerous body changes, such as alopecia, nausea, vomiting, mucositis, and change in mobility, must be dealt with in an open and caring manner. The potential or actual loss of a limb can be devastating. Initiating early contact with physical therapists facilitates rehabilitation and adjustment to using a limb prosthesis. The patient experiences a range of emotions, including anger, fear, resentment, guilt, shock, depression, and denial. Peer support groups are available at numerous centers, which are invaluable to young cancer patients who need to share their experiences.

18 Central Nervous System Tumors

CONNIE R. ROBINSON
SR. CALLISTA ROY
MARGARET L. SEAGER

BRAIN

The central nervous system (CNS) is composed of several major cell types that are important in understanding the function of the brain and spinal cord and the field of neurooncology nursing.

See the corresponding chapter in *Cancer Nursing: A Comprehensive Textbook*, by Baird, McCorkle, and Grant, pp. 608–636, for a more detailed discussion of this topic, including a comprehensive list of references.

Definition

Tumors that arise within the intracranial cavity have many unusual features. A discrepancy exists between their histologic nature and their biologic behavior. In addition, their location can be crucial because many vital structures may be involved. Also, the presence of the blood–brain barrier partially shields the tumor from the systemic circulation. All tumors of the CNS can pursue a malignant course to death because they grow within a unique environment, that is, a confined space. Even histologically benign and well-differentiated tumors require prompt diagnosis and management to ensure an optimal outcome for the patient. Intracranial and intraspinal tumors produce signs and symptoms primarily through expanding, compressing, and displacing vital neural tissue.

Unlike extracranial tumors, tumors of the CNS, even malignant ones (dedifferentiated or anaplastic tumors), rarely metastasize outside of the CNS. Tumors range from nonmalignant to highly malignant. Benign gliomas may recur as malignant ones. Outcomes depend not only on the nature of the tumor but also on its size and location at the time of diagnosis.

Incidence and Epidemiology

Overall, the incidence of primary brain tumors is approximately 10,000 cases per year (other sources report 15,000 to 17,000 cases per year), and the incidence of spinal cord tumors is approximately 4000 cases per year. Tumors of the CNS are found in excess of 16.1 per 100,000 population. The majority of these tumors are malignant and astroglial in origin. Brain tumors of all types represent the second leading cause of cancer deaths in children and the fourth leading cause of cancer deaths in middle-aged adult males.

Tumors occur in two major peaks across the life span: one in childhood between the ages of 3 and 12 years and the second in later life between the ages of 50 and 70 years. In children younger than 15 years, tumors of the CNS are the second most frequent type of cancer, exceeded only by leukemia. Most adult tumors are supratentorial cortical or within the cerebral hemisphere. The most common tumor type is glioblastoma. See Figure 18–1 for the incidence of brain tumors according to age.

Etiology

Convincing evidence is lacking for any particular factor (chemical, viral, or traumatic) as the cause of brain tumors in humans. However, some interesting research regarding causes is important to mention.

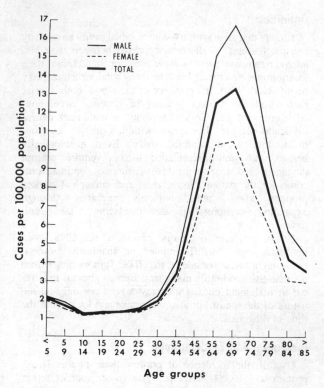

Figure 18–1. The incidence of all types of brain tumors in the United States in 1966 is shown according to 5-year age groups. (Data from U.S. Department of Health, Education and Welfare. Public Health Service [1968]. *Vital statistics rates in the United States 1940–1960*. Washington, DC: U.S. Government Printing Office, from Butler, A.B., Brooks, W.H., & Netsky, M.G. [1982]. Classification and biology of brain tumors. In J.R. Youmans [Ed.], *Neurological surgery* [Vol. 5, 2nd ed, p. 2682]. Philadelphia: W.B. Saunders Co. Reproduced by permission.)

Genetic

Evidence of genetic factors is weak but cannot be ignored. Some tumors have a hereditary component in three developmental disorders, of which von Recklinghausen's neurofibromatosis is an example.

Environmental factors

There is also little evidence that CNS tumors in humans are linked to environmental carcinogens, although many chemicals have carcinogenic activity in animals and produce CNS tumors in these animal models.

Viruses

Likewise, no evidence exists for viral causes of tumors in humans, although evidence for this in animals is of interest. Patients with primary CNS lymphomas have a high incidence of infection with the Epstein-Barr virus, and tissue from the tumors contains the Epstein-Barr virus genome.

In lymphoma and Epstein-Barr infection, immuno-suppression may play a role. Transplant recipients have a markedly increased risk of primary lymphoma of the brain, as do patients with AIDS.

Trauma

Trauma has been considered a cause of meningeal or glial tumors. A traumatic cause probably can be accepted for a small number of meningiomas. However, in most cases trauma probably initiates or aggravates clinical symptoms of a tumor already in existence.

Radiation

Sarcomas are reported to occur frequently after radiation therapy, carcinomas are rare, and gliomas are as yet unreported following radiation. The interval between radiation and symptoms of tumor ranges from 5 to 20 years. The mechanisms of radiation-induced tumors are uncertain.

Biology and Natural History
Biology of central nervous system tumors

Tumors grown by expansion, infiltration, or both. Growth by expansion is by proliferation of cells, fluid accumulation related to hemorrhage, increased permeability of blood vessels, and swelling and edema. Benign tumors, such as meningiomas, seldom infiltrate but expand surrounded by capsules of connective tissue. Malignant tumors both expand and infiltrate, especially around blood vessels in the brain. Generally, although not always, benign tumors tend to be more localized and malignant tumors more invasive.

The patterns of spread of tumors in the CNS differ from those of other tumors. There is no lymphatic system within the CNS. Spreading through the vascular system does occur but only rarely and mostly with operative intervention. Whether this phenomenon is due to the immunologically privileged status of the CNS or whether the short life expectancy of most patients does not allow time for metastases to become evident or whether some other factor is operative is unclear.

Tumors of the CNS spread locally and through cerebrospinal fluid (CSF) seeding. The intracranial astrocytomas are capable of invading normal tissue to a remarkable degree and can be found at sites distant from the primary focus. Some tumors seed through the CSF much more than others. Seeding occurs along the surface of the brain to local sites and by drop metastases, in which cells or groups of cells fall by way of the CSF to the spinal subarachnoid space and form secondary tumors. As a result, nerve roots and coverings of the cord may become involved. All sites in the spinal cord are vulnerable to this type of spread, but the lumbo-sacral area is most frequently involved.

Gliomas rarely metastasize at a distant location. They do invade locally to an extreme degree, grow relatively slowly, and have a varied cell population (heterogeneity).

Classification

The general principles that govern the statistical classification of tumors were established by a subcommittee of the World Health Organization (WHO) Expert Committee on Health Statistics. For flexibility and ease of coding, three separate classifications were needed. These are by (1) anatomic site, (2) histologic type, and (3) degree of malignancy.

One of the most commonly used and earliest developed classification systems for intracranial tumors is that of Bailey and Cushing, which was revised by them in 1920. Glial and neural tumors are classified and graded as well as intracranial tumors that arise from other types of cells found in the brain, for example, lymphomas, sarcomas, pineal tumors, and metastatic tumors.

When a cell begins the process of becoming a tumor of any type, it is said to undergo dedifferentiation. Generally, tumors are divided into two categories: benign or malignant. Tumors of the same cellular type are then divided into four grades, I through IV, based on the degree of cellular anaplasia (malignancy). In grade I tumor cells, differentiation ranges from almost 100% to 75%. In grade IV tumor cells, only 0 to 25% of the cells are differentiated. A single cell of astrocytoma can become a glioblastoma multiforme, as can oligodendrogliomas and ependymomas when they recur. However, the biology of the tumor—its invasiveness—rather than the histology is more important in determining the outcome for the patient. Usually, a patient with a better-differentiated tumor will live longer than a patient with a poorly differentiated one. Parenthetically, one must consider anatomic site as well.

In summary, CNS tumors may be classified as benign or malignant, as gliomas, neuromas, or sarcomas. Some may be graded I through IV according to the degree of dedifferentiation or anaplasia. Malignancy in the cranium is not, however, solely determined by cell of origin, and some tumors that are classified as benign may produce malignant responses. Therefore, clinical classification and consideration are also important. Further, the behavior of tumors of the same type varies in different patients.

The following discussion of major, commonly encountered tumors is from the WHO classification. For purposes of this chapter, the categories are collapsed, and a reasonable compromise of all classifications is used.

Gliomas. Approximately 60% of all primary CNS tumors are gliomas, which arise from glial cells. There are five distinct types of glial cells: astrocytes, oligodendroglia, ependymal cells, microglia, and neuroglial precursors. Each gives rise to tumors with different biologic and anatomic characteristics.

Astrocytomas, as a group, arise from astrocytes. Astrocytomas range from benign to highly malignant. The benign ones include cerebellar astrocytomas, juvenile pilocytic astrocytomas, and optic nerve gliomas. Malignant forms include the graded series of astrocytomas, with the last being the highly malignant glioblastoma multiforme. Progression from benign to malignant processes includes more rapid growth, tumor doubling, and loss of morphologic features.

Astrocytoma constitutes about 25% of cerebral gliomas and is the most frequent primary tumor of adults. It may occur anywhere in the brain or spinal cord but is most often found in the cerebrum, cerebellum, hypothalamus, optic nerve and chiasm, and pons. It grows slowly and infiltrates and has a tendency to form large cavities or pseudocysts.

In about half the patients, the initial symptom is focal or generalized seizure. Up to two thirds have recurrent seizures during the course of their illness. Headaches and other signs of increased intracranial pressure are relatively late phenomena. Temporal lobe lesions give rise to slight character and personality changes, moodiness, pseudoneurotic symptoms, and episodes suggestive of schizophrenia. Hemiparesis may be a symptom of frontal lobe glioma and may appear as only a slight drift of an outstretched arm, a mild limp, and enhanced tendon reflexes. It may remain slight for a long time. Language difficulties and sensory changes are also frequently slight. Symptoms may be present for 10 years or longer before the diagnosis is made. In cerebral astrocytoma, the average survival after the first symptom is 67 months. In cerebellar astrocytoma, the average survival is 89 months.

Optic nerve glioma of childhood is another example of a subgroup of astrocytoma and is characterized by slow growth over a period of years, with an evolution from benign to malignant. Eight-five percent occur before the age of 15 years and are twice as frequent in girls as in boys. Initial symptoms include visual problems. Treatment includes surgical excision and radiation. Survival is lengthy unless the tumor becomes dedifferentiated and invasive.

Glioblastoma multiforme (grade IV, astrocytoma) is a highly malignant, highly vascular tumor that infiltrates extensively. Necrosis, hemorrhage, and thrombosis often are present in varying degrees. It accounts for 20% of all intracranial tumors, for about 55% of all tumors of the glioma group, and for more than 90% of gliomas of the cerebral hemispheres in adults. Peak incidence is in midlife, and it occurs twice as often in men as in women. Approximately half of these tumors are bilateral, and a small percentage have several foci.

Symptoms are diffuse, and seizures occur in 30% to 40%. In most cases, symptoms have been present for 3 to 6 months before diagnosis is established. The tumor may become large and diffuse before deranging cerebral functioning. Less than one fifth of all patients survive for 1 year after the onset of symptoms. Approximately 10% survive more than 2 years. Surgery plus radiation extends median survival from only 14 weeks with surgery alone to beyond a year. Chemotherapy prolongs the median survival only slightly. The immediate cause of death is cerebral edema, increased intracranial pressure, and temporal lobe–tentorial herniation. Glioblastoma and malignant astrocytoma have the worst prognosis of any common solid tumor.

Oligodendrogliomas are most often found in the 40- to 50-year age group and constitute approximately 5% to 7% of all intracranial gliomas. Oligodendrogliomas grow slowly. Symptoms may appear from 28 to 70 months before surgical intervention. The first symptom in one-half the patients is focal or generalized seizures. Seventy percent of the patients eventually develop seizures. Fifteen percent may have early signs of increased intracranial pressure (IICP). However, at the time of surgery, only about one half have signs of IICP, and one third have focal signs, primarily those of hemiparesis. Mean survival time after surgery is 5 years. Half of the patients have recurrences within a few months following surgery.

Ependymoma is more complex and variable than the other gliomas. These tumors grow into the ventricles or adjacent brain tissues. In the brain, the most common site is the fourth ventricle; in the spinal cord, it is the lumbosacral region.

Approximately 5% of all intracranial gliomas are ependymomas (slightly higher in children, 8%). Forty percent of the infratentorial ependymomas occur in the first decade of life. Supratentorial ependymomas occur evenly throughout life.

Symptoms depend on location. For example, ependymoma of the fourth ventricle produces symptoms much like those of medulloblastoma. Cerebral lesions produce seizures in approximately one third of cases. Length of time from onset of symptoms to surgery varies from 4 weeks in the most malignant types to 7 to 8 years. Prognosis and survival depend on degree of anaplasia. In some stidues, 47% died within a year, but 13% were alive after 10 years. In the more benign group of ependymomas, 10-year survival can be as high as 55% to 60%.

Meningioma is a benign tumor and accounts for approximately 15% of all primary intracranial tumors. It is more common in women, with the highest incidence in the seventh decade. Persons who have had radiation to the scalp or cranium are particularly vulnerable to this tumor and develop it at an earlier age than those who have not had prior radiation. The cell of origin is not precisely known.

Meningiomas involve the dura and often erode cranial bones. The surface tumors often are found at autopsy in middle-aged and elderly adults and have caused no symptoms. Other patients may have neurologic signs 10 to 15 years before the diagnosis is made. Increased intracranial pressure eventually occurs but less frequently than with gliomas. Surgery may afford permanent cure if the tumor's location allows complete removal. For incomplete removal and inoperable cases, radiation is beneficial. Various series of studies report a 24% to 76% recurrence when removal is incomplete. If the meningioma becomes malignant, survival is less than 5 years.

Medulloblastomas are found primarily in children and are more prevalent in males than in females. The cell of origin was thought to be neuroglial, but recent evidence suggests that it originates from primitive neuroectodermal tissue. Therefore, it is a primitive neuroectodermal tumor (PNET). The tumor is aggressive and is always malignant. It is invasive and not encapsulated. It originates in the cerebellum and can spread by way of the CSF pathways to meningeal surfaces and around the spinal cord. Some fill the fourth ventricle and infiltrate the floor of that ventricle.

Symptoms may have been present between 1 and 5 months before diagnosis. Typically, the child becomes listless, vomits repeatedly, and has a morning headache. Later, stumbling gait, frequent falls, and squinting may occur. Papilledema, dizziness, and nystagmus are frequent. With surgery, radiation, and chemotherapy, two thirds of the patients survive 5 years. Extent of disease at diagnosis determines survival. Children considered at poor risk for survival are under 4 years of age, have less than 75% surgical resection, have positive CSF cytology, and have metastasis to the spinal cord, leptomeninges, or cerebrum or seeding of the cerebellum. These children have only a 25% to 30% chance of remaining disease free for 5 years. However, patients who are good risks have a 65% to 70% chance of remaining disease free for 5 years. Shunting of the CSF may be necessary. Surgical excision should be as complete as possible. The tumor is highly radiosensitive. The entire neuroaxis is radiated. Chemotherapy has been shown to be beneficial at recurrence.

Neural Tumors. The ganglion cell tumors—ganglioglioma and ganglioneuroma—are examples of neural tumors. They occur in young patients and range from benign to malignant. These tumors are extremely rare and are clearly demarcated but not encapsulated. Symptoms are related to the anatomic site. Surgery may be indicated. Survival statistics are unavailable, but Cobb and Youmans report one patient survived 23 years after surgery.

Lymphoma. Lymphomas arise probably from B lymphocytes and occur primarily in any part of the cerebrum, cerebellum, or brainstem. The lesions may occur singly or in multiple locations and are ill-defined and infiltrative. The same clinical course is seen in lymphoma as is seen in glioblastoma. The average length of time from first symptoms to diagnosis and surgery has been approximately 3 months. Focal signs are more common than are signs of IICP. These are personality change, dementia, seizures, and other focal neurologic symptoms.

Patients with immunodeficiency states are particularly likely to develop this type of tumor. Therefore, it is often seen in patients with AIDS and patients who receive immunosuppressive drugs for long periods of time, such as after renal or other organ transplants. Before the AIDS era, CNS lymphomas accounted for 1% of all lymphomas. Now, some estimate that it will become the most common primary CNS tumor by the 1990s. Lymphoma has always been more common in males, and it still is, although this may change. The peak incidence has been in the fourth, fifth, and sixth decades, but AIDS likely will lower the age of incidence. Some patients with lymphoma have been shown to have the Epstein-Barr virus.

Craniotomy for removal of single tumors may be done. A single biopsy specimen is taken for diagnosis when multiple tumors exist. Radiation and steroids are highly effective, although improvement is short-lived. Chemotherapy has produced variable results.

Sarcomas. Sarcomas of the brain are derived from connective tissue elements. These tumors are rare and account for 1% to 2% of all primary intracranial tumors. A few sarcomas have developed 5 to 10 years after gamma radiation for other tumors. These tumors are unique in their tendency to metastasize to nonneuronal tissue in the brain. They are slow to fast growing. Seizures occur in 25% of the patients. Headache, papilledema, and spontaneous hemorrhage also are symptoms. Surgery may be indicated. Survival has been reported to vary from 12 months to 5 years and is longer than 2 years if the tumor is nonanaplastic.

Metastatic Tumors. Metastatic tumors constitute approximately 10% of all intracranial tumors. The most common primary tumor is bronchogenic carcinoma, followed by carcinoma of the breast, kidney, stomach, and bowel.

The appearance of the tumor is that of any carcinomatous lesion. Usually, the tumor is circumscribed and solid. There may be more than one lesion with regional vasogenic edema. Presenting symptoms are those of cerebral lesions that are described later. Patients with metastatic carcinoma of the brain have a course similar to those with glioblastoma multiforme.

Systemic chemotherapy is ineffective against most cerebral metastases. The average period of survival is about 6 months, including patients who have had surgically treated single metastases. Patients with metastases to the bony structures live longer. For single lesions, surgery can be done and followed by radiation therapy. For multiple tumors, radiation and steroids are the treatment of choice.

Infiltration of the CNS occurs in patients with nonsolid tumors as well. There is a high incidence (about one third) of diffuse infiltration of the meninges, the cranial nerves, and the spinal nerve roots in patients with leukemia. The incidence is greater with lymphocytic than with myelocytic leukemia and is higher in children with acute lymphocytic (lymphoblastic) leukemia. The use of radiation therapy, vincristine, and intrathecal methotrexate has been associated with prolonged survival of children with acute leukemia. Unfortunately, there also has been a significant number of patients with necrotizing leukoencephalopathy (discussed later). This complication may appear within several days or months after completion of therapy. In most cases, death occurs, and most patients who die are under the age of 5 years.

Pineal tumors are unified by their location and include pineal area astrocytoma. Often, they are of low- or intermediate-grade malignancy. These tumors reproduce the structure of the pineal gland, enlarge the gland, become locally invasive, extend into the third ventricle, and seed along the neuroaxis. They resemble astrocytomas and may have varying degrees of malignancy. Obstructive hydrocephalus, headache, nausea and vomiting, lethargy, ataxia, and inability to look upward are the major symptoms. Survival rates vary with histology. Because of their location, pineal tumors are among the most difficult brain tumors to remove. However, surgery is important because some of these masses are radioresistant.

Teratomas—benign and arising from misplaced embryonic tissue from other parts of the body—occur here also and are treated with radiotherapy. Highly malignant embryonal tumors develop in the pineal location as well. The tumors are initially responsive to treatment but recur rapidly. Children, adolescents, and young adults are affected primarily. Males are affected more than females. Signs of IICP are present. Technical advances in surgery (use of the operating microscope) now make this tumor operable, although at a high risk. Shunting and radiation also may be used. Several patients have survived 5 years after the removal of the tumor.

Craniopharyngiomas are located in the suprasellar region

and because of the strategic location can behave as malignant tumors. They may press on or adhere to the hypothalamic structures. They are found primarily in children but may occur at a later age and are thought to be congenital tumors. Symptoms commonly include pituitary-hypothalamic-chiasmal derangement. Often, IICP is present. Symptoms are often subtle and long-standing. The tumor can be excised successfully in a majority of cases. After surgery, careful management of temperature and water balance is needed. Mortality ranges from 5% to 8%.

Pituitary tumors include both nonfunctional (producing their effect by pressure on surrounding structures) and functional hormonal tumors. They are age linked, becoming increasingly numerous with each decade. By the eightieth year, small adenomas are found in more than 20% of pituitary glands. Only a few enlarge the sella. Usually, they arise in the anterior pituitary. They may compress the optic chiasm and other surrounding structures. Usually, they are recognized because of endocrine abnormalities and visual problems. In both men and women, 60% to 79% secrete prolactin, 10% to 15% secrete growth hormone, and a few secrete adrenocorticotropic hormone. Proton beam radiation or transphenoidal microsurgery is used. Hormone imbalance must be treated. In many cases, a dopamine agonist, bromocriptine, is the only treatment needed or is used in conjunction with others.

The prognosis and outcome of the occurrence of any tumor is made by the informed opinion of the pathologist and clinician as a result of previous collaborative experience and joint correlative studies in neurooncology. Again, in this field it must be noted that two tumors of similar cellularity, mitotic rate, and other characteristics in fact usually do not exhibit the same biologic behavior.

Clinical Features
Pathophysiology

The cranial cavity has a restricted volume and contains three elements: brain, CSF, and blood. Because all are relatively incompressible, any increase in bulk in one means that one or both of the others must decrease in volume. The converse is also true: a decrease in volume of one results in an increase in volume of one or both of the other components. The pressures must remain constant at all times. When the bulk of one component increases beyond the compensatory capacity of the other components, IICP occurs, with some significant consequences for the patient.

Tumors first displace CSF from the ventricles and subarachnoid space into the spinal subarachnoid space and the perioptic subarachnoid space. Pressures are transmitted undiminished throughout the brain and spinal cord spaces. Lumbar pressure rises, and pressure in the optic nerve increases owing to diminished venous drainage, which results in papilledema.

Pressure in the microvasculature surrounding the tumor rises, and this increase along with the release of tumor factors damages the blood–brain barrier. Fluid accumulates around the tumor site in the brain (vasogenic edema). An increase in venous pressure and in CSF pressure results in diminished resorption of CSF and further edema. With an increase in venous pressure, arterial pressure also increases and is accompanied by bradycardia. Carbon dioxide accumulates in the vasomotor centers of the medulla and carotid bodies, resulting in cardiovascular changes and in respiratory changes (irregularity and arrest). The preceding changes occur in the sequence described—early to late.

Brain Edema. A prominent feature of cerebral tumors is brain edema. Malignant intracerebral tumors (specifically, glioblastomas and metastatic tumors) cause the greatest degree of cerebral edema. Vasogenic edema occurs as a result of the processes discussed earlier, that is, tumor growth and release of tumor factors. A third type of edema commonly identified is interstitial edema. Fluid seeps into the periventricular tissues and occupies space between cells. It occurs when pressure (specifically from CSF) is high.

Most patients with brain tumors have regional swelling of tissue (vasogenic edema). Regional pressure changes lead to displacement of structures, impairment of function, and possibly to herniation. Simultaneously, cardiovascular and respiratory changes occur.

Herniation. Herniation is important when considering brain tumor effects. The cranial cavity is divided into several compartments by sheets of relatively rigid dura. The falx cerebri divides the brain into right and left hemispheres, and the tentorium separates the cerebellum from the occipital lobes. Pressure from tumors shifts the brain tissue from an area where pressure is high to another where pressure is lower. This shifting may result in three well-known types of herniation: subfalcial herniation, tentorial herniation, and cerebellar-foramen magnum herniation.

Clinical manifestations of brain tumors are of three kinds: nonspecific effects of IICP, such as headache, secondary effects related to displacement of structures within the intracranial cavity, and focal effects related to direct involvement of the brain and cranial nerves.

Presenting Signs and Symptoms. These signs and symptoms may be classified into four categories: (1) hardly any symptoms and slight bewilderment, slowness in comprehension, or loss of capacity to sustain continuous mental activity, (2) early indication of cerebral disease in the form of a seizure or other dramatic symptom, yet evidence not clear enough for a diagnosis of brain tumor, (3) signs of IICP with or without localizing signs, and (4) symptoms so definite that an intracranial lesion is undoubtedly present.

Changes in Mental Function. These changes are often diffuse and vague and must be elicited from someone who knows the patient well. Signs and symptoms include a lack of persistence in tasks, undue irritability, emotional lability, inertia, faulty insight, forgetfulness, reduced range of mental activity, indifference to common social practices, and lack of initiative and spontaneity. The fact that all these complaints may be attributed falsely to worry, anxiety, and depression sometimes leads to a longer time between their onset and diagnosis. Patients usually accept these changes and complain only of being weak, tired, or dizzy. In fact, they may display inordinate drowsiness, apathy, equanimity, or stoicism. Within a few weeks or months, these symptoms become more prominent. The dullness and drowsiness may increase gradually and can progress to stupor or coma. Many of these symptoms are related to IICP and are unrelated to the site and nature of the lesion. In subjects older than 60 years of age, an even more skillful evaluation of symptoms must be done in collaboration with someone who knows the patient well.

Headaches. Headaches are an early symptom in about one third of patients with tumors. The symptoms vary, but what they may have in common is that they occur during the night or are present on awakening in the morning and have a deep, nonpulsatile quality. Sometimes CSF pressure is normal during the initial time that headaches are present.

Seizures. Twenty to fifty percent of all patients with brain tumors have either focal or generalized seizures. They may occur singly or in a series and may follow other symptoms or precede them by weeks or months.

Increased Intracranial Pressure. Classic signs and symptoms of IICP are seen initially in some patients with tumors. These signs include periodic bifrontal and bioccipital headaches that awaken the patient during the night or are present on awakening, projectile vomiting, mental torpor, unsteady gait, bowel and bladder incontinence, and papilledema. These signs and symptoms need immediate attention because they can result at any time in coma and death.

In summary, the most frequent combination of complaints in adults includes headache, weakness, personality change, and seizures.

Specific or Localized Signs and Symptoms. Such specific signs and symptoms of intracranial tumors may occur in addition to the more diffuse ones discussed earlier. With a knowledge of neuroanatomy and neurophysiology, the location of the lesion may be determined by neurologic findings. *Unilateral lesions of the right frontal lobe* can cause left hemiplegia, slight elevation in mood, difficulty in adapting to new situations, loss of initiative, and occasional primitive grasping and sucking reflexes. *Left frontal lobe lesions* can cause right hemiplegia and nonfluent dysphasia, with or without some apraxia of lips, tongue, or hand movements. *Bifrontal lesions* can cause variable degrees of bilateral hemiplegia, spastic bulbar palsy, severe impairment of intellect, lability of mood, dementia, and prominent primitive grasp, suck, and snout reflexes.

The effects of *temporal lobe syndromes* can range from impairment of perception and spatial judgment to severe impairment of recent memory. Auditory hallucinations and aggressive behavior can occur. Lesions of the *nondominant temporal lobe* can produce minor perceptual problems and spatial disorientation. Involvement of the *dominant temporal lobe* can produce dysnomia, impaired perception of verbal commands, and Wernicke-like aphasia. Bilateral disease of the temporal lobes is rare in comparison with that found in frontal lobes. *Parietal lobe syndromes* affect sensory more than motor modalities.

The *optic chiasm syndromes* often are produced by pituitary adenomas and less commonly by craniopharyngiomas and meningiomas. Sixty percent of patients with these syndromes have defects in the visual field when they seek medical care. The defect is usually partial or complete bitemporal hemianopia. The tumor presses upward on the optic chiasm and affects the upper temporal quadrants first.

Some *remote effects of neoplasia* on the nervous system have been identified. These are called *paraneoplastic disorders* and are linked with cancer more frequently than could be accounted for by chance. The nervous system has not been directly invaded or compressed by the tumor, yet symptoms occur. One example of this disorder is carcinomatous cerebellar degeneration. Carcinoma of the lung, ovarian carcinoma, and lymphoma, particularly Hodgkin's disease, and carcinoma of the breast, uterus, bowel, and other viscera have been implicated in the syndrome. Cerebellar symptoms have an insidious onset and progress over weeks to months. In about one half the cases, cerebellar symptoms are recognized before those of the associated neoplasm. The presence of antibodies to Purkinje cells of the cerebellum has been documented in patients with ovarian carcinoma. Little can be done to modify symptoms, although partial or complete remission has occurred with removal of the primary tumor.

Diagnosis

Diagnosis begins with a detailed review of the patient's history and observations by family members. A thorough neurologic examination follows. Then CT scans and radiographs of the skull are taken. Magnetic resonance imaging (MRI) and position-emission tomography (PET) are imaging procedures that have revolutionized diagnosis and treatment.

Other procedures that may be employed are audiograms, radionuclide scans, evoked potential studies, electroencephalograms, vestibular tests, psychometric tests, and others. Arteriograms are done if the CT scan has not clarified the problem sufficiently.

Skull radiographs

Radiographs of the skull may be done and are abnormal in 50% of patients with astrocytomas of the cerebral hemispheres.

Brain scanning

Brain scanning (radionuclide scanning or gamma encephalography) has been used for more than 20 years. The type of tumor affects the amount of radioactive nucleotide uptake. The timing of the scan is also important. Technetium-99m is the tracer most often used. Although CT has superceded brain scanning, the latter is useful in following patients who harbor primary or metastatic tumors and those who develop subarachnoid spread of tumor.

Chest radiographs

Chest radiographs are done routinely because bronchogenic carcinomas account for more cerebral metastases than any other primary malignant tumor.

Computed tomography scan

The CT scan is one of the first tests done after the potential patient has been identified. This test is extraordinarily useful, and more than 95% of all lesions are detected in the initial study. The location, appearance, and extent of peritumoral edema can be determined. In many cases, CT scans have allowed the designation of tumors as benign or malignant.

Magnetic resonance imaging

Nuclear MRI combines the anatomic precision of CT scans with some information about metabolic parameters of the brain. Gray and white matter can be differentiated with MRI, and thus greater anatomic detail is provided. This technique is a rapidly evolving one. MRI sees through bone and is done with the patient in a large magnet, which provides a uniform static magnetic field. Hydrogen nuclei are magnetized, and the recovery or relaxation to their original state induces an electric signal in a receiver coil surrounding the patient. This signal is measured, and the image of the brain is reconstructed.

MRI is useful also in imaging cysts, other fluid collections, hematomas, and vascular abnormalities. Acoustic neuromas can be well defined because the temporal bone essentially produces no signal. MRI is most applicable in imaging the CNS. Briefly, CT scans demonstrate calcification, and MRI shows water content of tumors. In 1988, a new contrast substance, gadolinium, was released for use in the United States for CNS enhancement only. Its use has resulted in a remarkable improvement in the resolution of the images produced.

Positron-emission tomography

Positron-emission tomography (PET) is not routinely available for diagnosis but has provided new insights in brain tumors. It does not compete with CT scanning or with MRI for anatomic localization of the tumor. Rather, PET scanning complements the other techniques by giving information on regional cerebral blood flow. In addition, some determinations of metabolic factors and oxygen use can be made with PET scanning. It is a noninvasive technique in which biologic tracers labeled with short-lived positron-emitting radionuclides are administered. A detector system or imaging device then shows the fate of the nucleotide in the brain.

Cerebrospinal fluid withdrawal

Cerebrospinal fluid withdrawal (lumbar puncture) is dangerous and could produce herniation. Under the appropriate circumstances, it is done, and pressure determinations are useful.

Electroencephalogram

An electroencephalogram (EEG) may be of considerable value, especially when the tumor is within the brain rather than extrinsic to it, as in meningioma, for example. There may be a localized dysrhythmia corresponding to the region of the tumor. A normal record does not necessarily exclude tumor, however.

Echoencephalography

Echoencephalography is done by applying a transducer first to one side of the head and then to the other. The transducer both emits and receives pulsed ultrasound waves. These are reflected from the side of the third ventricle and can demonstrate a shift from the midline by space-occupying lesions. This test is easily performed and requires relatively simple equipment. Often, it is done at the bedside when signs of deterioration are evident. However, CT would then be used for a more definitive assessment of progressive pathology.

Cerebral angiography

Cerebral angiography is often done when signs and symptoms of brain tumor are present. It can be helpful in localizing the tumor and determining its type.

Pneumoencephalography

Pneumoencephalography is done when air contrast studies are needed to visualize the fourth ventricle or the aqueduct, for example. A water-soluble iodinated contrast agent, metrizamide, is largely replacing air in most cases. These contrast studies are especially useful in the diagnosis of spinal cord tumors. Extradural tumors can be distinguished from intradural tumors, and often intradural extramedullary spinal cord tumors can be distinguished from intramedullary ones.

Chemical markers

Chemical markers in the blood and in the CSF have a role in some tumors. Patients suspected of having pituitary tumors, for example, may have serum prolactin and other serum hormones studied.

Stereotaxic biopsy

Stereotaxic biopsy may be done for diagnostic purposes so that the appropriate treatment can be matched to the tumor type.

Treatment

Treatment of brain tumors depends on the biologic behavior of the tumor. Benign tumors grow slowly, are non-invasive, and are amenable to total surgical removal in most cases. Rarely do they recur because of incomplete removal or conversion to a malignant tumor.

Malignant tumors are invasive but rarely metastasize outside the CNS. Often, these tumors grow slowly but can rapidly become fatal because they exist in a confined space and produce pressure changes inside the intracranial vault.

Malignant gliomas rarely metastasize distantly but do invade local tissue to an extreme degree, grow relatively slowly, and have a marked variation in cell population, or heterogeneity.

Tumor growth factors suggest that the tumors may become autonomous and self-stimulating. No means of limiting these growth factors exists. In addition, the fact that the cells are dividing slowly makes treatment difficult because therapy is aimed at the rapidly cycling cell population.

Unfortunately, treatment of malignant gliomas is mostly palliative. With regard to the host–tumor interaction, the tumor and its defenses are more effective than the host and its response to the tumor.

Surgery

Surgical removal is the treatment of choice for many tumors. Sometimes, however, surgery cannot be done because the tumor is located in vital tissue. Also, complete removal is often difficult owing to the invasiveness of the lesion. However, survival of the patient with medulloblastoma, for example, is correlated with the extent of the surgical resection. Often surgery is followed by radiation, as in the case of medulloblastoma, in which whole-axis radiation of the brain and spinal cord has been used.

Radiation

Differences in radiosensitivity of tumors exist. It is seen clinically that medulloblastoma is often rapidly responsive, whereas astrocytomas are not.

Whole-Axis Radiation. Frequently, the brain and spinal cord of patients with some types of tumors are radiated after surgical removal of the tumor to prevent subsequent seeding and because the entire tumor cannot be removed. An example is in medulloblastoma in children, noted previously. To achieve 50% to 75% 5-year survival for malignant astrocytoma in adults, a combination of surgery and radiation is required.

Interstitial Brachytherapy. The implantation of ribbons of seeds containing two frequently used isotopes is common. Iodine-125 and iridium-192 often are used. After the tumor type is identified, commonly by biopsy, and candidacy for brachytherapy is established, an extensive plan using CT scanning is developed by the neurooncology team. Maps for implantation of catheters into the tumor are drawn up. Using stereotactic surgery, the procedure usually is done in the operating room under local anesthesia. After the patient is stabilized, a repeat CT scan is done for verification of catheter placement and for potential intraoperative complications, such as bleeding or pneumocephalus. Finally, the radiation sources are brought to the intensive care unit, and under sterile technique, the dummy ribbons are replaced with the radioactive sources.

Chemical Sensitizers. Given along with radiation or chemotherapy, chemical sensitizers and *hyperthermia* of the tumor site are procedures that are being used to some extent and may enhance therapeutic outcomes in the future treatment of CNS tumors.

Radiation necrosis is a complication of this type of treatment and is not unique to patients with brain tumors. It also occurs in children who have leukemia and have been treated prophylactically by cranial irradiation. From 1 to 12 weeks (most often 6 to 12 weeks) after radiation, a transient encephalopathy can appear, with signs and symptoms of IICP, drowsiness, nausea, and exacerbation of preexisting neurologic deficit. Although uncommon with proper dosing, radiation necrosis can occur from 4 months to 9 years (most often from 1 to 2 years) after radiation therapy.

Chemotherapy

Systemic chemotherapy for CNS tumors presents problems because the tumors are at least partially shielded by the blood–brain barrier and because of other factors. The blood–brain barrier is an anatomic barrier that prevents large molecules from diffusing into the brain. The barrier consists of two components: tight junctions between endothelial cells of CNS capillaries and feet, or processes of astrocytes that encase the cerebral capillaries.

Chemotherapy is often polychemotherapy and is used in combination with other types of treatment. BCNU, a nitrosourea, has been in use for more than 10 years and has been employed widely in the treatment of malignant astrocytomas. It does cross the blood–brain barrier, as do most nitrosoureas. BCNU has been shown to have a membrane-specific effect. In some treatment centers, it is usually initiated at the conclusion of radiation for this tumor type. At other centers, BCNU may be reserved for use when the tumor recurs. The drug treatment may be discontinued if the patient becomes worse from the tumor growth. Patients may be monitored for interstitial pulmonary fibrosis, a complication of this treatment.

Other chemotherapeutic agents are used. These include CCNU, a nitrosourea that can be given in a single oral dose of 120 to 130 mg/m^2 body surface area at 6 to 8 week intervals. Procarbazine (a cell cycle nonspecific agent) does cross the blood–brain barrier. Vincristine does not cross it and is of limited use. Diaziquone (Aziridinylbenzoquinone, AZQ) has been found to have a specific effect on tumor cell mitochondria. Cisplatin appears to affect the cytoskeleton of the cell.

Clinical worsening may occur in some patients early in their treatment with chemotherapy. This occurs as a result of effective therapy when tumor cells die and lysed cells produce adjacent edema. The brain is inefficient in disposing of these dead cells.

Immunotherapy

The need for a specialized class of lymphocytes that can kill glial tumor cells has led to the discovery of autologous lymphocytes activated by interleukin 2 (IL-2) that are capable of destroying autologous tumor cells. Autologous cells are used in an attempt to boost the inadequate biologic defenses of patients with gliomas. Interferon has been used with patients who have gliomas. Some positive results were seen. Further evaluation is needed.

Corticosteroid therapy

Corticosteroids are used in patients who have CNS tumors and are effective in reducing the peritumoral edema. Recurrent malignant astrocytoma, for example, is often very sensitive to high-dose corticosteroid therapy (up to 100 mg of dexamethasone or 500 mg of methylprednisolone per day). There appears to be no direct oncolytic effect on the tumor per se.

Palliative therapy

Palliative treatment includes ventricular drainage—ventriculoperitoneal, ventriculocisternal, for example.

An Ommaya reservoir can be implanted in a tumor resection cavity or ventricle and can be used for intrathecal administration of cytostatic drugs. See Chapter 6 for a more in-depth discussion of the Ommaya reservoir.

Factors affecting the outcome of treatment

The prognosis for a person with a malignant brain tumor is not a good one in most instances. However, there are certain variables that affect the eventual outcome. The first is the histology of the tumor. The more aggressive tumors have a poorer prognosis. Glioblastoma multiforme grows rapidly, and long-term survival is virtually nonexistent. Low-grade astrocytomas, however, often have a survival of considerably more than 5 years.

The second factor is the age of the patient at diagnosis. In adults, the young patients are better able to withstand surgery and follow-up treatment. Their bodies may even use therapy more advantageously. The very young, under 3 or 4 years of age, are sometimes at a disadvantage because they may not be given as high a dose of radiation therapy.

Third, the higher the patient's performance or Karnofsky rating, the better the chance of doing well and surviving longer. Individuals who are debilitated and have severe neurologic deficits tolerate treatments with more difficulty. They are more susceptible to medical complications that may limit therapy.

Finally, the extent of surgical resection may influence the time to tumor progression. An extensive tumor resection decreases tumor burden, which may improve or limit the patient's neurologic deficits and thereby improve the patient's performance rating. It also allows for more effective radiation and chemotherapy. Although there is no way to predict how any given individual will respond to therapy or how long that person will survive, the previously mentioned factors can play a role in determining the answers.

SPINAL CORD TUMORS
Definition and Incidence

Primary tumors of the spinal cord have almost the same cell composition as intracranial tumors. However, the incidence of spinal cord tumors is vastly different. Both primary and metastatic cord tumors are less common than cerebral tumors with an occurrence of 1:7 to 1:10, depending on the population studied. The percentage of each tumor type also is different. Furthermore, the primary cord tumors tend to grow more slowly than their intracranial counterparts, thus providing the possibility for excellent survival with extensive and vigorous microsurgery.

One similarity among CNS tumors relates to their location

within bony structures. The spinal cord is contained within the bony vertebral column, just as the brain is contained within the skull, with little room for displacement. A small mass (1 to 10 g) may result in extensive dysfunction. Tumor growth creates a neurooncologic emergency with impending cord compression. Inattention invariably results in progressive paralysis, whereas prompt action may prevent or lessen such drastic effects.

Anatomically, tumors of the spinal cord are classified in relation to the dura. Extradural tumors are usually secondary, or metastatic, in nature, but sarcoma, lymphoma, myeloma, and choloroma occur as well. Intradural tumors may be of the cord itself, that is, intramedullary, or they may develop on the nerve roots or coverings of the cord, in which case they are called extramedullary. Tumors located in the substance of the cord are usually gliomas, including both astrocytomas and ependymomas. These present difficult problems in surgical removal. However, the extramedullary lesions are often removable when situated on the nerve roots (e.g., neurofibroma) or associated with the coverings (e.g., meningiomas).

Etiology and Epidemiology

For the most part, nothing is known about the etiology of spinal cord tumors, and the considerations related to ongoing research as discussed with respect to cerebral tumors apply. Primary spinal tumors have been associated with central von Recklinghausen's disease, and thus genetic influences are recognized for this tumor type.

The epidemiology of spinal cord tumors has not been studied separately from that of other CNS tumors. However, Levin and Wilson point out that meningiomas exhibit a striking dominance in females, arising at both the foramen magnum and the thoracic spine.

Natural History, Pathology, and Diagnosis

A tumor produces its effects on the cord or nerve roots in several ways that affect the clinical features of disease. Pathologically, the tumor may act by direct pressure on the neural elements, by interference with circulation, by pressure on veins or arteries of the pia, and, less commonly, by numerous extradural venous occlusions, that is, by metastatic infiltration or extradural encirclement.

The spinal canal itself is rigid and confining. Furthermore, there may be as little as 1 to 2 mm of space surrounding the normal cord. Nonetheless, the cord can adjust to a mass that grows slowly. It is common for cord tumors to grow slowly over several years, compressing the cord into a thin ribbon with minimal neurologic signs. In addition to speed of growth, softness of the tumor is an important factor in the type of damage to the spinal cord.

Symptoms of spinal cord tumors relate to two effects: those that are local, indicating the tumor's location along the spinal axis, and those that are distal, indicating the remote effects of involvement of motor and sensory long tracts within the spinal cord. Local spinal pain can be an important clue in making an early diagnosis, especially in metastatic tumors. Pain usually precedes progressive neurologic deficit. Such pain may be relatively diffuse over the involved area of the spine, but it often has a radicular component if one or more nerve roots are compressed, stretched, or infiltrated by the tumor. Radicular pain is encountered in the extremities or may be perceived as a bandlike pain across the dermatomes of the trunk. Distention of the dura from intradural or intramedullary tumors causes pain, but this pain is rarely as severe as that with extradural and extramedullary tumors.

Neurologic manifestations include motor and sensory deficits as well as loss of sphincter control. Motor weakness commonly begins unilaterally and develops asymmetrically, although with severe cord compression, the deficit tends to become symmetric.

Diagnosis usually can be made with a high degree of accuracy on the basis of a detailed history and neurologic examination. The use of CT scan and MRI complements the diagnostic value of plain radiographs and myelography. Spinal column films can demonstrate bony destruction or vertebral collapse, and vertebral lytic or blastic lesions are evident in 80% of metastatic spinal tumors. In the majority of spinal tumors, myelography indicates not only the tumor's location within the spinal axis but also its relationship to the dura and spinal cord. CT scanning in conjunction with metrizamide myelography is a particularly useful diagnostic tool. MRI has rapidly become a definitive test for delineating the extent of spinal lesions and their anatomic categories because of its ability to image through bone and to provide detailed views of soft-tissue changes.

Treatment

Treatment is determined by tumor type and location in relationship to the spinal cord and dura. If a lesion is likely to be of a primary type, surgical resection or at least biopsy usually is indicated. Microsurgery is used, and laser and ultrasonic suction has proved to be of value as well. Incomplete removal of primary tumors is often followed by postoperative radiotherapy. Chemotherapy has not shown consistent results.

Medical management of secondary tumors is largely determined by the origin of the tumor, the presence of other metastatic sites, and the general condition of the patient. In general, external-beam radiation is the treatment of choice. Surgical intervention for rapid decompression is employed for a patient evidencing acute spinal cord compression with quickly evolving dysfunction. Surgery may be indicated also for a patient with a radioresistant tumor.

In discussing the prognosis of spinal cord tumors, two major factors must be considered: (1) preservation and restoration of neural function and (2) local tumor control and survival. Prognosis for recovery of neural function is inversely proportional to the severity of the deficit at the time of therapy and the duration of neurologic symptoms. A slow-growing tumor generally has a better prognosis.

With metastatic tumors of the spinal cord, death likely results from the primary condition. Primary spinal cord tumors usually cause death by one of two mechanisms. High cervical cord tumors, that is, those at or above C4 level, may produce respiratory embarrassment, whereas tumors growing lower in the cord more often lead to chronic urinary tract disease.

NURSING CARE FOR PATIENTS WITH CENTRAL NERVOUS SYSTEM TUMORS

Caring for persons with tumors of the brain and spinal cord involves the full range of nursing knowledge and skill in neuroscience nursing, acute and long-term cancer care, rehabilitation, and care of the dying. Nursing has a long heritage of scientific and philosophic beliefs about the holism of the human being. The person is viewed as a perceiving, knowing, and feeling being who acts and relates with purposeful choice and values. The CNS is the key to these functions. Therefore, CNS tumors are seen as striking at the core of humanness and as having the most drastic effects on the person. Each unique human characteristic listed can be altered during the course of the diagnosis and treatment of the tumors. Accordingly, the challenges for nursing care are exceedingly complex.

This complexity can be approached by discussing the effects of CNS cancers and their treatment on the person and the family. The effects will differ and the types of nursing care required will change as human functions of the person change. The effects can be seen within what Roy refers to as modes of adaptation. For these patients, effects in the physiologic mode often require acute nursing care. The patient with a CNS tumor is dealing particularly with role changes during the rehabilitation and long-term care stages of illness. Effects on self and relationships are a prime concern in care of the dying patient.

Physiologic Effects: Acute Care

Tumors of the CNS have widespread physiologic effects that range from headaches and seizures to pain and incontinence. The implications of the physiologic effects for planning nursing care vary with the nature and course of the disease. Generally, the phases of diagnosis and initial treatment of these tumors are times of significant physiologic change, and thus the demand for acute care nursing is high. This care involves symptom monitoring and control as well as family support and patient advocacy activities.

These tumors may be slow growing. For persons with glioblastoma multiforme, there generally is an average of 3 to 6 months of symptoms before diagnosis. For those with meningioma or acoustic neuroma, there may be as many as 15 years of symptoms. In these cases, patients and families bring a long history of vague complaints, such as headache or sensory changes, that have not been definitively diagnosed and treated. The suggestion of the diagnosis of a CNS tumor brings some relief that an answer at last may be found, together with the horror of what this diagnosis might mean. Few persons, whether laypersons or health care professionals, can perceive initially the full impact that such a diagnosis holds.

For other patients, the onset of illness may be rapid. Seizures are not an uncommon presenting symptom of brain tumors, occurring in 30% to 40% of patients with glioblastoma multiforme and in more than 66% of patients with recurrent tumors. As brain tumors displace vital neural tissue, symptoms of increased intracranial pressure may occur with or without localization. Again, the nurse can help determine the symptom pattern and sequence of development. From the beginning of the diagnostic studies, the nurse helps the patient and family plan for the future in a confident and realistic manner.

When a diagnosis of brain tumor or spinal cord tumor—even a potentially benign lesion—is made, the patient and family are justified in seeking a second opinion, especially when the course of treatment outlined by the surgeon seems too aggressive or not aggressive enough. There is little doubt that surgery is the treatment of choice. However, the surgical procedures recommended vary from a biopsy to an aggressive resection. Also to be considered are the postoperative treatments of radiation and possibly chemotherapy.

Each individual, with the help and support of family members, must make an informed decision, which, of course, is true regarding all forms of cancer treatment. Patients with brain tumors may not be competent or may have a limited capacity to make these decisions, however. Such symptoms as decreased levels of consciousness, dementia, aphasia, and behavioral or personality changes may make it difficult or impossible for the patient to have input.

Once a decision has been made to proceed with treatment, an informed consent or a series of consents must be obtained. It is an awesome responsibility to sign a consent for surgery on the brain or spinal cord and for subsequent radiation and possibly chemotherapy. It becomes even more difficult for the patient, those responsible for the patient, and the health professional when the patient's judgment is questionable.

Often, patients do not realize that their capacity is diminished and will insist on making decisions. The professionals working with these patients want them to take an active role in all aspects of treatment that will affect their life and health. Nurses particularly are prepared to value these goals.

When the nurse knows the patient and family over time, changes in mentation can be noted, and the patient's wishes at a time of higher level cognitive functioning may be represented effectively at a later time by the nurse. In extreme situations, it may be necessary to apply for medical power of attorney or to obtain a court order for permission to proceed with potentially life-saving surgery and therapy.

Nursing care of patients undergoing surgical treatment for CNS tumors and radiation procedures, such as interstitial brachytherapy, requires the practice of advanced neurooncology nursing. Some key features of this practice can be highlighted here. In preoperative teaching, the nurse discusses intravenous fluids, anesthesia, catheters, pain, medications, and the intensive care setting. In addition, unique details are added, such as instruction regarding head shaving.

As in any preoperative situation, the nurse recognizes that learning is compromised by fear. In CNS surgery in particular, instruction requires careful assessment of the person's cognitive and emotional states as well as the crucial need for information. When tumors of the CNS are secondary to a primary cancer, the patient also may need help in the maintenance of altered body function due to prior surgical treatment, for example, tracheostomy care, ileostomy-colostomy care, and the like.

Following surgery, there are three broad fields of nursing responsibility: daily needs, recognition of neurologic deterioration, and rehabilitation. The nurse provides for food, fluids, cleanliness, comfort, bladder and bowel care, and drug administration with an awareness of the neurologic disability attendant to the disease and its treatment and the consequent limitations and expectations of function. Early recognition of signs of progressive cerebral or spinal cord compression caused by postoperative hematoma is crucial. Neurologic checks that must be done at regular intervals include level of consciousness, blood pressure, pulse, respiration, and sensory and motor function. Complications of craniotomy that the neurooncology nurse is prepared to recognize and assist in managing include IICP from hemorrhage, edema, and obstruction of CSF flow, respiratory complications of atelectasis, pneumonia, and pulmonary embolism, wound infection and meningitis, dural fistulas, imbalances of fluids, electrolytes, and hormones, steroid insufficiency, seizures, and common surgical risks, such as venous phlebitis, thrombophlebitis, abdominal distention, gastrointestinal ulceration, and urinary tract infection.

Neurooncology nurses at times will be responsible for radiation control and safety as patients undergo specialized procedures. Randall et al. described the basic principles of exposure reduction—time, distance, and shielding—as they apply to brachytherapy applications. Special attention is given by the nurse to the comfort and relaxation to be provided to these patients, who must remain essentially alone in one room for more than 2 days. In addition, nurses working in these situations are vigilant in providing the information necessary to make a decision to remove the radiation source prematurely—for example, rapid deterioration in neurologic, cardiac, or respiratory status that warrants constant assessment, intervention, or both, or procedures that require contact with the patient for longer than 15 minutes in close proximity to the source, such as intubation or central line placement.

Effects on Roles: Rehabilitation and Long-Term Care

The drastic physiologic effects of CNS tumors cause great changes in what a person is able to do in life, that is, the roles he or she can play. As neurologic symptoms appear, whether rapidly or slowly, and as treatment proceeds, the person shifts from being wife and mother, husband and father, sibling, son or daughter, person in the work force, or retiree to being a person in rehabilitation and long-term care.

These role changes are particularly dramatic in situations in which the patient is no longer able to make responsible decisions. A spouse or son or daughter may have to take on a more dominant role. This may mean a whole gamut of changes from doing all the driving to caring for the patient the way a parent cares for a child. The ability to drive an automobile seems to be considered a basic right in the United States. To take away that right, especially as it is symbolized by the possession of a state license, can generate open hostility and feelings of worthlessness for some people. However, seizure activity, visual field loss, lack of judgment, or motor paresis may mean the loss of ability to drive safely. In a highly mobile socity, the majority of adult roles are restricted by an inability to drive or to manage alone on public transportation. Often at this time, the patient has even greater transportation needs that are related to chemotherapy schedules, follow-up medical evaluations, and so forth.

For patients with CNS tumors, ongoing treatment involves rehabilitation that aims to restore and maintain function in regard to certain reasonable goals and to promote the maximum health possible. Rehabilitation nurses have expertise in providing care to individuals and groups with actual or potential disability that interrupts or alters function and life satisfaction. According to the Association of Rehabilitation Nurses, their specialized knowledge and clinical skills reflect the profound impact of disability on individuals and recognize its impact in the magnitude of disruption to physical, social, emotional, economic, and vocational status. Greenwood notes that after surgery for a CNS tumor, body and mental mobilization should be as rapid as the patient's limbs and mind will allow. The specialized skills of the physical and occupational therapists are of great importance, but the nurse provides both the coordination of the therapists' activities and often the challenge, motivation, and support that the patient needs.

After the drama of recovery from CNS surgery, it takes some refocusing to begin the long task of rehabilitation. Early return to familiar surroundings is encouraged to build the patient's ambition and determination necessary to regain maximum function and health. Although the resumption of as normal as possible a level of physical and intellectual activities is encouraged, return to work may be delayed lest minor temporary shortcomings damage the worker's reputation in the eyes of the employer. The nurse works with the patient, family members, and other associates to plan and implement the specific goals of rehabilitation.

Effects on Self and Relationships: Care of the Dying

All that has been written and said about the threat of malignant disease on the integrity of the person can certainly apply to persons with CNS tumors. In addition, these people suffer some unique threats to self and their relationships to others. Initially, patients fear that they are going to "lose their minds" or become "vegetables." Dementia and coma are very real aspects of many of these tumors.

It is probably those who fall between normality and coma who suffer most. These people and their families often become isolated from other family members and friends. Often, the patient does not realize what is happening, but the caregiver understands and may feel bitter. Familiar faces and routines can be important, and maintaining as normal an environment as possible can help to avoid the confusion and harm that can occur when the patient is isolated from others.

Throughout the course of CNS tumor disease, the nurse and the family assess when to initiate more support systems as patients move from an independent to a more dependent status, that is, as patients become less able to feed themselves, walk to the bathroom alone, get out of bed unaided, bathe, read, see, or swallow. The Karnofsky Rating Scale often is used to mark major changes in independent functioning.

It is not always easy for a spouse, an adult child, or a friend to relate to someone who is harboring a brain tumor. Children will have particular difficulty because of their limited understanding. Adults may resent the new duties that they have taken on because of the patient's illness at the same time that they grieve for the person whom they once knew but who has changed. All people relating to the patient need much help and support. Generally, many cancer support groups are available in major population areas. However, most of these groups do not deal with the specific problems generated by CNS tumors. Sometimes, families obtain more help from groups that deal with brain damage as opposed to cancer or from individual therapists. Ideally, support groups would exist that focused on the problems faced by patients with malignant CNS tumors and their families.

Eventually most patients with malignant brain tumors will succumb to their disease, as will many patients with spinal cord tumors. With increasing frequency, patients at the terminal stage are being cared for at home. As a tumor increases in size, the amount of cerebral edema also increases. Treatment with steroids may delay this process and enhance the person's feeling of well-being for a time. Given the structure of the brain within the skull, edema eventually causes IICP and shift of vital structures. The terminal course is one of slowly decreasing level of consciousness and increasing neurologic deficits. As hemiparesis progresses to hemiplegia or dementia progresses to coma, the need is for more constant care. The caregiver's need for support and assistance also increases. Again, if there has been a neurooncology primary care nurse involved with the family, the nurse can provide much help and guidance, often by telephone.

In addition, providing information about home care services is important. An increasing number of agencies are offering services from full-time nurses or aides to respite time help. Hospices are also available with direct care services as well as support and advice. The person caring for a comatose patient may need to learn how to turn, suction, tube feed,and safely medicate the person. However, just as important is ensuring that caregivers receive support and respite so that they can be as effective as possible in providing that care. The family will benefit from these services throughout the acute and long-term or rehabilitative as well as terminal stages of the person's disease.

SUMMARY

In this chapter, we have discussed tumors of the brain and spinal cord: their natural history, clinical features, diagnosis, and treatment. These particular disease processes have been noted to be complex and far-reaching in their effects on the person physiologically and in role functioning, self-concept changes, and relationships. Some key factors of nursing management at acute, long-term and rehabilitative, and dying stages have been highlighted, along with some notion of the range of advanced practice knowledge and skill that this care requires.

19 Aids and the Spectrum of HIV Disease

ANNE M. HUGHES
JEROME SCHOFFERMAN

The phenomenon known as acquired immunodeficiency syndrome (AIDS) was unrecognized before 1981. At that time, the first case reports of *Pneumocystis carinii* pneumonia and Kaposi's sarcoma in previously healthy homosexual men were described. These unusual illnesses were associated with profound cell-mediated immunodeficiency and became the harbingers of the AIDS epidemic.

By the end of 1992, an estimated 365,000 persons will be diagnosed with AIDS in the United States. Furthermore, it is estimated that between 1 and 1.5 million persons currently are infected with human immunodeficiency virus (HIV), the retroviral etiologic agent that causes AIDS. Evidence suggests that 50% of persons already infected with HIV will develop AIDS within 10 years.

EPIDEMIOLOGY
Transmission of HIV

There are three established routes of transmission of the HIV virus. Ninety percent of the reported cases of AIDS

See the corresponding chapter in *Cancer Nursing: A Comprehensive Textbook,* by Baird, McCorkle, and Grant, pp. 647–664, for a more detailed discussion of this topic, including a comprehensive list of references.

have been transmitted by only *one* of these three routes: (1) contact with secretions (semen, vaginal secretions) during intimate sexual activities (64%), (2) contact with blood while sharing needles during intravenous drug use (21%) and during blood or blood product transfusion (4%), and (3) contact via placental exchange or intrapartum or breast milk, in maternal–fetal/infant transmission (1%). Seven percent of the reported AIDS cases have *more than one route*, e.g., male homosexual contact and intravenous drug use. In the remaining 3% of cases, the route of transmission has not been established.

Although HIV has been recovered in tears, urine, saliva, cerebrospinal fluid, and alveolar fluid, no evidence indicates that these body fluids can transmit the virus from an infected person to another individual. Moreover, there is no evidence to suggest that HIV can be transmitted through casual contact.

Despite what appears to be a growing spectrum of disease associated with HIV infection, the groups most at risk for AIDS in the United States have remained largely unchanged. These risk groups include (1) homosexual and bisexual men, (2) intravenous drug users, (3) male or female heterosexuals who have sexual contact with persons infected with HIV, (4) hemophiliacs, and (5) persons who received blood or blood product transfusions before 1985 when widespread testing became available.

Demographic Profile of Persons with AIDS

Nearly 87% of all reported cases of AIDS have been in men and women from 20 to 49 years of age.

Females represent 10% of all AIDS cases and 50% of all pediatric AIDS cases. Women most at risk for AIDS are those who use intravenous drugs or who are sexual partners of infected men. More than 50% of all reported cases of AIDS in women are in women who are intravenous drug users. Women and sexually active adolescent females who are infected with HIV and become pregnant have a 50% chance of giving birth to children who will develop AIDS.

African Americans (27%) and Latinos (15%) account for 42% of all reported AIDS cases among adults and adolescents. African Americans (52%) and Latinos (20%) account for 72% of AIDS cases in adult and adolescent females. Among children reported to have AIDS, 77% are African American or Latino. African American infants and children represent 53% of all AIDS cases in children under the age of 13.

Children and AIDS

The diagnosis of AIDS in an infant is complicated by both the need to rule out a congenital immunodeficiency and the presence of passively acquired maternal antibodies, which may be detected for as long as 18 months after birth. In addition, the clinical presentation of AIDS in children may vary from that seen in adults. Children may have more bacterial infections, chronic swelling of the parotid gland, and lymphoid interstitial pneumonia, which are uncommon clinical signs in adults or adolescents. Developmental delays are common.

Of the 2055 pediatric AIDS cases reported to the CDC as of January 31, 1990, 58% (1199 cases) were related to intravenous drug use; that is, the mother of the child was an intravenous drug user (857, 42%) or had sexual relations with an intravenous drug user (342, 17%).

HIV Prevention Strategies

At the present time, no vaccine is available to prevent HIV infection.

All sexually active individuals are at risk for infection with HIV. Sexual transmission of HIV can best be prevented by avoiding anal or vaginal intercourse with persons infected with HIV or persons believed to be at risk for HIV infection. Using effective barrier techniques during intercourse (i.e., condoms) along with spermicides (which kill the virus) and dental dams during oral sex may decrease transmission of HIV.

Intravenous drug users are at particular risk for acquiring and transmitting HIV infection. Brickner et al. identified four strategies to prevent the spread of HIV in this population: (1) voluntary, confidential HIV testing, (2) free, but carefully controlled, distribution of sterile needles and syringes, (3) accessible drug detoxification and methadone maintenance programs, and (4) health education regarding safer sex techniques, perinatal transmission of HIV, and sterilization techniques for needles and syringes if sterile "works" are not available and continued drug use is likely.

Efforts by the CDC and blood banks have significantly reduced the risk of HIV infection from contaminated blood or blood products to between 1 in 100,000 to 1 in 1,000,000. As early as 1983, individuals at high risk for HIV infection were asked to refrain from donating blood. Beginning in 1985, all donated blood was tested for antibodies to HIV. Heat treatment of clotting factor VIII concentrates has further reduced the danger of HIV transmission to hemophiliacs.

Mother-to-infant transmission can best be prevented if women infected with HIV or women whose male sexual partners are infected do not become pregnant. Programs to identify, screen, and counsel women in high-risk groups (e.g., intravenous drug users, women with histories of multiple sexually transmitted diseases or multiple partners) are ways to reduce the vertical transmission of HIV infection from mother to fetus or infant.

Finally, reducing the risk of occupational exposure to HIV rests primarily in acknowledging the real risk (albeit low, < 0.5% prevalence rate) and its attendant fear. In 1987, the CDC recommended the adoption of universal blood and body substance precautions to reduce the risk of HIV transmission in health care settings. Basically, these precautions stress that *all* patients should be assumed to be infected with HIV and other bloodborne pathogens. Appropriate barrier protection (gloves, gowns, mask, goggles) should be worn based on the health care worker's judgment regarding the likelihood of contact with a body substance. *Needlestick injuries* while recapping or breaking needles *pose the greatest risk of accidental HIV exposure* for nurses and other health care workers.

PATHOPHYSIOLOGY
Human Immunodeficiency Virus

Human immunodeficiency virus belongs to a subgroup or classification of viruses known as retroviruses. The term *retrovirus* means that the virus carries its genetic code in RNA. Retroviruses have an enzyme called *reverse transcriptase* that transcribes RNA to DNA, which is incorporated into the genetic material of the host cell. The virus lives within the host cell, replicating itself and integrating with the host cell. As the cell divides, all progeny cells are infected also. Retroviruses characteristically are pathogenic for a long time. In the case of HIV, lifelong infection may be expected.

Human immunodeficiency virus has an affinity for a subclass of T lymphocytes called helper T cells or T4 (CD4) cells. After being infected, the helper T cell can produce more virus and can release HIV buds into the general circulation to infect more lymphocytes. Many HIV-infected T4 cells are dormant. When activated, however, the helper T cells can act like a virus factory. An invasion of HIV into a helper T cell eventually results in the death of that T cell. As the body produces more helper T cells to combat the invading virus, the virus infects more lymphocytes, and the viral burden, or viral load, is increased. It is the immune system's eventual depletion of helper T cells and its inability to produce more lymphocytes, or functional lymphocytes, that results in the development of diseases diagnostic of AIDS. Evidence suggests that HIV affects other components of the immune system, specifically B cells and macrophages. Macrophages serve as a reservoir of HIV. Some asymptomatic persons who are seropositive for HIV antibody show some immunologic and hematologic impairment.

Acute HIV Infection (CDC Group 1)

The initial manifestation of HIV infection may be a mononucleosis-like syndrome of sudden onset, lasting 2 to 3 weeks during the first few weeks after infection with HIV. This acute, self-limiting viral illness noted in various prevalence studies in 53% to 93% of subjects is associated with the individual's HIV infection seroconversion. Acute seroconversion illness is often characterized by neurologic and dermatologic findings (e.g., meningitis, neuropathies, affective or cognitive impairments, and rash or urticaria) in addition to the mononucleosis-like signs and symptoms: fever, pharyngitis, lymphadenopathy, arthralgia, myalgia, headache, lethargy, malaise, anorexia, nausea, and diarrhea. The availability of serologic HIV testing has made it possible to identify many symptomatic and asymptomatic persons who have been exposed to the virus and are assumed to be potential transmitters of HIV.

Screening Methods for HIV

Infection with HIV is confirmed by one of four methods: (1) detection of HIV antigen, (2) detection of HIV-specific antibodies, (3) viral culture of HIV, and (4) detection of HIV viral genome. Viral culture and viral genome testing (polymerase chain reaction, or PCR) are expensive and are used primarily for research purposes. Therefore, the most frequently employed screening methods are antibody testing and antigen testing.

Screening for HIV infection has been and still is extremely controversial because of the complex ethical and psychosocial ramifications.

The two most commonly used HIV antibody tests are enzyme-linked immunosorbent assay (ELISA) and western blot. Because the ELISA is more apt to give false positive test results, especially in populations with a low prevalence of HIV, the western blot is done routinely on all HIV-positive sera to confirm the positive test results. Because antibody tests require the presence of HIV-specific antibodies to confirm infection, there is a window of time—up to 3 to 6 months following infection—when these tests may give false negative test results in a person who is indeed infected with HIV.

Asymptomatic HIV Infection (CDC Group 2)

The incubation period from infection with HIV to emergence of symptomatic disease has been estimated to be as long as 10 years. However, not all persons infected with the virus develop AIDS. It has been suggested that the route of transmission and amount and frequency of viral inoculum may also influence the natural history of HIV infection.

AIDS-Related Complex (CDC Groups 3 and 4A–4E)

AIDS-related complex (ARC) is a term that was used to characterize persons with continuing, significant constitutional signs and symptoms, such as persistent fevers, persistent generalized lymphadenopathy, idiopathic thrombo-cytopenia purpura, chronic diarrhea, night sweats, and extreme fatigue, whose laboratory test findings indicated humoral and cell-mediated immune dysfunction. Despite these signs and symptoms, such persons lacked the diagnosis of an AIDS-index opportunistic infection or neoplasm. As the natural history of HIV became better elucidated, the HIV classification system was created, and it recategorized persons with ARC into group 3 or group 4.

Diagnosis of AIDS (CDC Group 4)

An AIDS diagnosis represents the most serious pathophysiologic consequence in the spectrum of HIV disease. The sensitive laboratory methods discussed earlier to determine HIV infection have been invaluable in confirming the diagnosis of AIDS. These laboratory tests were unavailable early in the epidemic. The CDC revised the case definition of AIDS in 1987 to incorporate laboratory evidence of HIV infection.

MEDICAL MANAGEMENT

The goals of medical treatment to halt the effects of HIV are fourfold. The first goal is the early detection of persons infected with HIV. The recent clinical trial that demonstrated the efficacy of zidovudine in delaying the onset of AIDS in persons who are asymptomatic but seropositive for HIV supports this goal. In addition, the CDC recommends primary prophylaxis against *P. carinii* pneumonia for persons without a history of it if they have evidence of severely decreased T4 (CD4) cell counts (less than $200/mm^3$). Finally, tuberculosis screening is recommended for all persons who are seropositive for HIV. If the individual has a reaction to purified protein derivative, it is recommended that tuberculosis prophylaxis be initiated to prevent reactivated disease.

The second goal is the continued development of safe and effective antiviral agents. Ongoing research continues to develop antiviral agents other than zidovudine that will act at various sites on the HIV molecule and at various stages in its replication. Zidovudine inhibits HIV replication. The initial clinical trials of AZT in persons with severe ARC or AIDS demonstrated improved survival, temporary increase in CD4 cell counts, fewer opportunistic diseases, weight gain, and decreased viral load as measured by the p24 antigen test. The initial recommended dose of 1200 mg/day was associated with significant toxicities, especially severe anemia and neutropenia, which often resulted in its discontinuance. The clinical trial 019 demonstrated that AZT both delayed progression to AIDS in persons who were seropositive for HIV and had CD4 cell counts of less than 500 mm^3 and was efficacious and safer (fewer toxicities) at a dose of 500 mg/day.

Because zidovudine may be carcinogenic, mutagenic, or both, its long-term safety is questionable. It has been suggested that zidovudine be given to individuals (e.g., health care workers who have sustained a significant exposure to HIV via needlestick injury) to prevent HIV infection at the time of exposure. The efficacy and safety of this practice are unknown.

The third goal is to restore normal immune functioning. Unfortunately, efforts to restore immune function in persons with AIDS, including bone marrow transplantation, have been unsuccessful to date.

The fourth goal is the early diagnosis and treatment of opportunistic infections, secondary cancers, and HIV-associated conditions.

Opportunistic Infections

According to the CDC, 86% of all persons with AIDS initially had an opportunistic infection at the time of diagnosis. Of these, 64% were diagnosed with *P. carinii* pneumonia, and the remaining 22% were diagnosed with other opportunistic infections. Five percent of the patients who were diagnosed with AIDS had both *P. carinii* pneumonia and Kaposi's sarcoma; 14% had only Kaposi's sarcoma. In general, persons with one or more opportunistic infections have a worse prognosis than persons with only Kaposi's sarcoma. Recurrent or multiple opportunistic infections also are poor prognosticators.

Volberding pointed out two confounding variables that complicate the medical management of the person with AIDS. First is the resistance of AIDS-associated opportunistic infections to conventional therapies, which means that patients with AIDS require longer courses of treatment than might be required for persons whose immune systems are not compromised. Second is the frequency of toxicities and complications related to treatment.

Glatt et al. identified six principles that influence the diagnosis and treatment of HIV-related infections. First, fungal, parasitic, and viral infections are rarely curable. Long-term suppressive therapy usually is required after the acute episode is controlled. Second, the majority of HIV infections are caused by the reactivation of previously acquired organisms and are not communicable. The only exceptions to this tenet are tuberculosis, herpes zoster, and perhaps salmonellosis. Third, multiple, concurrent infections are common. Fourth, certain fungal and parasitic infections are endemic to different locales. Therefore, travel history and place of origin may provide useful diagnostic information. Fifth, certain bacterial infections are now being recognized as HIV related, for example, pneumococcal pneumonia in young and middle-aged adults. Finally, HIV-associated infections are frequently severe, often disseminated, and characterized by a high density of organisms.

An understanding of the common opportunistic infections and malignancies associated with AIDS forms the physiologic basis of providing care to the person with AIDS.

Secondary Cancers

Forty percent of AIDS patients reported early in the epidemic had a cancer diagnosis as their AIDS-qualifying condition. Secondary cancers now account for only about 20% of cases as the AIDS-index diagnosis. The most common AIDS-related malignancy is Kaposi's sarcoma, but this AIDS-related disease varies from its classic and endemic forms that are seen in non-HIV populations and has been coined *epidemic KS*. This multicentric tumor that originates in blood vessels accounted for almost 90% of all AIDS-related malignancies.

Non-Hodgkin's lymphoma, especially as a primary brain tumor, accounted for an additional 10%. AIDS-related non-Hodgkin's lymphoma staging has documented bone marrow and gastrointestinal tract involvement as well as nodal involvement. These two cancers are reviewed later in this book.

Other cancers noted in persons infected with HIV have included Hodgkin's disease, squamous cell cancers of the head, neck, or oral cavity, cervical cancer, and cloacogenic anorectal cancers. These tumors are discussed later in this volume. They may be associated with other risk factors (e.g., age, sex, sexual activity, or substance abuse) because their link in the HIV spectrum of disease has not been established.

An interesting observation noted in persons who develop AIDS-related cancers is the prevalence of specific herpesvirus infections. Cytomegalovirus infection has been noted frequently in persons with Kaposi's sarcoma, and Epstein-Barr virus infection has been documented in persons with certain lymphomas. It has been suggested that HIV has oncogenic potential. If this hypothesis is accurate, the incidence of other cancers may be expected to increase in AIDS patients. Persons receiving cytotoxic cancer therapy for an AIDS-related cancer are at increased risk for developing an opportunistic infection.

NURSING MANAGEMENT

The complex medical, social, and psychologic issues that are linked to AIDS and the spectrum of HIV disease present care-intensive challenges to nursing.

Knowledge of the epidemiology, pathophysiology, and medical management of HIV disease can provide valuable basic information to nurses across practice settings. For example, sexually active adults and substance users are populations at greatest risk for acquiring and transmitting HIV. Risk reduction and health promotion programs should be targeted to these groups.

An understanding of the pathophysiology of HIV provides the basis for all nursing care. Expert symptom management requires this knowledge, as does the ability to coach and to support patients and their families through the long-term, variable, and uncertain HIV illness trajectory.

Finally, knowledge of the medical management of HIV is crucial: the diagnosis and treatment of HIV and diseases associated with it are core components of nursing care.

MARCIA GRANT
MARY E. ROPKA

See the corresponding chapter in *Cancer Nursing: A Comprehensive Textbook*, by Baird, McCorkle, and Grant, pp. 717–741, for a more detailed discussion of this topic, including a comprehensive list of references.

Alterations in nutritional status associated with the cancerous disease itself as well as with the antitumor treatments are common in cancer patients. Approximately two thirds of those patients who die from cancer experience anorexia and weight loss before death.

SIGNIFICANCE OF NUTRITIONAL ALTERATIONS

Weight loss is an important clinical composite indicator of nutritional status. A loss of weight more than 5% of total body weight in 4 weeks or more than 10% in 6 months is considered severe.

Anorexia and cachexia can lead to compromised immune status, as manifested by decreased macrophage mobilization, depressed lymphocyte function, and impaired phagocytosis. In such a compromised state, the patient is vulnerable to infections that may be life threatening. When the nutritional state is corrected, the immune state may also be reversed, improving the patient's response to disease and therapy.

If anorexia and a subsequent malnutrition occur during cancer therapy, the effect may be disabling and may even interrupt the therapy. Surgical patients with recent substantial weight loss may experience impaired wound healing. For patients receiving selected antitumor chemotherapy, nutritional compromise frequently occurs after other treatments associated with side effects, such as nausea, vomiting, and mucosal ulcerations. In combination, these side effects can be dose limiting, thus decreasing the amount of chemotherapy that was administered to levels below therapeutic doses.

The most devastating nutritional consequence associated with cancer is cachexia, a profound systemic abnormality in host metabolism that is characterized by weakness, wasting, general depletion, redistribution of host components, hormonal aberrations, and progressive failure in vital function. Cachexia is a common occurrence in progressive malignancy and is seen in as many as two thirds of terminally ill cancer patients.

DeWys et al. described the nutritional problems in patients with cancer, focusing on both the frequency of weight loss in a variety of tumor types and the prognostic importance of weight loss before survival. Data were collected from 3047 patients enrolled in 12 chemotherapy protocols of the Eastern Cooperative Oncology Group (ECOG). Weight loss, defined both as (1) percentage loss when current weight is compared with the patient's weight before illness and (2) loss within the previous 6 months, was collected by patient interview. Results revealed that 46% of the patients experienced no weight loss, 22% demonstrated less than 5% weight loss, 17% experienced a weight loss between 5% and 10%, and 15% experienced greater than

10% weight loss. For 9 of the 12 chemotherapy protocols, survival was significantly shorter in patients who had experienced weight loss when compared to those who had not lost weight. Furthermore, any occurrence of weight loss appeared to constitute the essential prognostic factor, not whether or not the patient dropped significantly below ideal body weight.

PHYSIOLOGIC FEATURES OF NUTRITION

Provision of adequate nutrition at the cellular level involves a number of processes, including ingestion of food, digestion, absorption, elimination, and metabolism. Each of these processes provides critical components in the chain of events that maintains cellular nutrition. Digestion and absorption occur throughout the gastrointestinal tract. Accessory organs, such as the liver and pancreas, provide substances critical to both digestion and metabolism.

Ingestion

In health, control of food ingestion includes physiologic, psychologic, and sociocultural factors. A functional gastrointestinal tract is essential.

Physiologic factors

Physiologic factors include central and peripheral components. The central components are located in the central nervous system and function as a central integrating and ingestion controlling center. For example, the glucostatic hypothalamic dual center hypothesis predicts a central nervous system component with two centers: (1) the feeding center, which activates feeding, and (2) the satiety center, which inhibits feeding behavior. It has been hypothesized that the source of stimulation for these centers is the blood glucose level. Peripheral components include a system of sensors for taste and smell in the oronasal region, a system of sensors that is primarily volumetric in the upper gastrointestinal tract, and a system of sensors (for example, in the liver) that is responsive to changes in metabolites and hormones in the blood.

Psychologic factors

Psychologic factors are influential in the control of dietary intake as well. Emotional states, such as depression and anxiety, have been known to result in decreased dietary intake. Stress has been associated with both decreases and increases in dietary intake, whereas other factors, such as time of day, have been associated with the initiation of feeding activity. Other factors associated with food intake include the pleasure of good meals enjoyed in an ambient atmosphere.

Sociocultural factors

Sociocultural factors are influential in determining the environment for eating, the companions with whom people eat, and the specific types of foods that are prepared and eaten.

Digestion

The mouth, esophagus, stomach, small intestine, and large intestine form the major anatomic structures of the gastrointestinal tract. The esophagus is a muscular, collapsible tube through which ingested food passes to the stomach. Digestion occurs primarily in the stomach and the small intestine. Other organs, namely the liver, gallbladder, and pancreas, facilitate digestion by secretion of enzymes and hormones. Enzymes contained in oral, gastric, and intestinal secretions initiate and aid the breakdown of ingested complex food substances into simpler components that are more readily absorbed, such as glucose, fatty acids, and amino acids.

Metabolism

Metabolism is the process by which energy is provided to drive the various vital body and cellular functions. This energy is provided as the digestive end products are used by various cells. Energy is used by cells to build tissue and secrete substances.

OCCURRENCE OF NUTRITIONAL DEPLETION IN CANCER AND DURING CANCER TREATMENT
Dysfunctional Gastrointestinal Tract

Diminished dietary intake in cancer patients is related to abnormalities of digestion and absorption in the gastrointestinal tract. Two potential processes may occur: tumors that impinge directly on the gastrointestinal tract and accessory organs and changes within the gastrointestinal tract that are associated with malnutrition.

Tumors that arise in or impinge on the gastrointestinal tract may directly affect nutritional status by interfering with the ingestion, digestion, or absorption of food. Tumors located at different anatomic locations affect nutritional status differently. For example, the difficulty resulting from tumors of the head and neck is primarily one of mechanical interference with food intake and chewing that results in decreased food ingestion.

When the malnourished state is present for a sufficiently long time to cause changes in the small intestinal lining, a vicious cycle of further depletion may occur. The migrating cells of the intestinal villi are shed into the intestinal lining, carrying with them enzymes used in the digestion of food. When a malnourished state persists, changes in this lining occur that include decreases in numbers of villi and result in reduction of available intestinal enzymes so that malabsorption occurs. This frequently is referred to clinically as the smooth bowel syndrome.

Central Nervous System Disturbances

Evidence has been found that links nutritional depletion with disturbances in the CNS. One mechanism involves the hypothesis that as brain tryptophan levels increase, serotonin synthesis increases. Because high levels of brain serotonin can cause anorexia, patients with cancer may experience anorexia when increased levels of tryptophan are present. The source of the tryptophan that leads to greater serotonin turnover has not been determined.

Other causes of CNS−related anorexia include the occurrence of distressing symptoms, such as nausea, vomiting, and pain.

Early satiety is yet another general symptom that leads to decreased gastric emptying, slow peristalsis, and complaints of feeling of fullness.

Peripheral Factors

Peripheral factors originating in the oral−gustatory system have been implicated in decreased intake experienced by cancer patients. Such disturbances include stomatitis or mucositis, xerostomia, taste and smell changes, and learned food aversions.

Bernstein hypothesized that tumor growth may suppress appetite indirectly by causing learned food aversions. These aversions are learned because they are associated with unpleasant internal symptoms that ultimately result in decreased dietary intake.

Dental problems may occur in a variety of cancer populations but can be particularly important when found in patients already experiencing eating problems. Dental problems lead to nutritional disorders because they frequently result in patients' limiting their dietary selections, especially to diets low in protein and total calories.

Changes in Metabolic Requirements

If decreased food intake alone accounted for the nutritional depletion frequently observed in patients with cancer, provision of excess calories should reverse the depletion. Although such an approach is sometimes successful, a large number of patients with cancer lose weight out of proportion to their intake. Provision of adequate calories by oral, enteral, or parenteral routes does not change median survival rates of patients with advanced cancer. Abnormalities in energy expenditure and in glucose, fat, and protein metabolism are hypothesized as additional factors that influence nutritional depletion in cancer patients.

ALTERATIONS IN CARBOHYDRATE, FAT, AND PROTEIN METABOLISM

Marked changes in the metabolism of carbohydrate, fat, and protein have been demonstrated in patients with cancer.

Alterations in Carbohydrate Metabolism

Several abnormalities in glucose metabolism have been observed in cancer, including increased occurrence of amino acid derived from glucose production via gluconeogenesis.

Two additional alterations are an increased cycling of energy-expensive lactate to glucose via the Cori cycle and a slower decrease in blood glucose levels during glucose tolerance tests. The latter finding is consistent with data on impaired glucose tolerance or insulin resistance that has been revealed by several studies.

Alterations in Fat Metabolism

Alterations in fat metabolism have been observed in cancer, but their exact mechanisms are not known. Profound wasting of body fat in cachectic persons occurs. A potential explanation for this wasting is the production by the tumor tissue of lipolytic substances that increase mobilization of fat.

Some studies have demonstrated the inability of the patient who has cancer to adapt to chronic starvation by utilization of fat stores. Instead, gluconeogenesis continues to occur from amino acid sources.

Alterations in Protein Metabolism

Studies of altered protein metabolism in cancer revealed increased glucose-to-alanine conversion, increased alanine levels, and increased flux of alanine from the circulation. These findings are consistent with the conversion of alanine to glucose via gluconeogenesis and illustrate the patient's inability during starvation to spare protein-derived glucose from being used as fuel.

One explanation of the nutritional depletion that occurs in patients with cancer focuses on alterations in energy expenditure and in carbohydrate, fat, and protein metabolism. Findings demonstrate abnormalities, but patterns are not consistent and the degree of abnormality demonstrated does not account for the extent of weight loss that occurs in most patients. It appears that although alterations in energy expenditure and carbohydrate, fat, and protein metabolism may account for some of the nutritional depletion seen in patients with cancer, decreases in dietary intake continue to play a major role in the continued and profound weight loss observed.

PSYCHOSOCIAL FACTORS INFLUENCING NUTRITIONAL DEPLETION

A number of psychosocial factors are thought to be associated with nutritional depletion in cancer patients. In the work reported by Holland et al., three general areas of anorexia have been identified: (1) anorexia that is transient and related to the initial diagnosis, recurrence, or prognosis of disease, (2) anorexia related to cancer treatment, and (3) anorexia related to the disease.

Social factors related to nutritional depletion that are experienced by patients with cancer include cultural differences reflected in choices of food during hospitalization, absence of usual eating companions, and the inability to consume usual foods. For example, if the normal diet includes spicy, highly seasoned foods and the patient is undergoing treatment that leads to a sore, inflamed mouth, these foods are no longer tolerated.

Examination of factors influencing dietary intake and feeding behavior reveals a multifactorial, redundant model, composed of physiologic, psychologic, and sociocultural factors. Interference with one of the factors may produce a temporary decrease in dietary intake, whereas interference with several of the factors over a period of time could result in devastating nutritional problems.

In patients with cancer, diverse physiologic and psychosocial factors influence food intake by decreasing dietary intake and increasing metabolic need. To prevent serious nutritional depletion, early and consistent interventions for the precipitating problems are needed. Although nurses' knowledge regarding what exact nutritional approaches are needed is incomplete, plans to help patients, especially those undergoing active treatment, must be comprehensive and individualized.

ASSESSMENT AND MANAGEMENT OF NUTRITIONAL PROBLEMS
Nutritional Abnormalities in the Person with Cancer

Nutritional abnormalities in patients with cancer occur as a result of the tumor itself or as a consequence of the effects of various cancer treatment methods, including surgery, chemotherapy, radiation therapy, and immunotherapy, used alone or in combination.

Definition

Malnutrition, or nutritional depletion, occurs when provision of energy and nutrients is inadequate to sustain the functioning of all physiologic systems. *Malnutrition, or macronutrient deficiency(ies),* commonly observed in some patients with cancer may be categorized as adult marasmus (chronic depletion of muscle and fat), acute visceral attrition (kwashiorkor-like), or a combination of the two (protein-calorie malnutrition). Malnutrition occurs when intake of nutrients is inadequate, in terms of either quantity or quality, to meet metabolic needs.

The term *protein-calorie malnutrition,* also called *protein-energy malnutrition,* includes a wide spectrum of general nutritional conditions that range clinically from almost undetectable symptoms to frank starvation and kwashiorkor. Protein-energy malnutrition results from a protracted period in which the patient fails to ingest or receive adequate amounts of energy and protein, resulting in a combination of marasmus and kwashiorkor. *Marasmus* occurs as a result of prolonged inadequate intake of energy sources during (metabolically) unstressed starvation. Marasmus is characterized by gradual wasting of body fat and skeletal muscle mass, with preservation of visceral proteins (serum albumin, transferrin, and prealbumin) and immunocompetence. The marasmic individual has minimal nutritional reserves and tolerates repeated or prolonged stress poorly. *Kwashiorkor* is the term used for another type of malnutrition that occurs as a result of stressed starvation and an inadequate intake of protein relative to energy. Kwashiorkor is characterized by preserved anthropometric measurements, especially fat stores, low visceral protein levels (serum albumin, transferrin, and prealbumin), and measures that reflect impaired immunologic function, specifically impaired cell-mediated immunity. In addition, muscle wasting may occur after prolonged catabolic conditions. The person suffering from kwashiorkor may not appear overly thin because of the presence of edema. Frequently, the patient with cancer experiences a combination of the two. Combined marasmus-kwashiorkor is characterized by skeletal muscle wasting, depletion of fat stores, low serum visceral protein concentrations, such as serum albumin and transferrin, and impaired immunocompetence. Persons with the combined form are at greatest risk of serious morbidity and mortality if nutritional support is not provided.

Causes of malnutrition

The degree of malnutrition that occurs is influenced by the anatomic site of the tumor, the extent of disease, and duration, amount, and combination of antitumor therapy. The frequency with which malnutrition is reported varies, but it tends to occur more commonly with tumors at certain sites, specifically tumors of the head and neck, CNS, gastrointestinal tract, and lung. In addition, highly malignant lymphomas also frequently are accompanied by malnutrition.

Surgery. Surgery is performed with both curative and palliative intent. Surgery can affect the development of malnutrition because of the normally expected increased metabolic demands that result simply from perioperative catabolism. Surgery is at times associated with undesirable prolonged periods (greater than 10 days) of inadequate nutritional intake resulting from preoperative diagnostic workups, surgery itself and its requisite healing period, or surgical complications. In addition, radical resection of specific anatomic sites is likely to impair the patient's ability to ingest, digest, or absorb nutrients, resulting in chronic nutritional consequences. These anatomic sites include the head and neck region and the gastrointestinal tract.

Radiation Therapy. Although radiation therapy has desired therapeutic effects in that it kills tumor cells, it also causes changes in or destruction of normal cells. Radiation therapy factors that are reported to affect the development of nutritional problems include (1) the part of the body in the radiation field, (2) the intensity of the radiation tumor dose, (3) the time period over which radiation therapy is delivered, (4) the volume of tissue that receives radiation therapy, (5) the nutritional status of the patient when he or she begins radiation therapy, (6) the sensitivity of the tissue to radiation, and (7) the person's general physical and psychologic status before treatment. Side effects and complications of radiation therapy may be fairly immediate, beginning as early as within 2 to 4 weeks after initiating radiation therapy or within 6 weeks after completing radiation therapy. Late effects of radiation therapy may be extensive and irreversible, occurring years after the culmination of radiation therapy.

Chemotherapy. Antitumor chemotherapy contributes to the development of malnutrition by interfering with the person's ability to ingest nutrients. As with radiation therapy, not only is chemotherapy therapeutic in that it kills tumor cells, but also it can cause side effects and toxicities, such as taste changes, nausea, vomiting, stomatitis, anorexia, and diarrhea, which interfere with intake. In addition, the subsequent development of malnutrition impairs the digestive and absorptive abilities of the gastrointestinal tract, especially as a result of mucosal atrophy that further compromises the bowel's absorptive function and as a result of dysfunction of major organ systems, such as the liver.

Nutritional Assessment in Cancer

Nutritional assessment is performed to determine a person's nutritional status or the degree to which his or her need for nutrients and energy is being met by present intake.

Goals of nutritional assessment

Nutritional assessment can be performed for a number of reasons, including (1) to screen for persons with cancer who are *at high risk* for developing nutritional problems, (2) to identify those patients with *existing* nutritional abnormalities, (3) to determine nutritional *requirements* so that appropriate nutritional interventions can be prescribed, and (4) to follow *responses* to nutritional therapies. Determination of which specific nutritional assessment methods are most appropriate must be made while considering the goal or goals of the nutritional assessment.

Methods of nutritional assessment

Unfortunately, there is no simple direct method or single datum by which the nutritional status of a person can be established accurately. Instead, measures that are thought to reflect nutritional status indirectly are used.

In the 1970s, a number of investigators proposed more technical and quantitative methods for nutritional assessment that were believed to reflect nutritional status indirectly. They can be categorized into five main areas: (1) biochemical, (2) immune function, (3) anthropometric, (4) dietary intake, and (5) clinical observation.

Biochemical laboratory measures proposed to reflect nutritional status include serum albumin, serum transferrin, and serum prealbumin levels, nitrogen balance studies, and creatinine-height index.

Measures of *immune function* associated with nutritional status include anergy panels reflecting cell-mediated immunity and total lymphocyte counts. Particularly in the patient with cancer, alterations in immune function may result from the disease or its treatment rather than from nutritional factors. *Anthropometric measurements* involve skinfold (SF) measures at various anatomic sites, midarm muscle circumference (MAMC), and body weight (WT). Body weight can be considered (1) as an isolated measure, (2) in relation to height (weight for height), or (3) in comparison to ideal body weight (percentage IBW), to usual body weight (percentage UBW) for that person, or to prior weight (percentage weight change).

Dietary evaluation can include both an assessment of what the person actually eats and drinks and an evaluation of knowledge about nutrition.

Clinical observation involves evaluation of the person's physical condition, consideration of psychosocial factors, including the ability to obtain and prepare food, determination of socioeconomic status, review of current medications (including vitamins), and information regarding comorbidity or other current health problems in addition to the cancer.

Reduced Assessment Schemes. Instead of using all of these potential measures related to nutritional status, some investigators have attempted to develop reduced schemes, or combinations, of nutritional assessment measures that could be useful clinically. The clinician wants to identify correctly those persons in whom nutritional intervention is indicated and for whom it will make a difference in terms of clinical outcomes.

One example of a reduced assessment scheme is the Prognostic Nutrition Index (PNI), developed by Buzby et al. The PNI is a statistical model developed to predict surgical morbidity and mortality from four selected nutritional parameters measured preoperatively.

General Management of Nutritional Problems

Two important considerations in approaching the management of nutritional alterations in the patient with cancer include (1) When does nutritional status make a difference in terms of clinical outcomes? (2) Who benefits from nutritional intervention, or when does nutritional intervention make a difference in clinical outcomes?

Ollenschlager et al. state two general indications for intensive nutritional therapy. The first indication is *apparent malnutrition,* characterized by current body weight less than 90% of IBW, weight loss greater than 10% over 6 months or 5% within 1 month, or serum albumin levels less than 3.5 g/100 ml. The second indication is *imminent malnutrition,* characterized by inadequate spontaneous oral intake less than 60% of predicted nutrient requirements for more than 1 week, administration of intensive antineoplastic therapy, or sepsis.

The second important consideration in approaching the management of nutritional alterations in persons with cancer involves determining which patients actually will benefit from nutritional intervention.

Evidence for the efficacy of nutritional support by TPN in decreasing radiation therapy- or chemotherapy-associated morbidity and mortality is weak. TPN may be helpful for three subgroups: (1) patients who are severely malnourished before undergoing major surgery, (2) patients who are well nourished before surgery but who develop complications that are expected to result in a prolonged period of ileus or inadequate nutritional intake, and (3) patients who are well nourished before undergoing surgery that usually results in prolonged periods of inadequate nutritional intake even if complications do not occur. These conclusions are further supported by the American Society of Parenteral and Enteral Nutrition (ASPEN) guidelines for use of TPN in hospitalized patients.

A similar ACP Clinical Efficacy Assessment Project position paper addressed the evidence for efficacy of nutritional supplementation by TPN to decrease morbidity and mortality during chemotherapy or combined chemotherapy and radiation therapy. This study recommended that the routine use of TPN for patients receiving chemotherapy should be strongly discouraged. The authors suggested that TPN may not be as detrimental to persons who were already malnourished, but the overall rate of complications from the TPN itself was troubling.

Determining energy and protein needs

Once it has been established that a patient requires nutritional intervention, the prescription must be based on individualized estimates of energy and protein requirements.

Energy Requirements. One pretreatment goal is the estimation of energy requirements to provide a nutritional regimen that replaces burned fuel and prevents loss of tissue mass. This is accomplished by estimating total caloric requirements on the basis of sex, height, weight, age, and disease state or by measuring oxygen consumption and determining actual metabolic requirements.

Energy expenditure estimates that provide a basis for determining caloric requirements can be obtained either by indirect calorimetry or by use of the Harris-Benedict formula to calculate basal energy expenditure. A third approach is use of a simple kilocalorie per kilogram formula to calculate estimated calorie needs. The goal in the metabolically stressed or catabolic patient is to maintain energy stores, whereas in the metabolically unstressed patient, it is to replete existing deficits.

In indirect calorimetry, estimated energy expenditure is calculated by measuring respiratory gas exchange. This method is impractical for routine clinical use and finds its primary application in research. For weight repletion, approximately 1000 calories per day should be added, for a total of 7000 calories per week.

The third method of estimating energy needs—which is by far the easiest to use in the clinical setting—is the kilocalorie per kilogram method. Daily calorie needs are determined by multiplying the current weight in kilograms by the suggested estimated kilocalorie levels. The suggested kilocalorie per kilogram levels vary slightly depending on the source, but are basically very similar. Recommendations for *maintenance* (anabolism) at rest range from 25 kcal/kg of current body weight per day for men and 20 kcal/kg of current body weight per day for women to a range of 30 to 35 kcal/kg of current body weight per day. Recommendations for *repletion* during catabolism are 40 to 50 kcal/kg of current body weight per day. Reports regarding hypermetabolism in patients with tumors have been inconsistent. These guidelines provide the average patient with 2000 to 2500 kcal/day for maintenance and with 3000 to 4000 kcal/day for repletion.

Protein Requirements. Requisite amounts of protein can be estimated from energy expenditure, such as from the Harris-Benedict formula. When the calculated energy expenditure is used to form the basis of the protein requirement calculation, the suggested ratio of nitrogen in grams to calories is 1:300 for maintenance and 1:150 for repletion. Alternatively, the actual mathematical conversion is 6.25 g of protein per 1 g of nitrogen. The recommended daily allowance (RDA) for protein is 0.6 to 0.8 g of protein/kg of body weight/day.

Nitrogen balance studies provide a means for verifying whether nitrogen intake is in balance with metabolic demands. They reflect the adequacy of protein supplied to maintain lean body mass. Eighty-five to ninety percent of nitrogen is lost through urinary excretion of urea. In addition, a small constant amount is lost through the skin and feces. Nitrogen balance studies can be particularly helpful when used intermittently to evaluate the protein intake of the critically ill patient receiving enteral or parenteral nutritional support. During treatment or recovery from illness, the daily goal is a positive nitrogen balance of 2 to 3 g.

Increasing oral intake

Although the symptoms that result from the cancer or its treatment perhaps do not obviously appear to be directly related to nutrition, their management is very important because of the impact that these symptoms can have on limiting the patient's ability to obtain, prepare, and receive adequate nutrition. This is especially true of nutrition by the oral route.

General measures that can help maintain adequate nutritional status involve (1) good oral hygiene, (2) moistening of the mouth with nonharmful agents, (3) careful dental evaluation to assess and correct gum disease, missing teeth, caries, poorly fitting dentures, and stomatitis, and (4) encouraging physical activity and exercise at a level appropriate for the patient.

Involving the patient and family in planning or providing meals and snacks that are appealing may increase the likelihood that the patient will be able to consume more. Food preparation and presentation can influence the ability to eat. Avoiding spicy or acidic foods and beverages and foods served at hot temperatures minimizes discomfort from stomatitis and oral lesions. Altering food texture may make it easier to chew or swallow when mastication or deglutition problems are present. When xerostomia (dry mouth) is a problem, serving foods with juices, liquids, gravies, or other sources of moisture may help. Decreasing portions and increasing the frequency of eating by serving small, frequent meals, six or more times per day, instead of three large meals may be more effective for the person who has difficulty eating, especially in the presence of anorexia. In addition, when the ability to consume adequate amounts through normal dietary approaches is significantly limited, the use of supplements becomes essential.

Enteral nutrition

When provision of nutrition is inadequate by the oral route because patients either cannot eat or will not eat but the gastrointestinal tract is functioning normally, the administration of nutritional support by the enteral route is preferable to the parenteral route. Enteral nutrition promotes more efficient utilization of nutrients and better preservation of intestinal functioning than administration by the parenteral route.

Enteral administration can be by bolus, intermittently by pump, or continuously by pump. Bolus feedings are much easier to provide as long as they are tolerated well and do not cause symptoms, such as nausea, vomiting, discomfort, or diarrhea.

A number of anatomic locations are possible for insertion of gastric tubes for enteral feedings, including but not limited to (1) nasogastric intubation, (2) a gastrostomy tube placed surgically through the abdominal wall, (3) an endoscopically placed percutaneous endoscopically guided gastrostomy (PEG) tube, or (4) cervical feeding esophagostomy or pharyngostomy. Occasionally, an enteral feeding tube called a jejunostomy is inserted into the small intestine, in which case bolus feedings are not tolerated, and a continuous infusion pump must be used.

Selection of enteral feeding products depends on the mode of administration, the patient's underlying nutritional difficulty, the route and rate of administration, product osmolarity, and nutrient content of the feedings.

Persons receiving enteral nutrition should be monitored for commonly occurring side effects, including nausea and vomiting, diarrhea, constipation, and metabolic complications. Tube feeding metabolic complications, listed in order of decreasing frequency, include hyperkalemia, hyponatremia, hypophosphatemia, overhydration, hyperglycemia, hyperphosphatemia, and zinc deficiency.

Parenteral nutrition

Use of the parenteral route for administering nutritional support is the least preferable. Because of the increased risk of mechanical, metabolic, or septic complications, the greater expense, and the potential difficulties in managing parenteral administration, especially by nonprofessionals, enteral approaches are preferred, regardless of whether they are delivered in the home or the institutional setting. Parenteral feeding is used when the gastrointestinal tract is inaccessible or not functioning or when it is functioning but is not capable of absorbing sufficient nutrients to meet metabolic requirements.

Parenteral nutritional support can be administered

peripherally or through a central line. Peripheral venous cannulation is indicated when intravenous administration of nutrient solutions with low osmolality is planned for limited periods of time. Peripheral intravenous nutritional support is used most effectively for weight maintenance in nonhypermetabolic patients (BEE less than 1800 kcal/day), for maintenance before initiating central parenteral feeding, or for supplementing tube feedings. It also is used to limit protein breakdown in stable postoperative patients whose oral intake is expected to return to adequate levels within 10 days.

All essential nutrients, including water, energy, protein in the form of essential amino acids, essential fatty acids, minerals, electrolytes, trace minerals, and vitamins, must be provided by TPN. Sixty to eighty percent of the calories are supplied by the dextrose solution. Twenty percent lipid emulsions provide 1.1 to 2.0 kcal/ml owing to their glycerol and lipid (9 kcal/g) content. Although the exact requirements in cancer patients are unknown, it is generally recommended that at least 20% of daily energy requirements be provided as lipid.

Administration of parenteral nutrition through a long-term venous access device—TPN—requires placement of a central venous line into the subclavian vein or an alternative anatomic site that can tolerate high-volume, high-osmolality infusions.

SPECIAL PROBLEMS ASSOCIATED WITH NUTRITIONAL DEPLETION
Early Satiety
Definition

Early satiety is experienced as a feeling of fullness shortly after beginning to ingest a meal. It may be caused by tumor directly infringing on the upper gastrointestinal tract and decreasing the size of the meal that can be ingested. Other causes of early satiety are delayed gastric emptying and decreased peristalsis. Early satiety frequently is absent at breakfast, mild at lunch, and severe by dinnertime.

Management

Interventions for early satiety include providing the largest proportion of required calories and protein for breakfast, when early satiety is minimal. Frequent small meals may allow for ingestion of adequate calories and protein. Empty calorie foods, such as diet drinks, coffee, and tea, should be avoided, especially at mealtimes. Ideally, every mouthful ingested should provide the maximum calories and protein possible. Use of nutritional supplements for patients suffering from early satiety is recommended.

Nausea and Vomiting
Definition

Nausea and vomiting are common symptoms experienced by cancer patients. Associated causes include radiation to the brain or the total body, fluid and electrolyte imbalances, chemotherapy or analgesic side effects, uremia, intestinal obstruction, brain and hepatic metastases, infections, and septicemia.

Nausea is an extremely uncomfortable sensation experienced in the back of the throat and epigastrium that generally ends with vomiting. It may be accompanied by pallor, cold clammy skin, increased salivation, faintness, tachycardia, and diarrhea. Frequently, decreased gastric activity accompanies nausea.

Vomiting is an involuntary reflex by which the contents of the stomach and the intestine are expelled. Vomiting is immediately preceded by widespread autonomic stimulation, resulting in tachypnea, copious salivation, dilation of the pupils, sweating, pallor, and rapid heartbeat.

Several types of vomiting occur in cancer patients. When associated with the administration of chemotherapy, vomiting varies depending on the emetic potential of the medications administered. Anticipatory nausea and vomiting (ANV) is a learned phenomenon that is stimulated by something that occurs in association with the true stimulant. Learned stimuli include thoughts, sights, tastes, and odors related to the treatment. Because ANV is a learned response, it occurs after the first chemotherapeutic dose has been administered. Occurrence of ANV may increase with each successive cycle of chemotherapy.

Pathophysiologic mechanisms

Nausea and vomiting occur after stimulation of a complex reflex coordinated by the vomiting center in the medullary lateral reticular formation. Neurologic stimulation may occur in one or more of several pathways. Pathways most frequently involved in cancer patients include the chemoreceptor trigger zone, which responds to circulating levels of chemicals, the vagal visceral afferents, which respond to gastrointestinal pathology, the sympathetic visceral afferents, which respond to hollow organ pathology, and the cerebral cortex and limbic system, which respond to stimuli from the senses, anxiety, pain, and increases in intracranial pressure. Mediation of stimuli is carried out by a variety of neurotransmitters, such as acetylcholine, dopamine, and serotonin.

Management

Clinical assessment of nausea and vomiting begins with a description of the patterns of occurrence and severity. As the patient moves from the potential for nausea and vomiting to the occurrence of moderate and severe symptoms, the assessment changes (Table 20–1). Interventions for nausea and vomiting include both pharmacologic and nonpharmacologic approaches. Selection of the most appropriate antiemetic regimen is related to the different mechanisms involved. Nonpharmacologic approaches include dietary interventions and behavioral interventions.

Taste and Smell Changes
Definition

Changes in taste and smell have been documented in studies of both humans and animals with cancer. Taste abnormalities may involve the development of a taste aversion, learned taste preferences, or changes in taste acuity. Development of taste and smell changes in cancer patients may be associated with administration of chemotherapy, radiation therapy, or tumor growth. Aversions may be stronger and may occur more quickly if new or novel foods are ingested. Aversions may disappear on completion of the therapy and when tumor growth has been stopped.

Common taste changes include aversions to meat and meat products, increased tolerance for sweet substances, and avoidance of foods taken during the time immediately surrounding treatment. Variations occur with individual patients.

Management

Interventions for taste and smell changes generally are individualized to the patient. However, some general guidelines are recommended. Protein sources should be derived from bland protein foods, such as milk and milk products, fish, and chicken. Beef and pork tend to taste bitter and should be avoided. When the "sweet" threshold is elevated, foods that ordinarily are considered too sweet will be acceptable. Some patients add additional sugar to sweeten foods more. Other patients have reported a decrease in sweet threshold and develop an intolerance for anything sweet. For these patients, complex carbohydrates can be substituted to meet needed energy and carbohydrate requirements.

If supplements are used, a taste test is advised. The patient can then select the supplement that tastes best. To avoid developing specific taste intolerances, favorite foods should be avoided during periods of nausea and vomiting.

Mood Changes
Definition

Changes in moods are common in cancer patients. Depression and anxiety may occur before the diagnosis is confirmed, after the diagnosis is made, during treatment, and at the time of recurrences. These mood states tend to

Table 20–1. NURSING CARE PLAN FOR THE PATIENT WITH POTENTIAL NAUSEA AND VOMITING

Assessment	Expected Outcomes	Interventions
Determine whether patient or family expects nausea and vomiting (N&V)	Expectations of patient or family are realistic	Determine whether patient has a high potential for N&V related to the disease present and the treatment
Determine what the patient or family believes about the occurrence of N&V	Myths about the occurrence of N&V need to be corrected	Teach patient or family what to expect regarding N&V
Determine what coping patterns patient usually uses to manage stress and discomfort	Patient manages to cope effectively with N&V	Describe the causes of N&V and its relationship to disease and treatment
		Identify previous successful coping behaviors; encourage patient to use these behaviors to manage N&V
Determine the potential for N&V depending on the treatment or stage of disease	Prevent or minimize N&V	Administer antiemetic agents as prescribed to prevent occurrence; institute nonpharmacologic measures
Identify patterns of occurrence, amount of distress, and effectiveness of interventions	Provide the most effective management of N&V	Evaluate effectiveness of interventions, revising approaches to provide the most effective relief of N&V and the associated distresses
Evaluate dietary intake	Maintain nutritional status	Provide for oral intake during times of least N&V; have patient avoid foods high in fat
		Provide frequent small meals
Identify environment most conducive to eating	Maintain adequate nutritional intake	Avoid areas with strong odors; provide a clean, pleasant environment for meals

319

be accompanied by decreases in food intake. Careful monitoring of the type and timing of dietary intake is an initial step in evaluating the effect of the mood on food intake.

Management

Improving the environment for eating and providing familiar foods and familiar settings can be used to make meals more appealing. Presence of friends or family members during mealtimes also makes the atmosphere more pleasant and homelike for the patient. Disruptive interactions with family members should be avoided, and the nurse may need to ask family members to leave if such a situation arises. Providing rest before mealtime may help the patient be better prepared for eating. A positive and supportive approach helps the depressed or anxious patient to ingest adequate calories and protein.

Dysphagia
Definition

Problems with swallowing can pose a severe threat to maintaining adequate nutritional status. *Dysphagia* is a term used to identify difficulty swallowing (as opposed to the term *odynophagia,* which refers to painful swallowing). Dysphagia is particularly likely to occur as a result of the local effects of tumors of the head and neck or the esophagus or secondary to treatment, especially with radiation therapy or surgical resection. Surgical excision of structures important to swallowing, such as the tongue, the soft or bony palate, the supraglottic larynx, or the esophagus, is particularly likely to result in dysphagia.

Management

Thorough assessment of potential or existing problems with dysphagia is an important first step, in addition to evaluation of the patient's current nutritional status. Signs and symptoms to observe for and report include (1) choking when swallowing liquids or solids, (2) drooling, regurgitation, or retention of food accompanying swallowing of liquids or solids, (3) food sticking in the pharynx or esophagus, (4) pain or discomfort when swallowing liquids or solids, (5) weakness of lips, tongue, or jaw, and (6) lesions in the oral cavity.

Some relatively simple interventions help minimize or eliminate dysphagia. The patient should sit with his or her head elevated at least 45 degrees while eating or drinking and should maintain that upright position for 15 to 30 minutes after finishing. Six to eight frequent, small feedings are more desirable than three big meals. Milk products should be avoided if mucus is copious. When aspiration is feared or likely, suction apparatus should be readily available. When the oral musculature is defective, bites should make use of the strong side of the mouth. If propelling the bolus to the posterior part of the tongue is a problem, food should be placed on the posterior part of the tongue with a syringe or long-handled spoon.

The following swallowing exercise or technique is helpful to prevent aspiration: (1) flex the neck, (2) inhale, (3) place a small amount of food on the tongue, (4) consciously hold the breath while swallowing, (5) exhale and gently cough or clear the throat, and (6) wait at least 30 seconds between swallows.

Dysphagia involving the oral musculature may be improved by providing semisolid foods (puddings, canned fruit, mashed potatoes) when chewing is impaired, by consuming thin, pureed foods, or by placing food on the posterior part of the tongue with a long-handled spoon. Dysphagia involving the pharyngeal phase of swallowing may be minimized by alternating solids and liquids, making postural changes, or performing the swallowing exercises described earlier. Esophageal dysphagia may require use of food supplements or ultimately enteral nutritional support.

Malabsorption and Diarrhea
Definition

Expressed functionally, diarrhea is too much of a too loose or liquid stool. Tremendous variation exists as to what different people consider to be "normal" in terms of their usual bowel function. A change in bowel habits is implicit in the identification of diarrhea as a problem for the patient with cancer. Clinically, significant alterations in stool frequency, fluidity, or abnormal constituents herald diarrhea. However, stool weight greater than 300 g on the usual western diet is an operational definition of diarrhea.

Pathophysiologic mechanisms

Understanding of the potential pathophysiologic mechanisms of diarrhea is essential to its identification and management. Diarrhea can be classified according to one of three predominant mechanisms—secretory, osmotic, or mixed.

Etiology. Diarrhea that is specific to the person with cancer can result either from the tumor itself or from its treatment. Each of the modalities employed in cancer treatment—surgical resection, chemotherapy, radiation therapy to fields including the gastrointestinal tract, or immunotherapy—potentially involves anatomic or physiologic alterations that can lead to diarrhea. When these treatments are used in combination, the results can be compounded. In addition, medications that are used to treat side effects of antitumor therapy, such as antacids, antibiotics, or colchicine, also can secondarily cause diarrhea. Lactose intolerance, occurring temporarily from radiation therapy or chemotherapy or permanently from surgical resection, also can cause diarrhea. Increased stress or anxiety can produce increased gastric motility that results in diarrhea. Malnutrition itself can contribute to the occurrence of diarrhea as a result of decreased functioning absorptive surface in the intestine. Finally, supplemental feedings with products whose osmolality is high can produce an osmotic diarrhea.

Management

Thoughtful evaluation to determine the cause of the diarrhea, as well as confirmation of it as a problem, provides a firm foundation for planning interventions for the cancer patient. A careful and thorough history that includes review of signs and symptoms, medications, dietary and nutritional status, usual patterns of elimination, prior surgeries, and concurrent medical conditions is essential. Management may emphasize, but is not limited to, dietary and pharmacologic measures. Treatment of underlying conditions, such as pancreatic insufficiency, hyperthyroidism, or diabetes mellitus, is essential when they are thought to play a significant role.

Assessment should include consideration of (1) ability to care for oneself, including food acquisition and preparation, (2) tolerance of activity and exercise, (3) gastrointestinal discomfort, (4) family and support systems, (5) sources of stress and anxiety, (6) usual patterns of elimination, (7) pattern of diarrhea (onset, duration, amount, appearance, frequency), (8) associated symptoms (cramping, flatus, abdominal distention), (9) possibility of partial fecal obstruction, (10) nutritional status and requirements, including fluid and electrolyte balance, (11) dietary patterns, (12) sleep–rest patterns and level of fatigue, (13) perineal–perianal skin integrity, and (14) effect on usual lifestyle.

Pharmacologic agents for control of diarrhea, such as Kaopectate (Upjohn), Lomotil (Searle), Immodium, low-dose codeine, or bulk-forming agents, should be administered as directed. Patients should be cautioned to observe for side effects or toxicities of these medications and should be advised about what to report to their health care provider.

Nutritional and dietary considerations are important in the management of diarrhea, both to decrease the occurrence of diarrhea and to ensure adequate nutritional status. They include the following: (1) eat low-residue foods that are high in protein and calories, (2) attempt small, frequent snacks rather than three large meals per day, (3) avoid foods that irritate or stimulate the gastrointestinal tract, (4) avoid extreme temperatures in foods or beverages, (5) eliminate foods that are highly spiced or greasy, (6) ensure adequate intake of uncarbonated fluids (2 to 3 quarts per day), best served at room temperature, (7) eliminate lactose-containing foods and beverages to prevent lactose intolerance, (8) use nutritional supplements to increase calorie and protein intake, and (9) consider a liquid diet or enteral nutritional support if diarrhea becomes severe.

Local and systemic measures that will increase comfort are essential. Heat may be applied to the abdomen to relieve the discomfort of cramping. Substances that protect skin and mucous membranes and promote healing, such as A & D ointment, Desitin, or Nupercainal can be applied to the perirectal area. Local anesthetics, such as Tucks, may be used around the rectum. Sitz baths may provide further comfort. The rectal area and perineum should be gently and thoroughly cleaned, followed by careful drying after each bowel movement. Anal or rectal stimulation should be avoided.

Constipation
Definition

The occurrence of constipation is common in cancer patients. Prevention of this symptom by active management in vulnerable patients is of utmost importance. Constipation occurs when the stool becomes hard, dry, and difficult to pass or when bowel movements are so infrequent that patients experience abdominal discomfort.

Etiology

Constipation in the cancer patient may occur as a result of decreased motility of the gastrointestinal tract, metabolic changes, such as hypocalcemia, inadequate food intake, decreased exercise, and medications, such as narcotics and vinca alkaloids. The environment of the cancer patient may have an effect on the occurrence of constipation because of hospital admission, the need for using a bedpan, a lack of privacy, and a change in normal daily routines.

Management

Management of constipation begins with a thorough assessment of the patient via a comprehensive history and physical examination. Evaluation should include a review of medications, diet, and liquid intake. Symptoms to look for include a distended abdomen with palpable colon, abdominal discomfort, hypoactive bowel sounds, and a history of no bowel movement for more than 2 days despite oral intake of food. A small amount of diarrhea may also be present, and hard stool may be palpable in the rectum.

Nutritional and dietary considerations effective in the treatment of constipation include increasing fluid intake to more than six glasses of water per day and increasing the fiber content of the diet. When pain medications are ordered, they should be accompanied by increased fluids, increased fiber, and specific medications, such as Peri-Colace or Doxidan. If fecal impaction is present, manual evacuation may be needed and can be preceded by a stool softener.

Patients and their families need to be educated to monitor

bowel movements, maintain fluid intake, increase fiber sources, and avoid constipating foods, such as dairy products and fried foods. The best approach to constipation is to identify a potential problem and vigorously implement approaches to prevent both constipation and impaction.

SUMMARY

Alterations in nutrition are common in cancer patients. They may occur at any stage of disease but are most common during treatment and when tumors are extensive. Anorexia and cachexia frequently are present in terminally ill patients. Skillful and creative nursing care is essential in individualizing approaches to maintaining patients' nutritional status.

21 Alterations in Oral Status

RYAN R. IWAMOTO

ANATOMY AND PHYSIOLOGY OF THE MOUTH

The mouth is composed of the lips, buccal mucosa, gingiva, teeth, hard and soft palates, and tongue. The epithelium of the oral mucosa is made up of stratified squamous cells. These cells have a high turnover rate of approximately 10 to 14 days. There are three types of oral mucosa: (1) the lining mucosa, which covers the labial and buccal regions, the soft palate, and the ventral side of the tongue, is a nonkeratinized epithelium, (2) the masticatory mucosa, which covers the gingiva and hard palate, is a keratinized epithelium, and (3) the specialized mucosa, which lines various areas of the oral cavity, contains the taste buds. The mucosa normally appears moist, soft, and pink. The oral mucosa serves as the first line of defense against infection and humidifies air as it is inhaled. The oral mucosa also facilitates ion exchange of sodium, potassium, chloride, and bicarbonate. Three pairs of salivary glands in the mouth,

See the corresponding chapter in *Cancer Nursing: A Comprehensive Textbook,* by Baird, McCorkle, and Grant, pp. 742–758, for a more detailed discussion of this topic, including a comprehensive list of references.

as well as other mouth glands, normally keep the mucous membranes moist and lubricate food for chewing and swallowing. The salivary glands also secrete the digestive enzymes ptyalin and amylase. The tongue is used for speech, chewing, and swallowing. Taste buds are located on the tongue as well as on the soft palate, glossopalatine arch, and posterior wall of the pharynx. The primary taste sensations are sweet, sour, salty, and bitter. An individual can perceive many different tastes that result from a combination of the different primary sensations.

STRESSORS IN THE ORAL CAVITY
General Stressors

There are many stressors in the oral cavity. Routine oral hygiene measures, such as brushing and flossing, can cause trauma to the tissues, which results in transient bacteremia.

Poor oral hygiene habits and consumption of tobacco and alcohol can damage the oral mucosa. When mouth care is neglected, plaque, calculus, and debris collect around the teeth, causing irritation of the gingiva. This irritation develops into an inflammatory response, and the gingiva separates from the teeth and forms pockets. Debris and bacteria collect in these pockets, causing more inflammation and proliferation of bacteria.

In persons with cancer, alterations in the oral status occur as a result of the disease, the treatment, or both.

Nutritional deficiencies can cause a thinning of the oral mucosa, an inflammation of the tongue, and a decreased ability to repair tissues. The incidence of anorexia and cachexia is well documented. Nausea and vomiting from the treatment or the disease, gastrointestinal obstructions and malabsorption, fatigue, and depression are often experienced by persons with cancer and can lead to nutritional deficiencies.

Chemotherapy

The nonspecific effects of chemotherapy on highly proliferating cells can result in alterations of the oral mucosa. The antitumor antibiotics, as well as the antimetabolites, are known for their toxic effects on the oral mucosa.

Stomatitis

Stomatitis (also called mucositis) is a generalized inflammation of the oral mucosa that may range from mild erythema to severe ulceration. Approximately 40% of persons receiving chemotherapy will develop some form of stomatitis. Chemotherapy interferes with cell production and maturation. Therefore, the basal cell layers of the oral mucosa are inhibited from replacing the superficial epithelium. The mucosa atrophies, which results in an inflammatory response—stomatitis. The development of stomatitis is varied and can occur on any mucosal surface, although ulceration usually occurs on nonkeratinized surfaces. Within 5 to 7 days of drug administration, changes in the oral mucosa are seen and may persist for 4 to 10 days. Initially, the oral mucosa may have a slight burning sensation and erythema. This reaction may resolve spontaneously or progress to superficial epithelial desquamation, severe ulceration and pain, glossal edema, and secondary infections. In addition, any minor, local trauma can disrupt the remaining thin layer of mucosa, leading to further inflammation and ulceration.

These changes in oral status that result from chemotherapy correlate with the timing of myelosuppression. Oral toxicity is observed 3 to 5 days before the initial drop in leukocyte counts following chemotherapy. The oral symptoms reach their most severe form before the peripheral granulocyte nadir. Subsequently, a complete resolution of stomatitis is found to occur 3 to 5 days before the full recovery of granulocyte counts.

Predisposing factors for stomatitis include poor oral hygiene, dental caries, improperly fitting dental prostheses, gingival diseases, chronic low-grade mouth infections, smoking and alcohol habits, and older age, which is accompanied by decreased salivary flow rates and mucosal atrophy. A significant relationship has been noted between the presence of dental plaque and stomatitis. Stomatis is graded according to level of severity, as shown in Table 21–1.

Infections

Chemotherapy inhibits the primary and secondary immune responses to antigens. This immune deficiency combined with chemotherapy-induced leukopenia results in increased incidence of infections. The infections are usually those of gram-negative opportunistic bacteria, such as *Pseudomonas* and *Klebsiella, Enterobacter, Escherichia coli,* and the fungus *Candida*. Persistent local oral infections can be transferred to the esophagus and stomach, become invasive, and lead to septicemia and death.

The two normal host defenses against gram-negative bacteria that are weakened by chemotherapy and antibiotics are a lessening of oral secretions and an alteration of the interbacterial inhibition of normal oral flora. As a result, oral bacteria increase in number and pathogenicity. Because chemotherapeutic agents diffuse into the oral tissues, the drugs may have a direct effect on the oral flora. Gram-positive infections may appear as dry, brownish yellow, purulent, circular eruptions. Gram-negative infections appear as creamy white, glistening, nonpurulent ulcers. These lesions are usually painful.

Candida is a common organism found in the mouth. Candidiasis tends to occur in persons who have received

Table 21–1. NURSING CARE PLAN FOR A PATIENT WITH STOMATITIS

Assessment	Interventions	Expected Outcomes
Nursing Diagnosis: Alteration in oral mucous membrane		
Grade 0		
No stomatitis Mucosa is moist, pink, and soft. No ulceration or lesions. No discomfort in mouth.	Instruct the client to stop smoking and reduce the intake of alcoholic beverages.	Minimization of mouth irritation.
	After each meal and at bedtime, brush teeth with dentifrice and floss (except during periods of thrombocytopenia and neutropenia). A plaque-disclosing dye can be helpful in identifying plaque to be removed by brushing or flossing. If client is edentulous, frequent oral irrigations should be performed.	Cleansing of oral cavity.

Grade I

Mild stomatitis

Whitish gingival area observable, or client mentions slight burning sensation or discomfort in oral cavity.

Every 2 hours, provide normal saline rinses.

Brush teeth after meals and at bedtime using dentifrice if not irritating.

Floss at least once a day. (except during periods of thrombocytopenia and neutropenia).

Use an ice massage to the web between the thumb and index finger of the hand on the same side as the painful area in the mouth.

Provide a soft, bland diet.

Cleansing of oral cavity.

Reported to be an effective measure to reduce pain, possibly because of the intense peripheral stimulation that activates the brainstem inhibitory fibers.

Less irritation to the oral tissues as result of a soft diet.

Continued

Table 21–1. NURSING CARE PLAN FOR A PATIENT WITH STOMATITIS *Continued*

Assessment	Interventions	Expected Outcomes
Grade II		
Moderate stomatitis Moderate erythema, shallow ulcerations, or white patches present. Client complains of pain but can continue to eat, drink, and swallow.	Every 1–2 hours, provide normal saline rinses. Brush teeth after meals and at bedtime using dentifrice if not irritating. Use Toothettes if toothbrushing is not tolerated. Floss once a day if tolerated (except during periods of thrombocytopenia and neutropenia).	Providing maximum oral care with least mucosal trauma.
	Topical anesthetics may be used if needed. Provide a soft, bland diet, especially cool foods. A dietitian can help plan meals to meet the nutritional needs of the client.	Decrease in pain. Increase in comfort while eating and minimization of mucosal trauma. (Cool foods are better tolerated.)

Grade III

Severe stomatitis

Severe erythema, full-thickness ulceration, mucosal necrosis, bleeding, white patches present. Client complains of severe pain and is unable to eat, drink, or swallow.	Every 1–2 hours, provide normal saline rinses. Toothbrushing and flossing may not be tolerated, so Toothette or gauze-wrapped finger is used to remove debris and plaque. Oral irrigations gently cleanse the mouth.	Providing maximum oral care with least mucosal trauma.
	An interim dental prosthesis to protect ulcerated mucosa and provide a surface for chewing has been described. It is worn while eating and at night while sleeping.	Prosthesis allows for immediate comfort and function.
	Topical anesthetics and systemic analgesics may be used as needed.	Pain reduction.
	Topical thrombin may be used.	Topical thrombin may stop oral bleeding.
	Tube feeding or parenteral nutrition may be needed.	Nutritional status of client will be maintained.

Note: Following resolution of stomatitis, clients should again brush their teeth after each meal and at bedtime and floss once a day.

331

intensive chemotherapy, experienced long periods of leukopenia and increased incidence of stomatitis, and received broad-spectrum antimicrobial therapy, steroid medications, or both. *Candida* usually appears as irregular, white plaques with multiple dome elevations, involves localized or large areas of the oral mucosa, and usually is preceded by stomatitis. Persons may notice a dry, burning sensation or tenderness in their mouths that is unrelated to xerostomia. *Candida* can be difficult to isolate and identify. Persons with oropharyngeal candidiasis are at significant risk of developing esophageal and systemic candidiasis.

Herpetic stomatitis has a wide range of manifestations and severity. Clusters of vesicles or lesions may appear within the oral cavity and extend over the lips. The person frequently experiences pain. The antiviral agent acyclovir is used for prophylaxis and treatment of oral herpes simplex infections.

The myelosuppressive and mucosal effects of chemotherapy can result in an acute exacerbation of preexisting periodontal disease. Periodontal disease, which includes gingivitis and periodontitis, is an extremely prevalent chronic inflammatory disease of the supporting structures of the teeth. The signs and symptoms of acute periodontal exacerbation are localized tenderness to palpation, temperatures higher than 38.3°C, and slight trismus.

People with dentures are susceptible to infection while receiving chemotherapy. Although removing the dentures during chemotherapy can lead to decreases in self-esteem, chewing ability, and nutritional intake, a poorly fitting denture can lead to inflammation, ulceration, and secondary infections.

Bleeding

Bleeding in the oral mucosa often occurs as a result of thrombocytopenia. The oral cavity may demonstrate an early warning of severe thrombocytopenia because oral petechiae often precede skin bruising. The person experiences oozing of blood in the mouth, which causes intermittent blood clots to form and break away. These blood clots may be aspirated and cause choking. Prolonged and spontaneous bleeding occurs mainly in the gingival interdental areas and can increase the person's susceptibility to infection. Spontaneous gingival bleeding can occur when the platelet count falls below 15,000. It tends to be more severe in persons with preexisting periodontal disease or poor oral hygiene. Petechiae and hematoma formation in the oral mucosa can occur when the platelet count falls below 20,000.

Xerostomia

Xerostomia related to chemotherapy has been reported. On examination, the oral membranes appear dry and atrophic. In severe cases of xerostomia, the tongue becomes heavily furred, and the oral mucosa and lips become cracked and painful. Medications taken by persons with cancer that can cause xerostomia include phenothiazines, tricyclic antidepressants, antihistamines, anticholinergics, and antispasmodics. Xerostomia is temporary and is treated palliatively with saliva substitutes.

Neuropathy

Chemotherapy-induced neuropathy may affect the oral cavity. The symptoms mimic those of odontogenic or periodontal origin. Vincristine sulfate has been reported to cause neuropathy of the trigeminal and facial nerves, which manifests as jaw pain, circumoral paresthesias, and weakness of the facial muscles.

Taste changes

An unpleasant taste in the mouth has been reported anecdotally while cyclophosphamide is being administered or immediately following infusion of the drug. Eating or smelling plain, white, soft mints during and after the infusion has been reported to be helpful in masking or eliminating the bad taste.

Radiation Therapy

Radiation therapy to the head and neck region causes several alterations in the oral cavity.

Stomatitis

Stomatitis occurs as a result of hyperemia and edema of the mucosa, which can lead to the formation of ulcers. These ulcers can appear after the oral cavity has received 1000 cGy (1 to 2 weeks). The early changes in the mucosa occur as a result of the effect of radiation on the fine vasculature of the tissues, which leads to vascular congestion and increased capillary permeability. The mucosa becomes whitish, and a pseudomembrane gradually forms. This membrane can slough off, leaving a reddish and friable underlying epithelium with ulcer formation. At 2500 cGy, the entire mucosa may become involved. Severe stomatitis occurs with treatment of tumors of the nasopharynx, soft palate, floor of the mouth, and retromolar area. The severity of the reaction depends on the area and volume treated, the radiation dose, and the individual. Persons who have a compromised oral mucosa as a result of alcoholism and who continue to consume alcohol and tobacco will have the most severe mucosal changes. With high doses of radiation to the head and neck area, chronic ulcers may form.

The peak of symptoms occurs at 6000 to 7000 cGy and may persist for 2 to 3 weeks after the completion of therapy. Mucosal reactions as a result of radiation therapy frequently are hastened or enhanced with concomitant chemotherapy.

Edema of the buccal mucosa and submental and submandibular areas of the mouth and tongue can occur. As a result, persons receiving head and neck radiation may have difficulty with the fit of their dental prostheses, impaired salivary control, and speech problems. The acute symptoms of radiation-induced stomatitis resolve within a few weeks after treatment is completed. However, long-term mucosal effects may occur and may include a thinned, overlying epithelium as a result of decreased keratinization and a less vascular and more fibrotic submucosa.

Taste changes

Taste changes as a result of head and neck radiation often occur. These changes can affect each of the primary taste sensations. Some people experience a decrease in all tastes, which has been termed *mouth-blindness*. A partial or complete taste loss may occur. In addition, unpleasant tastes sometimes are evident. An increased sensitivity for bitter tastes and a decreased sensitivity for sweet tastes are commonly noted. Changes in bitter and salty tastes occur earliest and last longest.

Degeneration and atrophy of the taste buds as well as damage to the microvilli of the taste cells are noted at 1000 cGy and can continue until the end of treatment. Although some return of taste may occur several months after treatment, some taste changes are permanent. The most commonly affected tastes are salty and bitter, and the least affected are sweet and sour. The presence of saliva may play an important role in regaining normal taste acuity.

Xerostomia

Xerostomia, or a decrease in saliva production, occurs when a dose range of 1000 to 2000 cGy is reached. Saliva is important for taste as well as for chemical digestion. People with xerostomia have difficulty with speech, chewing, and swallowing. Increased friction with removable oral prostheses and problems with retention of the prostheses also are noted. The serous acinar cells of the parotid glands are more affected than the mucinous acinar cells. Therefore, the saliva flow rate decreases, and the saliva becomes viscous and ropey and adheres to the oral mucosa. Xerostomia is initially worse at night (especially in mouth breathers) and better during the day.

The severity and chronicity of xerostomia are related to the type and dose of radiation, the area treated, and the age of the person. When the retromolar trigone, tonsils, soft palate, and nasopharynx are treated, severe xerostomia occurs. If the parotid and submandibular glands are within the treatment field, salivary gland function almost completely ceases. The parotid gland is less affected when the floor of the mouth and the base of the tongue are treated with radiation therapy, and an increase in saliva output can be noted 1 to 2 years after treatment.

Xerostomia seldom reverses completely and remains a chronic problem in people who receive a cumulative dose of greater than 4000 cGy to the head and neck region.

Caries

When xerostomia occurs, the pH of the saliva is lowered, and the saliva no longer acts as a buffering and lubricating agent. Therefore, an increase in caries formation is observed, and periodontal breakdown occurs.

Infections

Oral candidiasis frequently occurs during radiation therapy to the head and neck region. The tongue, buccal mucosa, and mucosal surfaces beneath dentures are prime sites for infection.

Osteoradionecrosis

All persons who receive head and neck radiation are susceptible to osteoradionecrosis. Poor oral hygiene and continued use of mouth irritants, such as alcohol and tobacco, are major contributing factors in the development of osteoradionecrosis. Osteoradionecrosis is progressive and irreversible and occurs more frequently in the mandible than in the maxilla because the blood supply in the mandible is less profuse than it is in the maxilla. The marrow becomes acellular and avascular, with increased fibrosis and fatty degeneration. Therefore, the bone structure is unable to respond to trauma or infection.

With severe osteoradionecrosis, the person experiences pain, trismus, fistula formation, and pathologic fractures, with loss of tissue and bone.

Following head and neck radiation, trauma in the oral cavity, such as extraction of teeth, oral surgery, and denture irritation, must be avoided. Tooth extraction and periodontal surgery can be the initiating factor in tissue breakdown. When osteoradionecrosis occurs, treatment involves gentle debridement with salt and soda rinses, antibiotic packs, and systemic antibiotic therapy.

Trismus

Trismus is a disturbance due to myositis of the muscles of mastication and occurs with unpredictable frequency and severity. The mouth opening may be restricted to 10 to 15 mm, which impairs chewing and oral access. Trismus occurs when the temporomandibular joint and masticatory muscles are within the treatment field. This treatment field is used for tumors in the nasopharynx, retromolar areas, and posterior palate. Trismus tends to be more severe when surgery and radiation therapy are combined.

Treatment for trismus involves the repetition of jaw exercises and the use of dynamic bite openers, which can increase the mouth opening by 10 to 15 mm.

Surgery

Surgery to the head and neck region disrupts the oral mucosa when the tumor and surrounding structures are removed. For the person who requires oral surgery for infectious complications during myelosuppression, preoperative, intraoperative, and postoperative care and planning can avert complications.

ORAL CARE

Systematic performance of oral care is most effective in minimizing the destructive effects of cancer therapy on oral mucosa. The purpose of oral care is to provide a comfortable and functional mouth, which is necessary for nutrition and communication, and to prevent infections. This is accomplished by keeping the oral mucosa and lips clean, soft, moist, and intact.

Assessment

Oral care starts with assessment, which includes an initial history that evaluates oral hygiene habits (flossing and brushing), history of gingivitis, use and fit of oral prostheses or dentures, other sources of irritation and infection, and previous complications with cancer therapy. The initial assessment should be done before the start of treatment. An examination of the oral cavity is necessary at least daily once treatment has started, and twice a day during periods of myelosuppression.

The equipment used in an examination includes gloves, pen-sized flashlight, and tongue blades. All mucosal surfaces within the oral cavity should be examined: hard and soft palates, buccal mucosa, dorsal and ventral surfaces of the tongue, gingiva, lips, and tonsillar fossa. Moisture, color, and texture of the mucosa and debris in the oral cavity are assessed during the examination. Teeth are evaluated for color, shine, and debris. The amount of saliva and the perception of changes in taste, voice, and comfort are noted.

An examination by a dentist is important before the start of cancer therapy. The dentist performs a clinical examination to evaluate the condition of the teeth and surrounding structures, identify possible foci of infection, and correct oral and dental problems. For the person about to start head and neck radiation, the dentist can provide initial fluoride therapy and instruct the person on the procedure for daily fluoride applications.

Careful assessment of denture use is necessary to reduce the oral complications. The denture wearer's mouth is inspected for signs of irritation. Dentures also need to be evaluated for stability, retention, and occlusion. Unstable or unretentive dentures can cause tissue irritation or ulceration. Xerostomia may cause problems with denture retention. Almost all persons with dentures report that their dentures do not seem to fit so well shortly after chemotherapy has started or on withdrawal of chemotherapy.

Intervention

The frequency of oral care is determined by the medical condition of the person and the status of the oral tissues. Oral care should be done at least after each meal and at bedtime. In addition, oral care before meals helps to freshen the mouth and stimulate the appetite. For those patients who have mild stomatitis (grade I), care is given at least every 2 hours. For those with moderate-to-severe stomatitis (grades II and III), oral care should be done at least every 1 to 2 hours. Omission of oral care for 2 to 6 hours can nullify the past benefits of care.

While a person is undergoing cancer therapy, meticulous denture cleansing habits are needed. Daily mechanical cleansing with a denture brush and an antimicrobial detergent, such as chlorhexidine gluconate, should be performed. Soft liners may be used to improve the stability of dentures and should be changed daily to minimize microbial growth. Dentures should be removed while sleeping and at other times to allow the mucosa to rest. Dentures should be soaked overnight, and the oral mucosa may be rinsed with chlorhexidine gluconate. If a person is unable to wear dentures because of pain, stomatitis, or bleeding, the dentures should be stored in a denture cup that contains a solution of Efferdent, Kleenite, or water. This solution should be changed daily. Before placing the dentures in the mouth, it is important to rinse the dentures well with water. If the neutrophil count is less than or equal to 1000, the platelet count is less than or equal to 50,000, and no other pathology is present, the prostheses should be worn only for meals.

Instruments for Oral Care

Plaque is best removed with toothbrushing and flossing. A small, soft, nylon-bristled toothbrush effectively removes debris and stimulates gingival tissue. The toothbrush is held at a 45-degree angle at the junction of the gingival margin and teeth and is moved in short, horizontal strokes. The teeth should be brushed for at least 3 to 4 minutes. Unwaxed dental floss is used once a day in conjunction with toothbrushing to remove dental plaque and debris. Although toothbrushing and flossing are the most effective means of removing debris and plaque, they are contraindicated during periods of severe stomatitis, neutropenia, and thrombocytopenia (platelet count less than 20,000) because of the potential for bleeding, bacteremia, fungemia, and septicemia.

During periods of thrombocytopenia and neutropenia, Toothettes are more appropriate to use. Unflavored Toothettes are recommended because the flavoring and dentifrice that sometimes are applied to the Toothette can further irritate the mucosa. For severe discomfort, a piece of gauze wrapped around the finger is useful and less painful to remove debris.

A gavage bag or gravity drip container with tubing is sometimes used to gently remove crusts and debris from the mouth. A red rubber-tipped catheter can be connected to the tubing to facilitate irrigation. A 500-ml normal saline IV solution bag with tubing attached to an 18-gauge angiocatheter also can be used to gently irrigate the mouth. A bulb syringe can serve the same purpose. The power spray or Water Pik used at a low-pressure setting is helpful in removing debris.

An atomizer may be used for mouth care. A small portable air compressor is connected to an atomizer with a long nozzle tip. The atomizer is filled with normal saline or other solution and delivers a fine mist to the oral tissues without damaging them.

Agents for Oral Care
Cleansing agents

A normal saline solution can be made with 1 teaspoon of salt mixed in 1 L of water. Daeffler, Segelman and Doku suggest the use of normal saline for persons with leukemia because it is not irritating or harmful to the mucosa. Sterile saline is used if the person is neutropenic or if ulcers are present. However, normal saline does not effectively remove hardened mucus, debris, or crusts.

Sodium bicarbonate is used as a cleansing agent and helps to decrease odor and relieve pain. This agent also helps to buffer acidity in the mouth and dissolve mucin. Sodium bicarbonate may be used after meals for general care and every 2 hours when ulcerations are present. A combination mouthwash of "salt and soda" is described in the literature. Salt and sodium bicarbonate in a 1:1 ratio are mixed in warm water (one-half to 1 teaspoon of each in 1 L of water) and used every 3 to 4 hours. This mouthwash is able to clean and lubricate tissues and provide moderate local pain control.

Hydrogen peroxide is a germicidal solution that is used for its mechanical cleansing, debriding, and effervescence. Passos and Brand evaluated the use of milk of magnesia, aromatic mouth wash, and hydrogen peroxide for oral care of persons who had had surgery. Although there was no significant difference in the efficacy of the three agents, hydrogen peroxide tended to maintain and improve mouth condition. However, hydrogen peroxide can also damage exposed bone, and caution must be used when ulcers or fresh granulation surfaces are present because the solution tends to break down this tissue. It is also irritating to the tongue and buccal mucosa. Elongation of the filiform and foliate papillae of the tongue has been noted. The elongated papillae serve as an excellent matrix for candidiasis. Therefore, hydrogen peroxide should be used with caution. The efficacy and safety of long-term use of hydrogen peroxide has been questioned. Cells are damaged when they are exposed to a high concentration of oxidants. With long-term use, peroxide may function as a cocarcinogen. Caution must be observed when a person has a compromised cough reflex because of the foaming action of hydrogen peroxide. The person who is unable to cough may have a problem with aspirating the foam. Fungal adherence may be increased with the use of hydrogen peroxide. Superinfections may occur as the normal oral flora balance is disturbed. In some people, oral use of hydrogen peroxide also causes nausea and subjective feelings of thirst and dryness of the mouth.

Hydrogen peroxide 3% should be used only if mechanical cleansing action is essential and should be diluted to one-fourth strength. Use of hydrogen peroxide must be followed with a normal saline or water rinse.

Pain control agents

Lidocaine viscous is frequently used 15 to 20 minutes before meals to provide comfort during meals. The anesthetic effect is brief. Dyclonine hydrochloride takes 10 minutes before onset of effects and lasts for approximately 1 hour.

CLIENT NEEDS AND NURSING INTERVENTIONS

Stomatitis

Assess the person's willingness and competence to perform mouth care. Instruct the client to stop smoking and reduce the intake of alcoholic beverages to minimize mouth irritation. Interventions for stomatitis vary depending on the degree of tissue damage.

Leukemic infiltration of gingival tissues

Nursing interventions are palliative. Frequent warm saline rinses five to six times a day will help to keep the mouth clean until the oral cavity and blood counts improve. Dietary modifications to a soft, bland diet may be necessary if chewing is difficult. If hemorrhage occurs, use nursing interventions for bleeding that are listed in the following section.

Bleeding

Monitor platelet counts. Provide systematic mouth care. Use bleeding precautions by reducing or eliminating mouth irritants, such as ill-fitting dentures or retainers. Toothbrushing and flossing should be discontinued if the platelet count falls below 20,000. A Toothette or gauze-wrapped finger may be useful to remove debris and plaque from teeth surfaces.

If active bleeding occurs, gently irrigate the oral cavity with normal saline to identify the areas that are bleeding.

Infections

Monitor neutrophil counts, and anticipate complications as the neutrophil count decreases. Inspect the mouth twice a day for local signs of an infection: erythema, pain, plaque formation, and candidiasis. Observe for systemic effects, such as fever, increased pulse, and malaise. Culture suspicious mouth lesions. Administer antibiotics as prescribed. If an oral fungal infection develops in a person who wears dentures, the dentures should be removed during the administration of topical antibiotics.

Taste changes

Assess changes in taste perception. Assess which foods have altered or disagreeable tastes and which foods taste the same.

Xerostomia

Saliva substitutes are convenient but temporary palliative measures to relieve xerostomia. Approximately 2 ml of the solution will provide some relief. Sugarless gum or mints can help to stimulate saliva production in persons with low salivary flow rates. Increasing fluid intake can help relieve dryness and moisten the mouth. Dry foods and foods that require an increased amount of saliva for chewing should be avoided. Foods need to be softened or moistened with gravy to make swallowing easier.

22 Alterations in Protective Mechanisms: Hematopoiesis and Bone Marrow Depression

DOUGLAS HAEUBER
JUDITH A. SPROSS

Hematopoiesis is a term used to describe the process of proliferation, differentiation, and maturation of blood cells. Although the process has been increasingly well defined through experimental research, much of what is known about human hematopoiesis remains speculative. Not all aspects of hematopoiesis observed in animal models have been confirmed in humans. The process of blood cell formation described here represents what has been demonstrated in humans plus what is likely to be true in humans on the basis of studies using animal models.

ORGANS OF HEMATOPOIESIS
Bone Marrow

The organs of hematopoiesis include the bone marrow, spleen, and lymphoid tissues. The bone is the principal site for production of blood cells. From birth until about the age

See the corresponding chapter in *Cancer Nursing: A Comprehensive Textbook*, by Baird, McCorkle, and Grant, pp. 759–781, for a more detailed discussion of this topic, including a comprehensive list of references.

of 4 years, most bones are involved in hematopoiesis. By the age of 18 years, much of the marrow has been replaced by fat cells, so that hematopoietic marrow is only found in the vertebrae, ribs, skull, pelvis, and proximal epiphyses of the femur and humerus.

Physiologic function of bone marrow depends on a number of factors, including the availability of selected micronutrients, a specialized microenvironment, normal stem cell function, regulation by specific hematopoietic and other hormones, and feedback inhibition from cell production. The reticular cells and stroma, which contain macrophages and fat cells, provide a hematopoietic inductive microenvironment (HIM), which is essential to blood cell production. The exact nature of the HIM in humans is unclear. The marrow is richly innervated, suggesting one mechanism by which the marrow may be activated on demand. These nerves may influence blood flow in the marrow and cellular release by responding to changes in intramedullary pressure and to extramedullary influences.

Spleen

The spleen contains both lymphoid and reticuloendothelial components. The spleen is an early responder to infection; it is a site of antibody and opsonin activity (opsonins prepare foreign material for phagocytosis). Other functions include phagocytosis, storage of platelets (20% to 30% of total platelet mass), iron metabolism, and mechanical filtration of cellular and noncellular debris.

Lymphoid Tissue

Lymph nodes are collections of lymphocytes, plasma cells, and macrophages existing in chains along the course of large blood vessels throughout the body. They drain regional tissue and empty into large, efferent lymph channels, clearing foreign material from the blood. Solitary lymph nodules found in certain parts of the body (such as the Peyer's patches of the ileum) produce a local response to antigen.

NORMAL HEMATOPOIETIC PROCESSES

Normal hematopoiesis results in the production of white cells, platelets, and red cells, and the processes of proliferation, differentiation, and maturation are mediated by various humoral factors. Predominant among these are the expanding set of so-called hematopoietic growth factors, also known as colony-stimulating factors (CSFs) or poietins.

The stem cell is the keystone of bone marrow hematopoiesis. *Pluripotential* stem cells, the youngest and most primitive, are capable of extensive, possibly lifelong self-renewal and of differentiation to all cell lineages, both myeloid and lymphoid. *Multipotential* stem cells are characterized by limited self-renewal capability. These cells, like pluripotential stem cells, are not irreversibly committed to a single cell lineage, but they are more differentiated than pluripotential stem cells. The best example of a multipotential stem cell is the CFU-GEMM. The term *colony-forming unit* or *colony-forming cell* (CFU or CFC) with the name of a cell line describes a specific stem cell or progenitor cell. CFU-GEMM is capable of differentiating to a more mature progenitor cell in any one of the following cell lines: granulocyte, erythroid, monocyte, or megakaryocyte. These cells provide offspring that are better differentiated and more responsive to poietins. *Bipotential* cells are progenitor cells capable of limited self-renewal and of differentiation to two cell lines. *Unipotential* cells are progenitor cells capable of limited self-renewal and of differentiation to one cell line, e.g., CFC-Eo (eosinophil), CFC-Mk (megakaryocyte). The progeny of these various progenitor cells are termed *precursor* cells. They are incapable of self-renewal and are morphologically recognizable as members of a single cell line.

Another important element in the process of normal hematopoiesis is the set of growth factors termed CSFs. These are highly specific proteins or cytokines that stimulate progenitor and precursor cells to differentiate and mature. Hematopoiesis is dependent on their presence. As with other cytokines, CSFs seem to act on target cells via receptors on cell membranes. Numerous types of CSFs have been identified. Some, such as multi-CSF, interleukin 2 (IL-2), and GM-CSF, seem to affect more than one cell line. Others, such as G-CSF and erythropoietin, are specific to a particular cell line or a group of precursor cells.

HEMATOPOIESIS
Leukopoiesis

The major function of white blood cells (WBCs) is to defend the host against infection. Circulating WBCs are classified as granulocytes or agranulocytes. Each of these two groups is further divided into specific cell types. WBCs are responsible for both cell-mediated immunity (CMI) and humoral immunity (HI). CMI refers to immune defenses that rely on a direct cellular activity (e.g., phagocytosis by a neutrophil). HI refers to immune defenses that rely on an indirect cellular activity (e.g., the elaboration of antibody by B lymphocytes).

Leukopoiesis or *granulopoiesis* refers to the development, differentiation, and maturation of granulocytes and monocytes. *Lymphopoiesis* is the term used to describe the process for lymphocytes.

The production and release of granulocytes and monocytes is mediated by various CSFs and influenced by the presence of infection and inflammation and by exercise, stress, and glucocorticoids. It seems to involve a feedback loop in which the presence of endotoxins and other bacterial byproducts causes increased production and release of CSFs by macrophages and endothelial cells, which in turn lead to the proliferation and release of neutrophils from the marrow.

The multipotential progenitors of granulocytes are GEMM-CFC or granulocyte-monocyte colony-forming cells (GM-CFC). During the proliferation stages, these cells divide and differentiate to myeloblasts, promyelocytes, and myelocytes. As these cells mature, they become metamyelocytes, bands, and finally neutrophils, basophils, or eosinophils. *Neutrophils* are the first line of defense against infection. They constitute 50% to 70% of the total WBC count. Immature neutrophils are referred to as bands or segmental forms because of the nature of their nuclei. *Left shift* is a term used to describe an increase in the percentage of neutrophils and bands (immature neutrophils) in response to infection. Granulocytes exist in the bloodstream as a circulating pool, where they have a lifespan of about 12 hours. They are quite mobile and can be attracted to the site of infection by a process called chemotaxis. Once there, they are capable of becoming attached to vessel endothelial cells (marginating) and can enter the tissues by diapedesis. In cancer patients, depressed neutrophil counts are often associated with cancer therapies or infiltration of bone marrow by cancer.

Less is known about *basophils* than about the other granulocytes. They are not phagocytic. The granules in the basophils are related to the granules in mast cells. *Mast cells* play a role in allergies, anaphylactic shock, and regulation of blood flow. Elevations of basophils are associated with some cancers, with postsplenectomy states, and with estrogen use, but their numbers seem unaffected by infection. *Eosinophils* detoxify foreign protein. They control the effects of mast cells and neutralize the products of mast cells. Their numbers become elevated in drug reactions, with steroid use, and in some cancers. *Monocytes* are active as mechanical barriers against organisms and play a role in the neutrophil feedback loop. Fixed monocytes *(macrophages)* are found in the spleen, lymph nodes, bone marrow, liver capsule, and adrenals. Macrophages influence antibody synthesis by lymphocytes. They are sensitive to steroids, and elevations in their numbers occur in persons with chronic infections, in those recovering from infection, and in those with neutropenia.

Lymphopoiesis

Although the development of lymphocytes occurs separately from that of other blood cell lineages, research indicates that like other cell lines, the lymphoid line has its origin in the pluripotential stem cells discussed earlier. At some early point after the initial division of the pluripotential stem cell into daughter cells, the lymphoid line follows a separate course, influenced by some of the same CSFs (e.g., IL-3 or multi-CSF) as well as by different ones (IL-2).

Development of lymphocytes depends on the migration of bone marrow precursors to specialized sites in the mononuclear phagocyte system (MPS) (formerly termed the reticuloendothelial system or RES), where further proliferation and differentiation occur. The lymphocyte stem cell gives rise to at least two types of cells: the T lymphocytes, which mature under the influence of thymic endothelium (a thymopoietin has been postulated), and the B lymphocytes, which differentiate and mature in the MPS in response to a postulated B cell growth factor.

Each of these cell groups has a variety of functions. Primarily they enable the immune system to distinguish self from nonself or foreign antigens and to respond to foreign antigens. These cells are responsible for the memory of the immune system, so that when exposed to the same antigen in the future, a quicker response can be mounted. T cells have both regulator and effector functions in the immune system. They are the primary effectors of CMI and immunoregulation. They mediate delayed cutaneous hypersensitivity reactions and transplant rejection. They seem to orchestrate the overall immune response to specific antigen as well as provide immunosurveillance against cancer. T cells protect against fungi and viruses and respond to bacterial diseases that have an insidious onset.

Lymphocytes are mobile and long-lived. Their life span may be measured in terms of years. They recirculate by passing from the thoracic duct into the bloodstream, which carries the cells to lymph nodes. These cells can also be transported to lymph nodes through lymphatic drainage. Lymphocytes constitute 20% to 40% of the total WBC count. Elevations in their numbers are seen in viral infections, and lymphopenia is often associated with the acquired immunodeficiency syndrome (AIDS).

Thrombopoiesis

The process by which platelets (thrombocytes) develop and mature are less well defined than those for leukocytes and erythrocytes. There does appear to be a growth factor, thrombopoietin, specific to the megakaryocytic line. Under the influence of this stimulus, the line differentiates in the following pattern: CSF-megakaryocyte (CSF-Mk), promegakaryoblast, megakaryoblast, promegakaryocyte, megakaryocyte, and platelet. Normal platelet values range from 150,000 to 400,000 per mm^3. Platelets, which are nonnucleated fragments of megakaryocytes, survive in the circulation for 7 to 10 days. They are responsible for clot formation and maintaining integrity of vascular endothelium by attaching to one another and adhering to blood vessel walls. Platelets are also a source of phospholipids for the clotting system and for plasma proteins.

Erythropoiesis

Red blood cells (RBCs) are derived from the pluripotential stem cells by way of a unipotential stem cell called the burst-forming unit (BFU-E, erythroid). Under the influence of a growth factor called burst-promoting activity (BPA), BFU-E gives rise to CFC-E, a more differentiated progenitor cell of the erythroid line. This group of progenitor cells in turn is influenced by one of the earliest identified of the hematopoietic growth factors, erythropoietin (EP). Both in vitro and in vivo studies suggest that EP accelerates RBC production by inducing the CFU-Es to differentiate into proerythroblasts. The primary factor influencing the production of EP is tissue oxygenation—cellular hypoxia initiates its production. Although it appears that EP is the predominant influence on the erythroid line, there is evidence that other growth factors, such as GM-CSF and G-CSF, may be involved in this process as well. Red blood cell production and metabolism require vitamin B_{12} and folic acid.

The major function of RBCs is to transport hemoglobin, which carries oxygen from lungs to tissues. Other functions include eliminating carbon dioxide, hemoglobin synthesis and maintenance, membrane maintenance, and buffering the blood. The normal values for RBCs range from 4.2 to 5.4 million/ml in women and from 6 to 6.2 million/ml in men.

PATHOPHYSIOLOGIC EFFECTS OF CANCER AND CANCER THERAPY ON HEMATOPOIESIS
Tumor Effects

Cancer may affect hematopoiesis directly or indirectly. Invasion and replacement of the bone marrow by tumor is called myelophthisis. Cancer cells compete with normal hematopoietic cells for nutrients and destroy hematopoietic cells. Anemia, thrombocytopenia, granulocytopenia, and impaired NK cell activity may result.

Cancer can alter hematopoiesis and immune regulation whether or not marrow invasion occurs. Roth has proposed four possible mechanisms of tumor-related immunosuppression.

1. An increase in the number or proportion of immunosuppressive cells
2. Elevated plasma levels of circulating antigen-antibody complexes
3. Increased levels of acute phase reactants with immunosuppressive properties (e.g., serum lipoproteins)
4. An unidentified humoral factor secreted by tumors that is immunosuppressive

Chemotherapy

The treatment most often associated with hematologic toxicity and marrow suppression is chemotherapy. The degree to which a patient experiences marrow suppression after chemotherapy depends on the agents used, the doses, schedules, and routes of administration, previous antineoplastic treatment, concomitant adjuvant therapy; and factors such as age, nutritional status, and tumor type and stage.

The hematologic toxicity of chemotherapy varies widely. Acute chemotherapy-induced myelosuppression is usually caused by the destruction of the proliferating progenitors (CFU-GM, BFU-E, and so forth) of mature cells. As progenitor cells are destroyed, preexisting mature cells are cleared at the end of their natural cycles, and the nadir of a person's blood cell counts occurs. Differences in lengths of the life cycle of blood cells account for the high incidence of granulocytopenia and thrombocytopenia.

Antineoplastic agents that are phase specific are myelosuppressive because of their impact on proliferating progenitor cells, which are in active phases when drugs are administered, but they do not destroy cells in the resting phase. Agents that are phase nonspecific destroy cells in the resting phase and can have a delayed, prolonged, and cumulative myelosuppressive effect. This is a consequence of the damage they do to nonproliferating stem cells, which are essential in the marrow response to a challenge such as chemotherapy.

Use of combinations of chemotherapeutic agents and sequencing may complicate myelosuppression. Other factors may influence the degree, severity, and duration of BMD. These factors include liver and kidney function, the presence of effusions, and exposure to other nonantineoplastic drugs that interact synergistically with the chemotherapeutic agents (e.g., nitrosoureas and cimetidine). In patients with malignant effusions, drugs may accumulate and slowly be released into the circulation—a factor that may delay BMD, prolong it, or make it more severe.

Chemotherapy has delayed and long-term effects on the bone marrow. Late effects include marrow failure secondary to atrophy and fibrosis or the appearance of second tumors. Three changes in the bone marrow seem to occur in the chemotherapy-treated patient. Initially, there is a hyper- or normocellular state with a large degree of ongoing phagocytosis. Then the marrow enters a stage characterized by edema, inflammation, and decreased hematopoietic activity. Finally, the marrow becomes hypocellular with small islands of normal hematopoiesis.

Testing of a new approach to the problem of BMD has begun in clinical settings. This involves administration of CSFs or hematopoietic growth factors. The most commonly used of the CSFs are granulocyte colony-stimulating factor (G-CSF), granulocyte-macrophage colony-stimulating factor (GM-CSF), and erythropoietin. These naturally occurring hormonelike substances stimulate one or more of the cell lines in the hematopoietic system, inducing proliferation and differentiation. Thus far four primary patient populations have been targeted.

- Cancer patients experiencing blood count nadirs owing to antineoplastic treatments
- Bone marrow transplant patients
- Persons with myelodysplastic syndromes
- Persons with AIDS

Radiotherapy

The effects of radiotherapy on bone marrow and immunity are similar to those of chemotherapy. Certain factors are present in radiotherapy that determine the degree of risk for BMD. Although total radiation doses and fractionation schedule are important, the most significant factor is the volume of productive marrow in the treatment field. Radiation to sites that include major blood vessels and lymphatic channels is toxic to lymphocytes. For this reason, mediastinal radiotherapy can be more immunosuppressive than radiotherapy to other sites.

Radiotherapy is not as destructive to progenitor cells as chemotherapy but is much more damaging to cells in the G_0 phase. Therefore, radiotherapy has a greater impact on pluripotential stem cells. Except for total nodal or total body irradiation, radiotherapy does not usually cause the nadirs in blood counts seen with chemotherapy. This is because radiation treatment is a local therapy that leaves substantial amounts of marrow intact and able to compensate for the damage to the radiated marrow (unless compromised by prior radiotherapy or prior chemotherapy). Radiated marrow recovers through a twofold process: (1) migration of stem cells from unirradiated marrow to the treated area and (2) conversion of mesenchymal cells in the haversian canal of the cortex of radiated bone into actively proliferating cells.

The destruction of the marrow microenvironment and the fact that radiotherapy is most damaging to the pluripotential stem cell pool that is not actively proliferating account for the potential long-term effects of this therapy. Residual effects include hypoplasia or aplasia of certain marrow segments and a propensity to various myelodysplastic syndromes. As a result, the radiotherapy patient may be relatively intolerant of further antineoplastic therapy, such as chemotherapy. It is apparent that the volume of marrow radiated is as important as the therapeutic dose in determining future treatment tolerance.

In addition to radiotherapy's effect on neutrophils, platelets, and RBCs, it is significantly more lymphocytotoxic than chemotherapy. The most significant effects occur when large parts of the lymphoid system are included in the treatment field, as in the case of total nodal irradiation (TNI) for Hodgkin's disease or radiotherapy to the chest with its large volume of circulating blood and lymph.

The precise effects of radiotherapy on lymphocytes have not been determined, but it is agreed that in radiation-induced lymphopenia, the T cell subset is particularly affected. Delayed-hypersensitivity immune responses are more depressed than antibody responses to antigen.

Chemotherapy and radiotherapy have synergistic effects on bone marrow. In general, chemotherapy should precede radiotherapy. When radiotherapy is administered first, as the marrow responds to the insult with increased proliferation and circulation of stem cells, bone marrow is more vulnerable to the impact of chemotherapy on dividing cells.

Surgery

Most studies of immunosuppression in surgical patients indicate that the most important effects are on CMI, as measured by delayed hypersensitivity skin test responses.

Possible effects of a depressed immune response after surgery include increased risk of infection, septicemia, and increased mortality. Because surgery is a common intervention in cancer patients, it is important to be aware of potential surgically induced immunosuppression during the postoperative period and of the prolonged recovery time that may be needed for cancer patients to return to a normal immunologic state.

Biotherapy

Biologic response modifiers (BRMs), including interferons (IFNs), tumor necrosis factor (TNF), monoclonal antibodies (MAB), and IL-2, exert potentially therapeutic effects through several possible mechanisms: (1) exerting a direct antitumor effect, (2) restoring, augmenting, or otherwise modulating the patient's immune system, and (3) demonstrating other biologic effects, such as interference with tumor cells' ability to metastasize.

Experience is too limited to be able to define the nature and severity of toxicities associated with specific BRMs. Considering that the mechanism of action of BRMs is to modulate the immune system, the potential for hematologic toxicity is apparent. In fact, those agents with which there is the most experience (IFNs and MABs) do demonstrate hematologic toxicities. Abundant evidence exists that IFN therapy causes a reversible fall in WBCs, and with continued treatment a patient may experience a mild anemia, thrombocytopenia (TCP), and lymphopenia. The hematologic effects are severe enough to warrant caution when IFN is given in conjunction with chemotherapy. Monoclonal antibody infusions have been associated with a substantial decrease in WBCs (reversible).

The mechanisms by which the BRMs cause their hematologic effects continue to be the subject of speculation.

Aging

Cancer is a disease of the elderly. Considering the myelosuppressive nature of antineoplastic treatments, it is essential to be aware of age changes that occur in the hematopoietic and immune systems. Platelets do not appear to be affected by aging. There is conflicting evidence regarding changes in the leukocyte count and the ability of aged persons to mount an adequate leukocyte response to infection. Anemia seems to be a fairly common change in the elderly.

Nutrition

Nutrition is a very important factor in determining a person's hematologic and immunologic status. The connection between nutritional intake and anemia from deficiencies of such nutrients as iron, folate, and vitamin B_{12} is well known. A relationship also exists between nutrition and immunity. It has long been recognized that an increased risk of infection occurs among persons suffering from protein-calorie malnutrition (PCM). PCM causes lymphopenia, cutaneous anergy, diminished levels of complement, and a diminution of certain immunoglobulins. As in the case of aging, T cells and CMI are substantially more affected by malnutrition than are B cells. Levy argues that malnutrition also impairs the killing activities of neutrophils and macrophages and that there is decreased production of lymphokines and chemotactic factors.

Psychoneuroimmunology

Specific associations between psychologic states and disease have been identified (e.g., stress and hypertension). Within the last 10 years, increasing attention has been directed toward an apparent relationship among stress and infectious diseases, autoimmune disorders, and cancer. This field of investigation, psychoneuroimmunology, postulates essential interconnections among the CNS and the neuroendocrine and immune systems.

Increasing evidence from clinical, epidemiologic and experimental studies suggests that the psychologic state of persons can affect their immune systems. Given the multiplicity of physiologic, financial, social, and emotional pressures experienced by cancer patients, it is important that this factor be considered in assessing overall risk of hematopoietic or immune system compromise.

Some of the factors that may be involved in the response of the immune system to stress include the actual or perceived severity of the stressor, its predictability, and its controllability.

OVERVIEW OF NURSING ASSESSMENT

The initial assessment of the person at risk of BMD should be comprehensive and includes the health history, physical examination, and laboratory tests. Subsequent assessments may be targeted to the specific hematopoietic impairment. A thorough health history is essential to determining potential or existing BMD, identifying needs for patient education related to BMD, and planning and implementing preventive and therapeutic nursing inverventions. Risk factors for specific complications of BMD are listed in Table 22–1.

COMPLICATIONS
Clinical Problem: Infection

Infection is the most common cause of morbidity and mortality in patients with cancer. Risk of infection is correlated with severity and duration of granulocytopenia (GCP). In addition, extremes of age, compromised host defense, and colonization with potential pathogens increase the risk of serious infection in persons with cancer.

In the cancer patient with GCP, infection may be difficult to assess because the usual response to infection, neutrophil mobilization, does not occur. The nurse has an important role in prevention and detection of infection and in monitoring the patient's responses to preventive and therapeutic interventions.

Prevention

Persons with cancer may have several coexisting risk factors for infection. Identification of risk factors from history, laboratory values, and clinical examination directs the nursing care plan. Prevention strategies are focused on patient education, avoiding damage to host defenses, bolstering host defenses, reducing acquisition of new potential pathogens, and supressing colonizing organisms (Tables 22–2 and 22–3).

The importance of patient and family education cannot be overemphasized. It is helpful to teach the patient as well as a family member or significant other.

Early detection

Because infection is the leading cause of morbidity and mortality in cancer patients, early detection is essential, particularly in the patient with GCP. An undetected, untreated infection often ends in death for the febrile cancer patient with GCP. Early detection of infection in febrile patients with cancer is complicated by a number of factors. Fever may result from tumor, chemotherapeutic and antimicrobial drugs, and transfusions.

In the patient with GCP, fever most often has an infectious cause. The absence of sufficient, functional neutrophils in

Table 22–1. RISK FACTORS FOR SPECIFIC COMPLICATIONS OF BONE MARROW DEPRESSION

Infection

Abnormal function of phagocytes (e.g., acute leukemia)
Insufficient phagocytes (e.g., postchemotherapy granulocyto-
  penia)
Abnormal antibodies (e.g., multiple myeloma)
Insufficient antibody (e.g., protein malnutrition)
Absent or damaged mechanical barriers (e.g., splenectomy)

Bleeding

Abnormal function of platelets (e.g., idiopathic thrombocytopenia)
Insufficient platelets (e.g., hemorrhage)
Defect in intrinsic or extrinsic clotting system (e.g., liver dysfunction due to metastases)

Anemia

Abnormal function of RBCs (e.g., RBC dysfunction)
Insufficient RBCs (e.g., postchemotherapy anemia)

Table 22–2. CONTENT FOR PATIENT EDUCATION REGARDING PREVENTION AND EARLY DETECTION OF INFECTION

Self-inspection of high-risk areas for signs of infection
Temperature-taking
Self-care of vascular access devices and other invasive equipment
Functions of white blood cells (WBCs)
Reportable signs and symptoms
Hygiene (skin, oral, sexual)
Prevention of exposure to communicable diseases
Expected time of WBC nadir
Self-monitoring for superinfection when on antibiotics
Health-promoting self-care practices (good nutrition, sleep, stress
  reduction techniques)

GCP means the clinician is unlikely to observe classic signs and symptoms of infection (e.g., no pus in lesions or urine). Pizzo and Young recommend that institutional criteria and policies should be established and adhered to to minimize infection-related morbidity. Such a policy and criteria for fever work-up in patients with granulocytopenia are outlined as follows. Any patient with a granulocyte count less than 1000 cells/mm³ who has a single temperature elevation above 38.3°C or two or more elevations above 38°C will have a fever workup. The fever workup includes two sets

Table 22–3. STRATEGIES FOR INFECTION PREVENTION IN THE IMMUNOCOMPROMISED CANCER PATIENT

Bolster Host Defenses

Rapid remission induction
Balanced, nutritional diet
Administer prescribed vaccines
Administer prescribed immunomodulators
Administer prescribed leukocytes
Transfusions
Encourage use of stress-reduction techniques

Avoid Damage to Body Barriers

Avoid invasive procedures (rectal thermometers and medications; urinary catheters)
Initiate pulmonary toilet and other measures to prevent bedrest complications for immobilized patients or those with limited mobility

Reduce Acquisition of New Potential Pathogens

Meticulous handwashing
Cooked food diet for granulocyte counts <500 cells/mm^3
No humidifiers
No cut flowers in room
Avoid exposure to communicable infections
Monitor environment for risk factors (e.g., inadequate housekeeping)
Inspect biopsy sites, sites of venous access devices (VADs)
Maintain asepsis when caring for patients with VADs, other invasive devices, and wounds
Maintain total protected environment procedures when prescribed

Suppress Colonizing Organisms

Administer prescribed antimicrobials; monitor serum levels; monitor patients on antimicrobials for superinfection
Monitor patient compliance with self-administration of antimicrobial drugs

---

Adapted from Pizzo, P.A. & Schimpff, S. C. (1983). Strategies for the prevention of infection in the myelosuppressed or immunosuppressed cancer patient. *Cancer Treatment Reports*, The National Cancer Institute, Bethesda, Maryland. *67*, 223–234.

of preantibiotic blood cultures, chest radiograph, and cultures of sputum, urine, wound, and other accessible sites suggestive of infection. If blood is drawn for culture from a vascular access device or indwelling Silastic catheter, additional blood for cultures must be obtained from a peripheral vein. Once the fever workup is completed, a regimen of empiric antibiotics usually is begun without waiting for culture results. Once culture and sensitivity test results are known, therapy can be adjusted to treat the identified organisms.

In addition to monitoring temperatures, daily assessment of high-risk areas is vital. High-risk areas include axillae, oral cavity, perineum (particularly anorectal area), intertriginous areas, and existing wounds or other integumentary changes (e.g., ingrown toenail). Anorectal pain in GCP may be the first sign of a perirectal infection. Neutropenic enterocolitis occurs in persons with severe GCP and is characterized by diffuse abdominal cramping and distention, fever, bloody diarrhea, and decreased or absent bowel sounds.

In some patients, pain or tenderness may be the only initial sign of infection. High-risk sites should be inspected at least daily in persons who are hospitalized. Some patients may simply have changes in personality and behavior or hypotension in the absence of a fever, which may signal a serious infection.

Treatment

Medical therapy of infections consists primarily of antibiotics and supportive therapy. Although antipyretics are often used to bring temperatures down, at least one investigator recommends against using antipyretics when temperature is below 105°F in the patient with GCP. Fever maximizes host defenses by several mechanisms: inhibition or destruction of microorganisms, diminishing certain trace elements, which further inhibits replication of microorganisms, increased production of antiviral interferons, and increased mobility and phagocytosis of polymorphonuclear leukocytes. Cunha identifies three situations in which physicians might consider antipyretics in the febrile patient with GCP: (1) if the patient is particularly uncomfortable, (2) if the temperature is 105°F or above, and (3) if the patient has serious cardiopulmonary disease that might be exacerbated by the fever. Prolonged fever in persons with limited ability to ingest food and fluid may increase the risk of metabolic complications from dehydration and malnourishment.

Clinical Problem: Thrombocytopenia

Thrombocytopenia, a reduction in the number of circulating platelets, is relatively common in persons with cancer. It may be a disorder of production, distribution, or destruction. Perhaps the most common cause of TCP among cancer patients is a disorder of production involving decreased megakaryocytopoiesis. This may be due to marrow replacement by tumor or to an acute or delayed effect of chemotherapy or radiotherapy.

The most common disorder of distribution that occurs in cancer patients is hypersplenism, in which more than the usual 20% to 30% of platelets are sequestered in the spleen and not available in the circulation. If this type of TCP disorder is suspected, the spleen should be assessed carefully for splenomegaly because the absence of a palpable spleen will rule this out.

Several disorders of destruction may cause TCP in the person with cancer, including coagulopathies (e.g., disseminated intravascular coagulation, DIC), tumor effects that may release factors that activate coagulation, and effects of infection in which bacterial endotoxins and leukocyte response to them can enhance platelet consumption.

The role that nurses play in clinical assessment of the patient with TCP and in patient education is an important one. A person's risk of bleeding cannot be determined solely from the platelet count. Other factors that influence this risk include the presence of infection, potential sources of bleeding, the direction in which the platelet count is moving, and the cause of TCP. Potential bleeding sites may be observable (e.g., wounds or the site of an invasive procedure) or hidden (e.g., necrotic tumor masses, mucositis, or intracranial bleeding). The direction in which the platelet count is moving is significant because a patient is at greater risk for hemorrhage when the count is still falling than when it is rising, even when the absolute number is the same. The reason appears to be related to the fact that the platelets in circulation when the count is returning to normal tend to be younger and larger and, therefore, clot more effectively. Treatment-induced TCP tends to be of shorter duration and is associated with less risk of bleeding than that resulting from a myelophthisic marrow.

A grading system developed at the University of California, Los Angeles, uses the following values to assess risk of bleeding in TCP patients, with 0 being normal, and 4 indicating the most risk.

0 = 100,000 platelets/mm³
1 = 75,000 to 100,000 platelets/mm³
2 = 50,000 to 75,000 platelets/mm³
3 = 25,000 to 50,000 platelets/mm³
4 = less than 25,000 platelets/mm³

A patient with more than 50,000 platelets/mm³ is thought to have a slight risk of hemorrhage. The risk of spontaneous hemorrhage is much greater when the count is fewer than 20,000/mm³. However, spontaneous hemorrhage may occur at values higher than that when other factors compromise platelet production or function (such as infection, fever). In addition to platelet count, the nurse should monitor the CBC and measures of coagulation, such as prothrombin time (PT), partial thromboplastin time (PTT), bleeding time, and DIC screens when indicated.

Physical assessment of the person with TCP should be thorough. Bleeding may occur in any organ. However, sites in which it may be life threatening are priorities for assessment. These include the brain, the respiratory system, and the gastrointestinal system. Reportable neurologic observations include history of a recent fall or blow to the head, headache, blurred vision, pupillary changes, and changes in mental status, such as confusion or disorientation. Respiratory bleeding may be heralded by hemoptysis or by changes in respiratory status, such as congestion or wet cough. Hematemesis or blood in the stool may signal gastrointestinal tract hemorrhage. All gastrointestinal output, including emesis, nasogastric tube drainage, and stool, should be checked by guaiac test for blood. Changes in vital signs, such as hypotension and tachycardia may be the nurse's first clue to a spontaneous hemorrhage. Depending on the acuteness of the patient's condition, physical assessment and vital signs should be done every shift or more often.

Other areas that may require daily or more frequent assessment include the skin, mucosa, and eyes. Petechiae, purpura, and easy bruising are hallmarks of a low platelet count, and changes in the number or extent of such signs should be followed closely by head-to-toe inspection. A careful oral assessment should be done to detect petechiae or hemorrhagic blebs on the palate or oral mucosa as well as for bleeding from sites of mucositis. Occurrence and duration of epistaxis should be documented. Retinal hemorrhage may also occur.

In addition to assessment and monitoring, the nurse may use preventive interventions. The nurse can ensure that other providers know the patient's condition so that invasive procedures that may cause bleeding (such as enemas and biopsies) are avoided, or, in the case of important invasive diagnostic procedures, that preprocedure or postprocedure interventions (e.g., platelet transfusion, pressure to venipuncture sites) are initiated. Constipation, nausea, and vomiting are clinical events that increase intracranial pressure and may precipitate bleeding in a person at risk. Interventions to prevent these problems are essential in the patient with TCP. Menstrual bleeding in women with TCP should be monitored (e.g., by counting pads). Administration of hormones to inhibit menses may be needed to minimize profound blood loss. Patient education information for TCP is found in Table 22–4.

The treatment of choice for TCP (usually at levels less than 20,000 platelets per mm^3) is platelet transfusion. Some clinicians maintain that patients will tolerate a platelet count of 10,000 to 20,000 if there is no evidence of bleeding. Usually six to eight units of platelets are transfused depending on the initial degree of TCP and the patient's weight. One unit of platelets is the number of platelets obtained from 500 ml of whole blood. The response or "bump" obtained by a patient after transfusion is determined by a 1-hour posttransfusion platelet count.

Table 22–4. CONTENT OF PATIENT EDUCATION REGARDING THROMBOCYTOPENIA (TCP)

Function of platelets and normal laboratory values
Pathophysiology of TCP and expected course of recovery
Reportable signs and symptoms of bleeding
Preventive measures (e.g., eliminating environmental hazards;
    using an electric razor instead of a safety razor)
Avoiding invasive procedures (e.g., enemas, suppositories)
Development of a bowel maintenance program
Prophylactic antiemetics for nausea and vomiting
Avoidance of drugs that impair platelet function

The usual expected increase is 5000 to 10,000 platelets/mm^3 unit transfused. If the increment is substantially lower than this, the patient is likely to be alloimmunized, that is, to have developed antibodies against histocompatibility locus antigens (HLA) transfused with the platelets.

If the patient does develop a sensitivity to random platelets, it becomes necessary to find donors whose platelets are as closely matched in terms of HLA antigens as possible. In some cases, a family member may be able to give multiple units through platelet-pheresis. In other situations, a match that is close will have to suffice.

Clinical Problem: Neutropenia
Case study

Neutropenia is possibly the most problematic aspect of myelosuppression, whether the marrow failure is due to antineoplastic treatment, disease extension, or other causes. Appropriate and timely supportive care of the febrile neutropenic patient is essential and may involve standard antibiotic therapy, the use of controversial approaches, such as granulocyte transfusions, and, more recently, the administration of hematopoietic CSFs.

Clinical Problem: Anemia

Anemia is a common condition in cancer patients. Dutcher estimated that it occurs in 50% of cancer patients. Usually, anemia is relatively mild and does not require treatment. In more severe cases, intermittent transfusion is required. Several mechanisms underlie anemia: hypoproliferation, ineffective erythropoiesis, and hemolysis. Most anemias in cancer patients result from one of the first two mechanisms. The most frequent cause of anemia in cancer patients is a poorly understood condition called *anemia of chronic disease,* a hypoproliferative state. This type of anemia is rarely debilitating or progressive and does not require treatment as the hematocrit value usually remains above 30%.

Although the anemia of chronic disease does not imply

marrow invasion by tumor, myelophthisis can cause anemia, either by itself or in conjunction with anemia of chronic disease. Myelophthisis is a hypoproliferative state because replacement of marrow by tumor causes a decrease in both stem cells and erythroid precursor cells. The severity of this anemia depends on the extent of the primary disease, and although the patient can be supported with transfusion, the therapy of choice is to control the cancer.

Antineoplastic therapies also can cause hypoproliferative anemia because the erythrocyte line recovers more slowly than other cell lines. Thus, some chemotherapy schedules that are planned primarily around the granulocyte and platelet counts can lead to a chronic anemia. The erythroid line also can be involved in the prolonged or delayed pancytopenia caused by certain drugs, which strongly affect pluripotential stem cells.

Ineffective erythropoiesis is associated with nutritional deficiencies, particularly of iron, vitamin B_{12}, and folate. This may be a significant problem in persons with cancer cachexia and anorexia.

The classic symptoms reported by the person with anemia include fatigue, lassitude, and weakness. Palpitation, dyspnea, increased sweating, and pounding headache also may occur. Other symptoms associated with anemia may be anorexia or other gastrointestinal tract disturbances owing to diminished oxygen supply to this system and insomnia, decreased concentration, and confusion. All of these symptoms may be exacerbated in the elderly, who may have preexisting age-related or pathologic cardiovascular conditions.

The examiner should pay particular attention to two features in the client with anemia: color of skin and mucous membranes and cardiovascular status. Examination of mucous membranes is particularly important in clients whose skin color precludes adequate assessment. Other areas that may demonstrate the pallor of anemia are the nailbeds, the conjunctivae, and palmar creases of the hands. In severe anemia, patients may have evidence of increased cardiac output, such as tachycardia, powerful apical impulses, and murmurs that result from increased contractile force and blood turbulence.

In addition to assessing the foregoing symptoms, laboratory evaluation includes at least a CBC and may also require other tests, such as for plasma iron, total iron-binding capacity, and serum ferritin. The reticulocyte count is an indicator of RBC turnover and marrow response to anemic conditions. The mean corpuscular volume (MCV) and mean corpuscular hemoglobin (MCH) are useful indicators of impaired hemoglobin synthesis. A bone marrow aspirate and biopsy may be performed after an abnormal blood smear to further define abnormal morphology as well as indicate decreased overall marrow cellularity owing to neoplastic or fibrotic processes.

It is preferable to attend to the underlying cause of anemia (e.g., with radiation or chemotherapy). When that is not possible, the anemia itself is treated. Patients may require supportive packed cell transfusions while undergoing marrow suppressive therapy to keep the hematocrit level above 25%. A number of potential hazards exist, including transfusion reactions, circulatory overload (especially in the elderly and those with cardiac disorders), alloimmunization to HLA antigens, and the contraction of non-A, non-B hepatitis or AIDS. The risks of acquiring AIDS from blood transfusions have received much attention in the last several years. These risks have led to the increased use of direct donor transfusions and the practice of storing one's own blood for future use. Clearly, this approach is not feasible for many cancer patients.

23 Alterations in Comfort: Pain

NESSA COYLE
KATHLEEN M. FOLEY

Early and aggressive management of pain is among the highest priorities for the nurse when working with cancer patients. Unrelieved pain can strip people of their dignity, make them wish for an early death, destroy a family's ability to remain with the patient, and leave the staff feeling angry, ineffectual, and frustrated. Paradoxically, the patient may be blamed in some way if the pain remains severe despite the unstinting efforts of staff and family.

See the corresponding chapter in *Cancer Nursing: A Comprehensive Textbook,* by Baird, McCorkle, and Grant, pp. 782–805, for a more detailed discussion of this topic, including a comprehensive list of references.

More than 70% of patients could have their pain controlled satisfactorily by pharmacologic approaches alone, and the combination of drugs with other methods could control most of the remaining 30%. However, estimates from the World Health Organization and other sources suggest that cancer pain treatment is often inadequate. To improve this situation, the complex nature of pain must be addressed and barriers to appropriate pain management must be defined and corrected. Nurses have both the opportunity and the responsibility to play a significant role in these areas.

PREVALENCE OF PAIN IN CANCER PATIENTS

Data describing the incidence, prevalence, and severity of pain in the cancer population suggest that moderate to severe pain is experienced by one third of patients in active therapy and by 60% to 90% of patients with advanced disease.

CAUSE OF PAIN IN CANCER PATIENTS
Definition of Pain

Pain has been defined as "an unpleasant sensory and emotional experience associated with actual or potential tissue damage or described in terms of such damage." Pain is a subjective experience and may be either acute or chronic. The best measure of pain is the patient's report. Chronic pain draws attention to itself by its persistence. Suffering associated with the meaning of this pain may be profound.

Major Pain Types

Acute and chronic pain may be associated with somatic pain, visceral pain, and neuropathic pain.

Somatic pain

Somatic pain occurs as a result of activation of nociceptors (sensory receptors) in cutaneous and deep tissues. The pain is described by the patient as gnawing and aching, and it is usually constant and well localized. This is the most common type of pain experienced by cancer patients, and it is frequently associated with tumor metastasis to the bone, postsurgical incisional pain, and myofascial or musculoskeletal pain.

Visceral pain

Visceral pain results from activation of nociceptors in the cardiovascular and respiratory systems and in the gastrointestinal and genitourinary tracts. Unlike somatic pain, visceral pain is poorly localized, is frequently referred to a cutaneous site distant from the lesion, and may be associated with tenderness in the referred cutaneous site.

Neuropathic pain

Nuropathic pain results from neural injury, either peripheral or central. The injury may result from tumor invasion, surgery, radiation therapy, chemotherapy, or other factors. Neuropathic pain appears to be less responsive to opioid drugs than somatic or visceral pain. Combining an opioid with adjuvant drugs, such as a tricyclic antidepressant or anticonvulsant, is often more effective.

Common Pain Syndromes and Sites of Pain

In many patients with advanced disease, the pain originates from multiple sites and sources. The most common pain syndromes found in cancer patients fall into four major categories: pain associated with direct tumor involvement of pain-sensitive structures, such as bone, nerve, and hollow viscus, pain associated with cancer therapy, such as surgery, chemotherapy, and radiation therapy, pain associated with immobility, and pain unrelated to cancer or to its treatment.

Epidural spinal cord compression

Epidural spinal cord compression, in which pain is the presenting complaint in 96% of patients, requires special emphasis. Paraplegia can result if the early signs and symptoms of cord compression are not recognized and appropriate treatment carried out. Although any patient may develop this neurooncologic complication, it is more commonly seen in patients with cancer of the lung, prostate, and breast. Spinal cord damage results from compression by tumor in the epidural space or from direct invasion of the cord. Pain may be present for days or weeks before other neurologic signs and symptoms appear. The pain is of two types. *Local pain,* which occurs near the site of the involved vertebral body, is described by the patient as dull, aching, and constant. This pain is made worse by lying down and may be relieved by sitting or standing. *Radicular pain* is more common when the cervical or lumbosacral spine is involved. Cervical and lumbosacral radicular pain is usually unilateral, whereas thoracic radicular pain is usually bilateral. The patient frequently describes this pain as constricting, bandlike, as though he or she were "in a cast," and radiating around the abdomen or chest. If left untreated, neurologic signs and symptoms progress to include weakness, sensory changes, and bowel and bladder dysfunction. Once neurologic symptoms other than pain occur, rapid progression to complete paraplegia may occur over a period of hours or days.

PSYCHOSOCIAL FACTORS INFLUENCING THE PAIN EXPERIENCE

Both psychosocial and physiologic variables have a major impact on the pain experience.

Profile of Patients with Cancer Pain

The pain of cancer is experienced not only as the response of an organism to tissue damage but also as the response of a person with a life trajectory of pain and pleasure and of present and future hopes and despair. This may be described as the *suffering* component of cancer pain and is tightly woven into the pain experience.

Patients with acute cancer-related pain

The first group includes those patients with acute cancer-related pain. The pain may be associated with tumor growth or with cancer therapy.

Patients with chronic cancer-related pain

The second group includes patients with chronic cancer-related pain. As with the acute pain group, the pain may be associated with disease progression or with its treatment. In patients with chronic pain associated with tumor progression, the escalating pain is caused by tumor infiltration of pain-sensitive structures. Suffering plays a major role in the total pain these patients experience, and both physiologic and psychologic fatigue is common. These factors must be addressed if therapy is to be managed adequately.

Chronic pain also may be associated with cancer treatment (e.g., postmastectomy, postthoracotomy, and phantom limb pain). The cause of the pain may be secondary to nerve injury and development of a traumatic neuroma. It is essential that the cause of the pain be explained to the patient and family as being unrelated to tumor progession. This has a major effect on the patient's psychologic state. Methods of treatment of this type of pain concentrate on physical therapy and the use of the cognitive behavioral approaches.

Patients with preexisting chronic pain and cancer-related pain

The third group includes patients with a history of chronic pain unrelated to cancer, who then develop cancer and have cancer-related pain. These patients already have a compromised functional and psychologic state because of their previous chronic pain. With the added stress of cancer and its accompanying pain, the risk is high for further psychologic and functional deterioration. Early identification of this group of patients enables appropriate supportive intervention.

Patients with a history of drug abuse and cancer-related pain

The fourth group includes patients with a history of drug abuse who develop cancer-related pain. Three subgroups of patients can be identified within this heading. These are (1) patients who are actively using street drugs, (2) patients who are in methadone maintenance programs, and (3) patients who have not used illicit drugs for many years.

Patients with pain who are dying

Patients with cancer and pain who are dying constitute the fifth group. The primary focus of care is comfort, and treatment is no longer directed toward curing the disease. At no time is pain more destructive than in the dying patient. Families are left with a lasting memory of the pain of the person's death, which is difficult to erase. Both pain and suffering must be vigorously addressed in the dying patient through consistent, competent, compassionate support and appropriate analgesic titration.

Environmental Settings and Their Influence on Pain Management

The environment within which the patient with cancer pain receives care affects both response to pain management and adequacy of pain control. Professional variables also affect adequacy of pain management. These include the knowledge of pain control and the nurse's and patient's cultural backgrounds, social class, and age.

ASSESSMENT OF PAIN

Knowledge of the basic anatomy and physiology underlying pain, as well as an awareness of common pain syndromes, multiple sites of pain, and profiles of patients with cancer-related pain, is a necessary background to the nursing assessment of the pain complaint. It is important to remember that pain is a symptom, not a diagnosis. Pain perception is not merely a reflection of the amount of tissue damage a patient sustains but also a complex state determined by many factors, including age, sex, cultural and environmental influences, and multiple psychologic variables. Belief in the patient's pain and acknowledgement of the devastating effect that pain can have on the lives of both the patient and the family are critical not only to the assessment of pain but also to its management.

The Pain History: General Principles
Current pain complaints

The first step is to take a careful history of the current pain complaints. Patients frequently have more than one site and source of pain. Each needs to be evaluated to ensure appropriate management. Included in the evaluation are the onset of the pain, its site and characteristics, the referral patterns, exacerbating and relieving factors, and any associated symptoms.

Onset

The onset (temporal classification) of the pain includes questions relating to when the pain started, how long the person has had pain, and what were the precipitating events.

Site(s)

The site(s) (topographic classification) of the pain may be best illustrated by the patient's demonstrating on his or her body, or on the nurse interviewer's body, where the focus of the pain is felt and its pattern of radiation to other areas. Another useful approach is for the patient to use a body chart and shade in each area of pain.

Characteristics

Characteristics of the pain are learned by asking the patient to describe it.

Exacerbating and relieving factors

Exacerbating and relieving factors of pain frequently are recognized by patients and either used or avoided in the attempt to control pain. The nurse obtains this information not only as additional data for understanding the source of the pain but also as support for effective patient-initiated pain management approaches.

Associated symptoms

Associated symptoms occurring on a background of pain require critical attention, as they may signal an acute complication in the patient.

Psychosocial history

After eliciting a careful history of the present pain complaint, the next step is to obtain a psychosocial history. This will provide information about how pain influences the patient's day-to-day living and psychologic and social functioning. It is also important that the nurse direct questions toward the patient's previous experience with both pain unrelated to cancer and to cancer-related pain. Questions are aimed at gaining an understanding of the place of anxiety and depression in the patient's pain complaint. Questions are asked about how the person has dealt with stress in the past, so that appropriate behavioral techniques can be taught or reinforced.

Past pain relief management approaches

The nature and effectiveness of past pain relief management approaches the patient has undergone are reviewed. These include chemotherapy, surgery, radiation therapy, and behavioral modification techniques. Questions are asked about the current analgesic regimen, including the drug(s), route of administration, dose, time interval between doses, effectiveness of pain relief, and side effects, if any, such as sedation, nausea, constipation, or feeling "mentally hazy." Questions are also asked about prior exposure to narcotics on the part of the patient, family, or friends. Fears and misconceptions concerning the use of narcotics for pain frequently surface at this time, and unless they are dealt with in an open and forthright manner, they will interfere with the appropriate use of these drugs.

Examining the site of pain and possible referral sites

Examining the site of pain and possible referral sites is part of the nursing assessment. A critical factor for the nurse to remember is that normal results on physical examination do not negate a patient's pain complaint.

MEASUREMENT TOOLS TO EVALUATE PAIN AND PAIN RELIEF MEASURES

Pain by its nature is a subjective experience. A problem arises when doctors and nurses, who are used to basing their treatment decisions on objective data, are asked to base their decisions to a large part on the patient's verbal report of pain and pain relief. If the patient is given tools to translate the subjective experience of pain into a more objective form, communication among the patient, doctor, and nurse is enhanced. Asking the patient standardized questions also lessens the likelihood that valuable information will be omitted.

A variety of instruments are available to evaluate pain and the effectiveness of pain relief measures. The McGill Pain Questionnaire is the most widely used of such tools. To address the need for a more concise clinical tool, Daut, Cleeland, and Flannery developed the Brief Pain Inventory. This tool evaluates the following dimensions: history of pain, site of pain, intensity of pain, medications and treatments used to relieve pain, relief obtained, and the effects of pain on mood, activities, and interpersonal relationships.

Assessment and reassessment is an ongoing process. Changing parameters must be monitored by the nurse on a regular basis and are a useful measure of the effectiveness of pain management techniques. The Memorial Pain Assessment Card, designed specifically to assess the effectiveness of a particular analgesic dose for a particular patient, is being evaluated for use in this more global way.

Two simple measures used frequently in the clinical setting to evaluate the effectiveness of a treatment approach are numerical estimates (0 = no pain, and 10 = the worst possible pain) and categoric scales (none, mild, moderate, and severe). Documenting the amount of pain relief a patient is receiving is a critical part of assessment.

MANAGEMENT OF PAIN

The management of pain flows directly from its assessment. Inadequate assessment of pain usually results in inadequate pain relief. Because of the multidimensional nature of both pain and suffering in the cancer patient, a multidisciplinary approach is most effective. As patient advocate, the nurse frequently coordinates such a multidisciplinary approach for the patient and family and must, therefore, be familiar with the various pain management techniques used.

Nonnarcotic Analgesics (Nonsteroidal Anti-Inflammatory Drugs)

Nonnarcotic analgesics have four major pharmacologic properties: analgesic, antipyretic, antiplatelet, and anti-inflammatory. They have a peripheral site of action and produce analgesia by inhibiting prostaglandin synthetase. Prostaglandins sensitize peripheral nerve endings to the pain-producing effects of chemical substances, such as bradykinin. Nonsteroidal anti-inflammatory drugs (NSAIDs) are most effective in treating mild to moderate pain when an inflammatory component is present. In the patient with cancer, they frequently are used in combination with a narcotic. Unlike the narcotic drugs, the NSAIDs have a *ceiling effect* (a dose beyond which added analgesia is not obtained) but do not produce tolerance, physical dependence, or psychologic dependence. The major adverse effects of this class of drugs are hematologic (e.g., interference with platelet aggregation), gastrointestinal (e.g., dyspepsia and ulcer formation), hypersensitivity reactions (e.g., severe breathing restriction and hives), and renal (e.g., edema and renal insufficiency). Prostaglandins mediate these adverse affects. The most commonly used NSAIDs are ibuprofen (Motrin), fenoprofen (Nalfon), diflunisal (Dolobid), and naproxen (Naprosyn). Choline magnesium trisalicylate, a less widely known anti-flammatory drug, does not interfere with platelet aggregation and is, therefore, especially useful for patients with decreased blood counts. Acetaminophen, although lacking anti-inflammatory effects, is also helpful in managing pain in this group of patients. The major adverse effect of acetaminophen is hepatotoxicity, and this drug must be used with caution in patients with severe liver dysfunction.

Narcotic Analgesics

Narcotic analgesics produce their analgesic effects by binding to the opiate receptors at the peripheral and central nervous systems and altering the perception of pain. Misconceptions concerning tolerance, physical dependence, and psychologic dependence (addiction) by doctors, nurses, and patients are a major reason for the undertreatment of cancer pain.

Tolerance. Tolerance means that a larger dose of a drug

is needed to maintain the same effect. It may occur in any patient receiving narcotic analgesics on a regular basis and is related to dose, frequency of administration, and route of administration. The first sign of development of tolerance is the patient's complaint that the analgesic effect of the drug does not last as long, and the pain starts returning. In the cancer patient, increasing analgesic requirements frequently are associated with progressive disease. Lack of understanding of tolerance by doctors and nurses reinforces two basic patient fears: (1) that they have become addicted to the drugs and (2) that if "too much" of the drug is used now, when they "really need it," the medication will not work.

The effects of tolerance in the patient with chronic cancer pain can be minimized by using a combination of narcotic and nonnarcotic drugs and by switching to an alternative narcotic (cross-tolerance is not complete among narcotics), starting at one half to one third of the equianalgesic dose of the previous drug.

Physical Dependence. Physical dependence is an altered physiologic state occurring in patients who use opioid drugs on a long-term basis. If the drug is stopped abruptly, the patient exhibits signs of withdrawal but without exhibiting drug-seeking behavior unless specifically related to pain. Signs of abrupt opioid withdrawal in the tolerant patient include anxiety, alternating hot flashes and cold chills, salivation, lacrimation, rhinorrhea, diaphoresis, piloerection, nausea, vomiting, abdominal cramping, and insomnia. The time course of the withdrawal syndrome depends on the half-life of the drug. For example, in drugs with a short half-life, such as morphine or hydromorphone (Dilaudid), symptoms may occur within 6 to 12 hours of stopping the drug and be most severe after 24 to 72 hours. In drugs with a long half-life, such as levorphanol (Levo-Dromoran) and methadone (Dolophine), the symptoms may not occur for several days. Gradual reduction of the opioid drug in the tolerant patient who no longer has pain will prevent the withdrawal syndrome. An appropriate tapering schedule is suggested by the American Pain Society.

The use of an antagonist, such as naloxone, in the drug-tolerant patient will precipitate acute withdrawal symptoms unless carefully titrated. Patients to whom this has happened describe the sensation as feeling as if they had been plugged into a live electric socket, and pain recurs promptly. Such patients may become extremely fearful of falling asleep, fearing a repeat of the abrupt awakening with excruciating pain. As the half-life of naloxone is considerably shorter than that of the majority of the opioid drugs, an infusion of naloxone, carefully titrated to respirations and level of pain, may be the safest approach once the patient has become responsive. In the comatose patient, an endotracheal tube should be inserted before administration of naloxone to prevent aspiration.

Psychologic Dependence. Psychologic dependence (addiction) is defined as a pattern of compulsive drug use characterized by a continued craving for a narcotic and the need to use the narcotic for effects other than pain relief. Drug-seeking behavior is characteristic, the person using any means to obtain the drug. Psychologic dependence is rare in cancer patients, but it is cited frequently as the reason why doctors underprescribe narcotics, why nurses administer smaller amounts than are prescribed or at longer time intervals than are appropriate, and why patients are reluctant to take adequate amounts of a narcotic to control their pain.

Guiding Principles. The guiding principles for the oncology nurse in the use of narcotic analgesics to manage cancer pain are shown in Table 23–1. Tables 23–2, 23–3, and 23–4 give more information on narcotic analgesics.

Adjuvant Analgesics

Adjuvant analgesics are a third group of drugs used to treat patients with pain. This group includes several different categories of drugs, including tricyclic antidepressants, anticonvulsants, phenothiazides, and corticosteroids. These drugs produce analgesia in certain painful states by mechanisms not directly related to the opiate receptor system.

Tricyclic antidepressants (e.g., amitriptyline, imipramine, desipramine) are used frequently to treat pain with a neuropathic component. This pain is often described by patients as having a dysesthetic burning quality and may be associated with surgical trauma, radiation therapy, chemotherapy, and infiltration of the nerve by tumor. The mechanism of action of the tricyclic antidepressants is believed to involve enhancement of the descending pain modulation system by blocking the reuptake of serotonin and norepinephrine.

Anticonvulsants (phenytoin, carbamazepine, sodium valproate, clonazepam) are useful in treating paroxysmal lancinating pain arising from peripheral nerve damage. This pain is frequently described by patients as having a sharp, shooting component. Examples are postherpetic neuralgia or glossopharyngeal neuralgia. The mechanism of action is believed to be suppression of spontaneous neuronal firing.

Phenothiazides, with the exception of methotrimeprazine, do not relieve pain or enhance opioid analgesia. Methotrimeprazine may be useful in the management of the patient who is highly tolerant to opioids or experiences dose-limiting side effects. It lacks both the respiratory depressant and constipating effects of the opioids. The drug also has anxiolytic and antiemetic properties. This drug, however, is available only in parenteral form and has significant orthostatic and sedative side effects.

Table 23–1. PRINCIPLES TO GUIDE THE ONCOLOGY NURSE IN THE USE OF NARCOTIC ANALGESICS TO MANAGE CANCER PAIN

Select a drug appropriate to the patient's level of pain, previous analgesic history, metabolic state, and extent of disease
Know the pharmacology of the selected drug(s)
    Drug class (agonist, agonist-antagonist, antagonist)
    Duration of analgesic effects
    Pharmacokinetic properties of the drug(s)
    Equianalgesic doses for the drug and its route of administration
Know the difference and clinical significance among tolerance, physical dependence, and psychologic dependence
Suggest a route or routes of drug administration geared to the patient's needs (i.e., to maximize the analgesic effects and reduce adverse effects)
Administer the analgesic(s) on a regular basis; make sure "rescue" doses are available
Use drug combinations to provide added analgesia (e.g., NSAIDs)
Avoid drug combinations that increase sedation without enhancing analgesia (e.g., most phenothiazines)
Anticipate and treat side effects
    Respiratory depression (not usually a problem in the tolerant patient)
    Nausea and vomiting
    Sedation
    Constipation
    Urinary retention
    Multifocal myoclonus
Prevent and treat acute withdrawal
    Taper drugs slowly
    Use diluted doses of naloxone (0.4 mg in 10 ml of saline) to reverse respiratory depression in the tolerant patient
Respect individual differences in pain and response to therapy

Corticosteroids have specific and nonspecific effects in the management of acute and chronic cancer pain. They may directly lyse some tumors (e.g., lymphoma) and ameliorate painful nerve or spinal cord compression by reducing edema in tumor and nervous tissue.

ANESTHETIC APPROACHES

Anesthetic approaches are most useful in treating patients with well-defined localized pain. Short-acting and long-acting anesthetics are used for temporary and diagnostic nerve blocks, whereas phenol, alcohol, and freezing cryoprobe are the common neurolytic approaches for permanent blocks. The limitation of these procedures is that each peripheral nerve subserves sensory function over multiple

Table 23–2. PLASMA HALF-LIFE FOR NARCOTIC ANALGESICS

Drug	Plasma Half-Life (Hours)
Morphine	2–3.5
Meperidine	3–4
Methadone	15–30
Levorphanol	12–16
Heroin*	0.05
Hydromorphone	2–3
Pentazocine	2–3
Nelbuphine	5
Butorphanol	2.5–3.5
Codeine	3
Propoxyphene	12

*Biotransformed to acetylmorphine and morphine (Foley & Inturrisi).

levels, requiring multiple nerves to be blocked for adequate pain control. The use of an autonomic nerve block, such as the celiac plexus block, to manage midabdominal pain associated with cancer of the pancreas can be very successful and is often considered the procedure of choice for such patients.

Epidural and intrathecal nerve blocks with neurolytic agents can produce motor weakness and autonomic dysfunction. However, intermittent or continuous epidural infusions of local anesthetics have been used for management of severe pain associated with lumbosacral plexus or sacral lesions without interruption of motor or autonomic function.

Two anesthetic approaches used to manage the patient with diffuse pain are a chemical hypophysectomy and intermittent inhalation therapy of nitrous oxide. Chemical hypophysectomy, which involves the injection of alcohol into the sella turcica under radiologic guidance, is used to control pain in patients with widespread metastatic disease. The result in some patients can be dramatic. Nitrous oxide is most useful in managing acute incident pain, especially in the patient with advanced cancer who is comfortable at rest but not on movement. It is also a useful tool for managing procedure-related pain.

Trigger point injections may be useful for almost 15% of cancer-related pains reported to be musculoskeletal in origin. A focal injection of saline solution or local anesthetic is made into a painful muscle, often providing dramatic relief. When relief is temporary, further blocks may relieve pain for longer periods of time.

NEUROSURGICAL PROCEDURES

Cordotomy and the placement of epidural and intrathecal or intraventricular catheters are the most common neuro-

Table 23-3. ANALGESICS BOTH NARCOTIC AND NONNARCOTIC COMMONLY USED ORALLY FOR MILD TO MODERATE PAIN

Drug	Equanalgesic Dose* (mg)	Starting Oral Dose Range (mg)	Comments	Precautions
Nonnarcotics				
Aspirin	650	650	Often used in combination with narcotic-type analgesics	Renal dysfunction; avoid during pregnancy, in hemostatic disorders, and in combination with steroids
Acetaminophen	650	650	Like aspirin	
Ibuprofen (Motrin)	ND	200–400	Higher analgesic potential than aspirin	Like aspirin
Fenoprofen (Nalfon)	ND	200–400	Like ibuprofen	Like aspirin
Diflunisal (Dolobid)	ND	500–1000	Longer duration of action than ibuprofen; higher analgesic potential than aspirin	Like aspirin
Naproxen (Naprosyn)	ND	250–500	Like diflunisal	Like aspirin

Morphinelike Agonists

			Comments	
Codeine	32–65	32–65	"Weak" morphine; often used in combination with nonnarcotic analgesics; biotransformed, in part to morphine	Impaired ventilation; bronchial asthma; increased intracranial pressure
Oxycodone	5	5–10	Shorter acting; also in combination with nonnarcotic analgesics (Percodan, Percocet), which limits dose escalation	Like codeine
Meperidine (Demerol)	50	50–100	Shorter acting; biotransformed to normeperidine, a toxic metabolite	Normeperidine accumulates with repetitive dosing causing CNS excitation; not for patients with impaired renal function or receiving monoamine oxidase inhibitors

*These are the recommended starting doses from which the optimal dose for each patient is determined by titration and the maximal dose limited by adverse effects.
ND, not determined.

For these equianalgesic doses (see also Comments) the time of peak analgesia ranges from 1.5 to 2 hours and the duration from 4 to 6 hours. Oxycodone and meperidine are shorter-acting (3 to 5 hours), and diflunisal and naproxen are longer-acting (8 to 12 hours).

From Foley. K. M., & Inturrisi, C. E. (1987). Analgesic drug therapy in cancer pain principles and practice. *Medical Clinics of North America, 71,* 210–211.

Continued

Table 23–3. ANALGESICS BOTH NARCOTIC AND NONNARCOTIC COMMONLY USED ORALLY FOR MILD TO MODERATE PAIN *Continued*

Drug	Equianalgesic Dose* (mg)	Starting Oral Dose Range (mg)	Comments	Precautions
Morphinelike Agonists cont'd				
Propoxyphene HCl (Darvon) Propoxyphene napsylate (Darvon-N)	65–130	65–130	"Weak" narcotic; often used in combination with nonnarcotic analgesics; long half-life biotranformed to potentially toxic metabolite (norpropoxyphene)	Propoxyphene and metabolite accumulate with repetitive dosing; overdose complicated by convulsions
Mixed Agonist-Antagonist				
Pentazocine (Talwin)	50	50–100	In combination with nonnarcotics; in combination with naloxone to discourage parenteral abuse	May cause psychotomimetic effects; may precipitate withdrawal in narcotic-dependent patients

374

Table 23–4. NARCOTIC-TYPE ANALGESICS COMMONLY USED FOR MODERATE TO SEVERE PAIN

Drug	Equianalgesic Intramuscular Dose* (mg)	Intramuscular Oral Potency	Starting Oral Dose Range (mg)	Comments	Precautions
Morphinelike Agonists					
Morphine	10	3–6	30–50	Standard of comparison for narcotic type analgesics	Lower doses for aged patients and those with impaired ventilation, bronchial asthma, increased intracranial pressure, liver failure
Hydromorphone (Dilaudid)	1.5	5	4–8	Slightly shorter acting HP intramuscular dosage form for tolerant patients	Like morphine

*These doses are recommended starting in doses from which the optimal dose for each patient is determined by titration and the maximal dose limited by adverse effects.
†Irritating to tissues on repeated administration.
HP, high potency.
For these equianalgesic intramuscular doses (see also Comments) the time of peak analgesia in nontolerant patients ranges from ½ to 1 hour and the duration from 4 to 6 hours.
The peak analgesic effect is delayed and the duration prolonged after oral administration.
From Foley, N. M., & Inturrisi, C. E. (1987). Analgesic drug therapy in cancer pain principles and practice. *Medical Clinics of North America, 71,* 210–211. *Continued*

Table 23-4. NARCOTIC-TYPE ANALGESICS COMMONLY USED FOR MODERATE TO SEVERE PAIN *Continued*

Drug	Equianalgesic Intramuscular Dose* (mg)	Intramuscular Oral Potency	Starting Oral Dose Range (mg)	Comments	Precautions
Morphinelike Agonists cont'd					
Methadone (Dolophine)	10	2	10–20	Good oral potency; long plasma half-life	Like morphine; may accumulate with repetitive dosing causing excessive sedation
Levorphanol (Levo-Dromoran)	2	2	2–4	Like methadone	Like methadone
Oxymorphone (Numorphan)	1		See Comments	Not available orally	Like IM morphine
Heroin	5	(6–10)	Not recommended	Slightly shorter acting; biotransformed to active metabolites (e.g., morphine); not available in United States	Like morphine

Meperidine (Demerol)	75	4	Not recommended	Slightly shorter acting; used orally for less severe pain	Normeperidine (toxic metabolite) accumulates with repetitive dosing causing CNS excitation; not for patients with impaired renal function or receiving monoamine oxidase inhibitors[†]
Codeine	130	1.5	See Comments	Used orally for less severe pain	Like morphine
Mixed Agonist-Antagonists					
Pentazocine (Talwin)	60	3	See Comments	Used orally for less severe pain; mixed agonist-antagonist; less abuse liability than morphine; included in Schedule IV of Controlled Substances Act	May cause psychotomimetic effects; may precipitate withdrawal in narcotic-dependent patients; not for myocardial infarction[†]

Continued

Table 23–4. NARCOTIC-TYPE ANALGESICS COMMONLY USED FOR MODERATE TO SEVERE PAIN *Continued*

Drug	Equlanalgesic Intramuscular Dose* (mg)	Intramuscular Oral Potency	Starting Oral Dose Range (mg)	Comments	Precautions
Mixed Agonist-Antagonists cont'd					
Nalbuphine (Nubain)	10		See Comments	Not available orally; like intramuscular pentazocine but not scheduled	Incidence of psychotomimetic effects lower than with pentazocine
Butorphanol (Stadol)	2		See Comments	Not available orally; like IM nalbuphine	Like intramuscular pentazocine
Partial Agonists					
Buprenorphine (Buprenex)	0.4		See Comments	Not available orally; sublingual preparation not yet in the United States; less abuse liability than morphine; does not produce psychotomimetic effects	May precipitate withdrawal in narcotic-dependent patients

surgical procedures for pain relief. A cordotomy involves the interruption of the anterolateral spinothalamic tract in the cervical or thoracic region. It may be performed by an open surgical approach or by a percutaneous stereotactic procedure. This technique is most useful in managing unilateral pain below the waist. Initial complications in a small percentage of patients include paresis, ataxia, and urinary dysfunction. Although initial pain relief from cordotomy occurs in 70% to 90% of patients, this levels to 80% in 3 months, and at the end of 1 year, about 40% of patients report a return of pain.

A phenomenon that is beginning to be recognized clinically is the depression that occurs in patients who receive complete pain relief after a neuroablative procedure, such as a cordotomy. Pain has left abruptly, and suddenly the implication of having advanced disease is the overwhelming force. The oncology nurse plays a major role in working with these patients and families both before and after such procedures.

NEUROAUGMENTATIVE APPROACHES

Neuroaugmentative techniques include counterirritation (for example, systematic rubbing of a painful part or applying alternating heat and cold), transcutaneous nerve stimulation, acupuncture, dorsal column stimulation, and deep brain stimulation. Such approaches are thought to provide pain relief by activating endogenous pain-modulating systems. The most commonly used neuroaugmentative approaches for cancer patients are counterirritation and transcutaneous nerve stimulation. These approaches are most effective for nerve injury pain (including deafferentation pain and postherpetic neuralgia). Frequently, they are used in combination with other pain management techniques.

BEHAVIORAL APPROACHES

Behavioral interventions are particularly helpful to the patient in developing a sense of mastery over incident pain and procedure-related pain. A sense of uncertainty and loss of control can overwhelm a patient, increasing the suffering and level of pain.

The assessment phase, as in the general pain assessment, is the first step in these therapeutic interventions. During the process of discussion with the nurse, the patient gradually develops an awareness of the multidimensional nature of the pain and suffering. Through keeping a pain diary or by noting the fluctuating levels of the pain, the patient begins to recognize the relationship of stress and anxiety to increased pain. In the next step, the patient learns self-monitoring, so that signs of stress are recognized. The behavioral techniques most helpful to this group of patients are focused breathing, muscle relaxation, and guided imagery.

CONTINUITY OF CARE AND SUPPORTIVE CARE

Continuity of care and supportive care with a multidisciplinary team approach are increasingly being recognized as an integral part of the care of a patient with chronic pain and cancer. A variety of models of continuing care have been developed. Such models include (1) hospice, which may consist of home care with brief periods of hospitalization for symptoms poorly controlled at home or institutional care away from the hospital environment, (2) palliative care service within a general hospital, in which the resources of the hospital are readily available to the patient, family, and community, (3) the use of a mobile van unit directed by the staff of a general hospital, in which frequent team visits are used to provide care for extremely ill and dying patients at home, and (4) a supportive care model, which can be developed as part of a pain service within a comprehensive cancer center and which attempts to integrate family and community resources to provide the patient with continuity of care from home to hospital.

24 Alterations in Patient Coping

ANNE JALOWIEC
SUSAN DUDAS

THE STRESS OF CANCER

It is widely acknowledged that cancer is one of the most feared and stressful of all diseases. Therefore, cancer is a severe threat not only to the physical welfare of patients but also to their psychologic well-being, and it can cause such reactions as anxiety, depression, despair, helplessness, guilt, and anger. Until fairly recently, much of the literature on cancer had emphasized coping with the stress of impending death. With improvements in treatment methods and increased survival rates, however, the focus has changed to coping with cancer as a chronic disease. Coping can be defined simply as using various behavioral and cognitive means to deal with the physical and psychologic threats imposed by a stressful situation—in this case cancer.

The importance of coping in the cancer experience is reflected in the identification of coping as one of the ten standards for cancer nursing as developed by the Oncology Nursing Society. This standard is stated as follows: While living with cancer, the client and family manage stress within their physical, psychological, and spiritual capabilities and their value systems. Populations at risk for inef-

See the corresponding chapter in *Cancer Nursing: A Comprehensive Textbook,* by Baird, McCorkle, and Grant, pp. 806–820, for a more detailed discussion of this topic, including a comprehensive list of references.

fective coping are persons who have diagnostic workups and receive a positive diagnosis of cancer, those undergoing initial treatment for cancer, persons with relapse or unsuccessful treatment of cancer, and those under stress because of perceived vulnerability to cancer.

Cancer patients have to cope with a wide variety of stressors, including loss of function in numerous body systems, pain, nausea and vomiting, anorexia, fatigue, mutilation and disfigurement, decreased mobility, social isolation, uncertainty regarding the future, loss of self-esteem, fear of death and dying, loss of control over one's own body and over numerous aspects of daily living, adjusting to the hospital environment, fear of dependency, need to understand new medical terms, dealing with a variety of health care providers, sexual problems, strained interpersonal relationships, diminished work capacity or loss of job, cognitive impairment, financial problems, inability to perform various social roles, and fear of recurrence of the cancer. Obviously, some of these stressors may be more dominant at certain stages of the illness than at others, and they may vary in their intensity depending on the individual characteristics of both the person and the situation.

This chapter focuses on a domain very salient to nursing—that of patient coping with the stresses of cancer. The aim is to foster in the oncology nurse an appreciation for the complexity and the primacy of the coping process in cancer patients.

MODELS OF STRESS AND COPING
Lazarus's Psychologic Model of Stress and Coping

Lazarus's theory of stress and coping can be seen as having special relevance for oncology nursing because it is a transactional model that allows for feedback between the person and the environment; it places primary emphasis on the particular meaning of a situation to the individual; it takes into consideration the many person-related and situation-related factors that can affect the stress and coping process; and it focuses on the dynamic nature of adaptation. The dynamic nature of stress and coping is especially germane to oncology patients because they must constantly cope with the many different demands of their illness as it progresses and as new therapies are tried. Thus, Lazarus notes that any time nurses are examining the coping process in cancer patients, they should identify very specifically what the patient is actually having to cope with at that point and how the coping process is changing over time.

Weisman's Cancer-Specific Model of Stress and Coping

Weisman identified 15 major coping styles that patients use to handle the stresses of cancer. In addition, he proposed what he called *countercoping* strategies used by health professionals to help patients cope more effectively. Countercoping is seen as complementing the patient's coping efforts by strengthening good strategies and minimizing harmful ones. Weisman identified four countercoping tasks: clarification and control, collaboration, directed relief, and cooling off.

The extensive work done by Weisman on the coping process in cancer patients has much applicability for oncology nursing. Weisman's model can prove useful for nurses in understanding what the cancer patient is experiencing, in anticipating the needs of patients at various stages of the illness trajectory, and in planning for holistic cancer care.

CLINICAL ASSESSMENT OF COPING BEHAVIOR

Nurses have increasingly incorporated assessment of the coping behavior and adaptive potential of clients into their clinical practice, using both formal tools and less structured assessment approaches. To determine which patients are at risk for ineffective coping, nurses need to identify specific stressors in the patient's life, assess the patient's perception of those stressors and attributional beliefs about their causes, and evaluate the available coping resources and social support systems. Psychosocial adjustment can be further assessed by obtaining information on the patient's previous ways of dealing with stress, the patient's perception of illness, and prior relationships with people who had cancer. The last-mentioned factor can exert either a positive or a negative influence on the patient's outlook on the diagnosis, depending on the types of experiences the patient has had with other cancer patients. Such an assessment also should include information on family history, interpersonal relationships, and the patient's expectations of nursing care.

Further, Weisman suggested that by listening well and learning to ask tactful questions, health professionals can better elicit information on the patient's psychologic status. The use of open-ended questions can provide an elaboration of the patient's views and emotional states, so that psychosocial vulnerability can be recognized and appropriate interventions instituted.

These assessment techniques are necessary to obtain information on the patient's available coping strategies and to determine the patient's problem-solving ability. These aspects are then incorporated into the nursing care plan, so that appropriate interventions can be planned to allay the patient's anxiety, decrease stress, and facilitate more effective ways for coping with the stresses of cancer.

Weisman's Coping Interview

Weisman (a psychiatrist) uses a coping interview to elicit information on the problems and concerns of the cancer patient, what the patient is doing about the problems, and who the patient turns to for help. The predominant concerns identified by cancer patients through these interviews fall into seven categories: health, self-appraisal (as self-esteem, proficiency, approval), work and finances, relationships with family, relationships with friends, religion, and concerns about death.

On the basis of these interviews, Weisman identified the 15 major coping styles used by cancer patients to deal with these concerns. Persons who cope well with cancer, according to Weisman, are those who confront reality, consider alternatives, focus on problem solving when the situation is amenable to problem solving but turn to problem redefinition when it is not, avoid excessive use of denial, communicate openly with significant others, are largely self-reliant but can accept help when it is offered, make use of available resources, are flexible and realistically hopeful, and try to maintain morale and self-esteem.

Weisman also uses a scale that indicates how vulnerable the cancer patient is to high emotional distress. On the basis of the results from this scale, Weisman identified correlates of vulnerability for high emotional distress in cancer patients. The oncology nurse can use this vulnerability profile as an assessment checklist to identify patients who are at high risk for suffering extreme emotional distress from having cancer.

Cancer patients are especially prone to high emotional distress at certain times in the illness process. These have been identified as the time of diagnosis or recurrence of the disease, after loss of a bodily function or part, when repeated complications occur, when effective treatments have been exhausted, and when social support fails. Therefore, health care providers need to monitor cancer patients vigilantly for increased distress at these times.

ENABLING AND HINDERING FACTORS IN PATIENT COPING

Reports in the literature have indicated that many coping factors can influence adjustment to cancer; some coping activities facilitate the adaptation process (enabling factors), whereas others hinder it. Enabling factors include social support, control, hardiness, positive appraisal, hopefulness, humor, positive comparisons, religiosity, healthy self-esteem, good body image, information seeking, open communication, social skills, and problem-solving ability. In contrast, coping factors that hinder adaptation include denial, avoidance, helplessness, powerlessness, hopelessness, despair, depression, erosion of autonomy, isolation, withdrawal, fear, anger, hostility, guilt, blaming others, wishful thinking, and noncompliance.

Enabling Factors in Coping with Cancer
Social support

Ample evidence has documented the essential importance of an adequate social support system when trying to cope with almost any formidable stressor, including serious illness. Social support can include both formal and informal systems of support and can emanate from a diversity of sources, such as spouse, parents, children, siblings, relatives, friends, supervisors and co-workers, clergy, teachers, counselors, health care providers, and members of self-help groups with the same type of problem. Social support systems can provide help of many different kinds to stressed persons. This help can come in the form of providing an avenue for the ventilation of feelings, affirming the person's importance and place in the world, encouraging the open expression of thoughts and feelings (especially negative ones), acknowledging the appropriateness of a person's interpretation of events, providing feedback on the person's behavior, having someone to confide in, supplying needed information and advice, acting as an advocate for the person, and providing more tangible types of support, such as materials, money, and physical help with chores and responsibilities.

Social support can facilitate adaptation by altering the use of coping strategies, by influencing the occurrence and appraisal of stressful events, by enhancing the motivation for health-promoting behaviors, by increasing self-esteem and altering mood states, and by synergistically interacting with other resources that promote adaptation. Hence, social support may have both direct and indirect (i.e., buffering or mediating) effects.

Evidence abounds in the literature of the beneficial impact of social support in promoting various types of positive outcomes in cancer patients. The evidence is overwhelming that patients who are able to maintain close relationships with family and friends, despite their illness, are more likely to cope effectively with cancer. Hence, it is imperative that the nurse help cancer patients to mobilize their social supports by including significant others in the plan of care and by informing patients of the various types of programs available that have supportive functions.

Programs have been designed to provide more formal types of support groups for patients with various kinds of cancer, thereby supplying both educational and psychosocial resources to help patients and families cope more effectively. Peer groups with similar cancer experiences, such as mastectomy patients and Reach to Recovery, have proved useful primarily as a function of modeling—that is, as a method of learning better ways to cope by sharing and knowing someone else who has successfully coped with cancer. "WE CAN" weekends, a family-oriented program for persons experiencing the crisis of terminal illness, have been designed to help cancer patients and their families improve problem-solving techniques, strengthen self-esteem, and increase interactional skills. This program also tries to combat the social isolation that often occurs in families unable to cope with the reality of the cancer diagnosis.

Although most writers overwhelmingly laud the beneficial effects of social support, Wortman and Dunkel-Schetter and Tilden and Galyen remind us that social support can also have negative aspects, which can then increase stress rather than buffer it. For example, social support can have a negative impact when a person's privacy is invaded, when promises are made that are not kept, when unwelcome or misleading advice is offered, when the other person discourages compliance with the treatment regimen, when a feeling of extreme dependency is created, or when the other person extracts more from the relationship than is given in return. Hence, some social relationships can cost more than any positive benefits that might be gleaned from the association. Therefore, oncology nurses need to be cautious in evaluating the quality and adequacy of social support systems of their cancer patients. Just because a patient has a large network of significant others, it should not be taken for granted that the person is deriving solely positive benefits from that network.

Control

Writers have for a long time promulgated the beneficial impact of the factor of control on the stress and coping process. Langer points out that control is such a primary and motivating force in life that it is perceived even in situations that are determined by chance (such as lotteries) and that people selectively filter information that enhances their perception of control. It is usually thought that having personal control over a situation reduces feelings of threat and helplessness and gives a person a sense of mastery over the situation, thereby leading to better adaptational outcomes.

Overall, research seems to indicate that persons with an internal locus of control show a preference for constructive coping strategies that work toward altering the stressful situation, whereas those with an external locus of control prefer more palliative types of coping behavior. Knowing that a cancer patient has an internal locus of control has relevance for anticipating the types of coping behavior that may be displayed by such patients, and it also has implications for the teaching and promotion of more action-oriented coping skills.

Folkman and Lazarus found that persons used more problem-focused coping if they felt they had some control over health-related situations, but they used more emotion-focused coping if they had little or no control. Therefore, if nurses encourage cancer patients to control as many aspects of their disease and treatment regimen as possible, they can promote the greater use of problem-oriented coping strategies that can lead to more successful resolution of the problems encountered during illness. Moreover, because patients' feelings of personal control are sometimes eroded by the lack of improvement in their condition, nurses need to constantly reinforce patients' efforts to exert control to foster confidence in their ongoing ability to maintain control over their lives. Silberfarb and Greer hypothesized that patients' feelings of reduced control may partly account for the increasing popularity of less orthodox treatments for cancer (e.g., mental imagery). Therefore, nurses should reinforce patients' control efforts by encouraging an active role in the treatment process, by letting patients know what alternatives they have related to the many aspects of the treatment regimen, by allowing and promoting decision making, by providing the information necessary for sound decision making, and by giving positive feedback on patients' appropriate efforts to control their environment (Table 24–1).

It should also be kept in mind that, depending on the particular situation, control can be more stress inducing than

Table 24–1. WAYS TO INCREASE PATIENTS PERCEPTION OF CONTROL

Encourage problem-solving behavior

Foster confidence in ability to control situation

Encourage information-seeking behavior

Let patient know what to expect

Encourage active role in treatment program

Inform patient of alternatives or options

Allow decision making in care

Provide necessary information for decision making

Promote self-care activities

Identify personal assets that facilitate control

Identify elements in environment conducive to control

Discourage excessive or inappropriate dependency

Give positive feedback on appropriate efforts to control environment

Encourage action-oriented coping activities when appropriate to situation

Encourage cognitive control activities when behavioral control not possible

Help patient differentiate between controllable vs uncontrollable situations

Help patient identify things he or she wants to control vs things the patient does not wish to control stress alleviating, especially in relation to the questions of desired control and the necessary skills to control. In this regard, Dennis points out that nurses should not insist that patients control things that they are not equipped to handle, nor should they deprive patients of controlling-type coping strategies if patients desire them.

Hardiness

Related to the factor of control is the concept of hardiness, which was developed by Kobasa in her work on stress and illness in business executives. She found, both retrospectively and prospectively, that executives who experienced a large number of stressful events but who possessed this hardiness factor, were less prone to illness than executives who were exposed to high stress but did not possess hardiness. Kobasa conceptualized hardiness as a stress-moderating personality style composed of three essential characteristics: commitment, challenge, and control. Thus, hardy persons feel committed to something that is important in their lives (as work or family), and therefore they feel that their lives are meaningful. They feel challenged rather than threatened by change, stress, and problems, and they feel that they have some control over their lives and their environment. Underlying all of this is a pervasive optimistic bent that hardy persons feel they will be successful in whatever dealings they have with the world. Therefore, hardiness moderates stress by influencing both the cognitive appraisal of stressful situations and the choice of coping strategies.

Identifying a patient with cancer as hardy can allow nurses to anticipate the patient's reactions to cancer and treatment and to plan patient care more effectively. For example, hardy patients with cancer might need to be given more latitude in decision making regarding their illness and treatment because they tend to be more independent and assertive. In the same vein, it is important to keep hardy patients actively involved in what is going on because they tend to feel a deep commitment to what they value in life. These hardy patients might seem to have a higher pain threshold owing to their need to control their environment. Because hardy persons like a challenge, it is wise to phrase information regarding cancer and treatment so that the patient sees that such factors can also help to foster development and inner growth. Furthermore, hardy cancer patients might be expected to be efficient problem solvers, to feel that they can handle almost anything, and to tend to see things in a positive light.

On the other hand, oncology nurses should keep in mind Lee's warning that hardiness could also possibly have negative effects on cancer patients because the strong sense of independence and personal control in hardy persons may cause them to ignore professional advice regarding treatment. It is also important to remember Pollock's finding that hardiness did not have a stress-moderating impact in arthritic patients because of insufficient control over their pain. This point can have implications that the stress-buffering effect of hardiness could be less in cancer patients who have severe and unrelenting pain.

Hopefulness

A feeling of hope is paramount for patient adjustment to cancer and indeed for survival itself. In fact, hope is probably the single most important factor needed for living with cancer. Hope enables patients to cope with problems in ways that make possible the desired outcomes. Thus, hope can figure prominently in the dynamics of self-fulfilling prophecies, for being hopeful may cause goals to be realized owing merely to the fact that people work harder toward those goals when they are motivated by hope.

Nurses can bolster the patient's sense of hope by communicating confidence in the efficacy of therapy, by helping patients identify those aspects of life that are important to them and therefore worth living for, by helping patients develop an awareness of the small things in life that can be enjoyed, by setting realistic goals that will promote a sense of accomplishment and thereby generate further hope when they are attained, by being enthusiastic in interactions with the patient, and by helping patients to incorporate religion and humor into their lives. When patients can no longer realistically hope for a long life or for a cure from cancer, hope can then be redirected toward short-term, more tangible goals, such as a week with less suffering or a chance to see spring come again, or ultimately a hope for a comfortable death.

Information seeking

An important enabling factor in coping with cancer is that of seeking information. For example, information-seeking behavior was significantly correlated with less distress and better social adjustment in breast cancer patients, and patients who received systematic information on chemotherapy drugs and side effects were able to undertake more self-care. Encouraging the patient to seek accurate information also will facilitate development of the patient's decision-making abilities. Patient education materials often reinforce the idea that the patient is responsible for asking questions if he or she wants more information. Therefore, patients should be advised that they are free to ask direct questions about any aspect of their illness. Detailed information about cancer and its treatment is needed to reduce the uncertainty inherent in the cancer experience and to allow the patient to feel a sense of control over the situation. However, it is important to evaluate how much information is desired by the patient. Some patients may not want detailed information at certain times because it may be overwhelming and thus may interfere with their ability to cope. Facilitating patient acquisition of needed information about the illness and about how to cope with the cancer experience is the basis for various educational programs offered to patients with cancer (e.g., the American Cancer Society program I Can Cope).

Problem-solving ability

Problem-solving ability is a necessary prerequisite for adequately coping with any serious illness, especially cancer. For example, Scott, Oberst, and Bookbinder found that men with genitourinary cancer who had better problem-solving ability were able to cope more effectively with their cancer, as measured by resolution of cancer-related problems and less dysphoria. Patients at risk for ineffective coping by virtue of few problem-solving skills can be taught to accurately identify problems and to consider choices for handling stressful situations. Sobel and Worden have demonstrated that problem-solving behavior can be taught systematically. Points covered in their problem-solving approach are defining the highest priority problems, identifying the patient's feelings, thoughts, and behaviors in response to those problems, relaxing before confronting the problem, taking into consideration all possible solutions, identifying the advantages and disadvantages of all options, and choosing the best solution.

Hindering Factors in Coping with Cancer
Denial

Denial has long been considered one of the worst things to do when trying to cope with a stressful situation, especially a situation as serious as a life-threatening illness. However, denial is not an all-or-none phenomenon, for many cancer patients show some degree of denial, which may fluctuate during various phases of their illness. In addition, patients may show acceptance of some aspects of their illness but reject other aspects. For example, patients may acknowledge that they indeed have cancer but may ignore certain evidence indicating that the cancer is incurable. Accordingly, Weisman has identified three orders of denial in cancer patients. First-order denial is repudiation of the diagnosis itself. Second-order denial is dissociation of the diagnosis from its therapeutic implications. Third-order denial is renunciation of deterioration and decline in status.

Extremes in denial have been shown to be an obstacle to adjusting to the many demands of the cancer experience. For example, excessive denial has been associated with indifference toward serious symptoms, delay in seeking treatment, noncompliance with therapeutic regimens, nonuse of existing resources for information and support, blaming others for self-induced problems associated with the illness, and poorer long-term adjustment to cancer.

Although denial has long been considered a hindering factor in coping with a serious illness, more recent research suggests that the role of denial is more complicated than was originally thought. Therefore, denial may in fact be beneficial at some points in the coping process. For example, denial of the seriousness of the illness when the person first learns of a diagnosis of cancer can often give the person time to get used to the idea of being ill. Therefore, the person can have some breathing space to muster the energy and resources needed to cope with the problems that will follow. Also, denial that he or she is going to die soon from the cancer may allow the person to keep living life as fully as possible and not dwell morbidly on what is to come. In addition, denial has been found in some studies to be associated with less depression, lower levels of both physiologic and psychosocial disruption, and, surprisingly, with increased rates of survival in cancer patients. Denial does cause problems, however, when it interferes with taking the necessary steps to see a doctor, continue treatment, or make plans for the future that might be indicated (e.g., to plan for the financial welfare of dependent children). Therefore, denial might work well in the short run in handling the distress associated with cancer and treatment, but it is not as effective in the long run for resolving problems and for adjusting to the demands of the illness.

As Weisman points out so well, "the proper balance between denial and acceptance cannot be packaged into the proper dosage for everyone." Therefore, nurses should not make snap judgments that denial is bad for all cancer patients at all times. Too often in the past, nurses have believed that it was their responsibility to make sure the patient accepted the stark reality of the situation so that they could help prepare the person to die in the right way. However, knowing what is now known about denial, nurses should instead examine the particular characteristics of a patient's situation and see if denial might not be doing the patient some good, at least for the time being.

Helplessness or powerlessness

Patients with serious illnesses often experience a sense of helplessness and powerlessness related to the loss of both physiologic control over their body and psychologic control over the events in their lives, as well as to the loss of control over their environment. Contributing to helplessness in cancer patients are feelings of uncertainty, ambiguity, indecisiveness, despair, and the expectation that nothing can be done to change the ultimate outcome of the situation. The phenomenon of *learned helplessness* was first identified by Seligman as a precipitating factor in depression. The cancer experience too readily fosters learned helplessness because of its devastating implications for the patient's welfare, its chronic nature, the recurring acute episodes, the need for long-term adherence to a treatment regimen, the debilitating side effects associated with treatment methods, and the patient's previous experiences with others who have died from cancer.

Observing patients for vulnerability during crucial periods of their illness is useful for detecting signs of helplessness that require treatment. Interventions recommended for preventing or relieving helplessness include setting realistic goals, sharing information about what can be expected, pointing out varying degrees of success achieved by therapy (no matter how small), helping the patient accept a realistic explanation of why uncontrollable events have occurred, identifying elements in the patient's environment that are more conducive to control, allowing patients to make decisions about different aspects of their care, and eliminating any activities that encourage undue or inappropriate dependency and diminish control.

Hopelessness and depression

Along with helplessness, feelings of hopelessness have been identified as one of the major characteristics of depression. The uncertainty so prevalent in the cancer experience may be detrimental to keeping the patient hopeful and involved in treatment plans. Therefore, perceived unpredictability concerning the course and outcome of an illness has been shown to have a strong negative effect on the patient's attitude and adjustment during diagnosis and treatment. For example, uncertainty has been associated with a loss of motivation, sadness, depression, fatalism, passivity, giving up, poor expectations about the future, and a pervasive pessimistic attitude. Hopeless and depressed persons also display a sense of worthlessness and lowered self-esteem. Therefore, they feel that they do not matter at all and should not be bothered with.

Hopelessness can be detected through an assessment of patients' lack of self-esteem and of their unrealistic or distorted negative expectations about the future. Using a tool such as the Beck Depression Inventory early in a cancer treatment program can detect those persons needing structured positive experiences to foster more optimistic attitudes and feelings of personal control. Positive and control-promoting experiences are necessary to counteract these patients' expectations that nothing they do can change the outcome of their cancer situation. Otherwise, the feelings of hopelessness and depression can prove to be a monumental impediment to adjustment because of the immobilizing effect on patient progress in all aspects of treatment. In fact, a long-term study on breast cancer even showed that those patients who felt hopeless, helpless, and depressed had lower rates of survival at both 5 and 10 years after testing. The same was found in patients with testicular cancer after a 7-year period.

In identifying depression, the nurse should keep in mind that sometimes it is hard to sort out some of the physical symptoms of depression (e.g., anorexia, fatigue, weight loss, sleep disturbance) from symptoms of the cancer itself or from side effects of therapy. Therefore, assessing the presence of the psychologic concomitants of depression (hopelessness, helplessness, worthlessness, despair) is important in differentiating symptoms attributable to organic and therapeutic causes from those resulting from depression.

Anger and hostility

Anger or hostility may be a generalized response to cancer not specifically directed toward anyone or anything in particular, or it may be focused on someone specific or on some particular aspect of the disease or therapy. Feelings of anger may be accompanied by a sense of frustration and unfairness at being stricken with cancer. Persons who especially tend to display feelings of anger and hostility are those who have followed all the precautionary measures that are promulgated as protective against serious illness (e.g., eating right, exercising, avoiding known carcinogens, and living life in moderation) but nonetheless develop cancer. Conversely, anger directed inwardly might be found in persons who failed to heed the advice of the health community and subsequently developed cancer—for example, those who continued to smoke despite warnings from health care providers. In addition, people who have been very active and athletic before the diagnosis of cancer also might become angry at the thought of the dependency enforced by chronic illness. Thus, anger sometimes serves to mask the feelings of powerlessness that patients with serious illness often experience.

The persistence of anger in patients with cancer can lead to a diversion of energy away from constructive coping with illness-related problems to inappropriate blaming of others for existing problems. It also can cause significant others to shy away from contact with the patient, thereby adding the problem of social isolation. Patients need to be helped to identify the reasons for and objects of their anger, to learn to express anger in nondestructive ways, and then be helped to redirect hostile feelings into more constructive channels. The patient needs to know that anger is a normal reaction to cancer.

Health professionals have long held the belief that repressed anger is more dangerous than ventilated anger. This led to the development of various cathartic techniques, both verbal and physical, for promoting the expression of anger. However, ventilatory techniques for handling anger have been found to be more effective when they are combined with cognitive restructuring techniques in which the person is taught to reinterpret feelings and events in a new light. Although most health professionals see anger as an undesirable reaction to stress (often because the patient seems more difficult to handle), it should be pointed out that two studies have indicated that breast cancer patients who expressed anger and hostility (i.e., displayed a fighting spirit) had better survival rates. Therefore, "getting up the patient's dander" may help by stimulating the emotional energy needed to motivate the patient to deal with problems more actively rather than handling problems with passive avoidance or a feeling of helplessness.

METHODS FOR PROMOTING EFFECTIVE PATIENT COPING

A primary role for oncology nurses is to facilitate a functional coping process in patients under their care. Therefore, nurses should help patients to use their coping abilities more effectively. The need for periodic alterations and adjustments in coping should be kept in mind and monitored because of the chronic nature of cancer with its recurring acute episodes. Further, nurses need to recognize the uniqueness of the individual cancer patient and to encourage and support those constructive coping activities that seem to work best for that patient.

For cancer patients with a nursing diagnosis of ineffective coping, Doublsky suggests that nurses focus on stressors and responses to them during therapeutic interactions and also try to reinforce positive self-care behaviors. For those persons with severely impaired coping and incapacitating psychoemotional behaviors, Doublsky recommends setting limits while at the same time showing positive acceptance of the patient, as well as collaborating with mental health workers to develop individualized therapeutic plans. For the more severe case of ineffective coping, referral to a professional counselor is the appropriate nursing intervention.

In addition to verbal communication with cancer patients about coping strategies, written materials can be used to teach patients new coping skills. Carey and Jevne have developed an effective teaching program for postmastectomy patients to help them cope with breast cancer. The program includes specific guidelines on dealing with emotions, handling changes in family roles and relationships, encouraging family involvement in care, dealing with problems in sexuality, discussing cancer with other patients, communicating with physicians and family, and developing specific coping skills. The educational materials also advise patients to help friends and family to be comfortable with the cancer diagnosis by giving accurate information without dwelling on the matter and by sharing their feelings and needs.

This teaching program indicates that it helps the patient to know that denial, anger, frustration, guilt, worry, depression, sadness, and fear are all normal reactions to cancer. Suggestions are offered to patients for dealing with these emotions by distracting themselves through activity, by talking with someone with whom they feel comfortable, by solving everyday problems as they arise and not letting them build up, and by learning specific relaxation techniques. For example, to handle anger in an appropriate way without alienating needed social support resources, Carey and Jevne advise that patients write down their feelings, confide in someone they feel close to, and even hang up some sort of punching bag to serve as a tension-release mechanism. Furthermore, patients are encouraged to use all the support resources they can muster. Other useful suggestions, such as considering a shift in or reduction of responsibilities for a period of time if feeling tired or overwhelmed, are provided in this helpful educational program.

To enable health care providers to facilitate patients' coping by accomplishing the countercoping tasks of clarification, collaboration, relief, and cooling off, Weisman suggests the following activities appropriate for nurses: clarify problems for the patient, help patients maintain control by encouraging them to exercise whatever options they have available to them, try to discourage emotional extremes by offering a willing and noncritical ear so that patients can relieve pent-up tensions without fear of retribution, redirect the patient to more constructive channels for releasing anxiety, reduce the problem to manageable size, share concern but without further aggravating the patient's feelings of anxiety, discourage hasty actions, and at times just be comfortable with sharing periods of silence with the patient. In these sometimes small but nonetheless effective ways, the nurse can promote the patient's positive adaptation to the stresses of cancer.

In addition, nurses should encourage patients to take advantage of the many resources available for cancer patients, such as the multiple services offered by the American (and regional) Cancer Society and often by local hospitals and community groups. Patients need to be provided with timely information on all such resources. While still hospitalized, patients should be given for future reference a list of the addresses and phone numbers of important local agencies that can serve their many needs. However it should be kept in mind that patients might not be ready to avail themselves of certain resources when they first learn of them. Therefore, patients need to be reminded on an ongoing basis of current resources available in the area, either through newsletters, phone calls, posted notices, pamphlets, or meetings. Any such protocol for informing patients should be systematized so that the distribution of information is not happenstance and left to serendipity.

Patients should be advised of the various support groups available for cancer patients generally and for their specific type of cancer or operation, such as ostomy patients, laryngectomy patients, and mastectomy patients. Patients should be encouraged to attend such meetings with a partner or friend, so that they can link up with the appropriate self-help support groups available in their area. Again, patients may not be ready for this immediately, so they need to be reminded later that such groups exist and how to contact them.

Furthermore, patients should be informed of the diversity of cognitive and behavioral methods available for controlling the extreme emotional distress and various other problems associated with cancer. These methods include progressive relaxation, meditation, biofeedback, hypnosis, stress inoculation training, systematic desensitization, mental imagery, and various kinds of cognitive restructuring (thought-changing) techniques. Not all patients may be attuned to using such techniques, nor do all patients benefit equally from them. Nevertheless, patients should be apprised of the existence of such methods for handling tension and anxiety. Preliminary studies indicate that some of these methods also seem useful for controlling the pain of cancer and the nausea and vomiting associated with chemotherapy.

SUMMARY

Owing to the complexity of the coping process and to the magnitude and diversity of stressors with which patients with cancer have to deal, oncology nurses have a substantial challenge facing them if they are to help their patients cope more effectively with their illness and its treatment. The oncology nurse is indeed one of the most significant professional support systems available to the patient with cancer because the nurse has the most frequent contact with the patient, possesses the critical skills and knowledge for facilitating the adaptive process in patients with cancer, and is wholeheartedly invested in the premise of holistic cancer care. Therefore, no nursing care plan should be without specific goals and activities directed toward helping the patient with cancer achieve the highest adaptive level possible in dealing with illness and its treatment.

25 Alterations in Body Image

NANCY BURNS
BARBARA C. HOLMES

Body image changes probably occur in most individuals with cancer, and if these changes are not effectively integrated with the self system, they can greatly diminish the quality of life. Nursing actions, based on a thorough knowledge of body image theory, may be able to facilitate healthy management of body image changes by the person with cancer, the family, and the patient's social system.

THE DEVELOPMENT OF THEORETIC THOUGHT ABOUT BODY IMAGE

The body image develops gradually as the person matures. From experiences that begin in childhood, persons learn to place different values on various parts of their body.

Body image is related to self-esteem, self-concept, and identity. High self-esteem is a feeling of worthiness. Body image and self-esteem have been found to be highly correlated. Individuals who have poor body image also tend to have low self-esteem. Self-concept has been defined as the composite of all the feelings a person has about the self. From this point of view, body image and self-esteem are considered elements of self-concept.

Of importance is the need to identify those persons at risk of being unsuccessful in integrating body image changes. Depression and emotional lability before the surgery may be predictive of poor adjustment in the following year. Those patients who experienced phantom breast syndrome also

---

See the corresponding chapter in *Cancer Nursing: A Comprehensive Textbook,* by Baird, McCorkle, and Grant, pp. 821–830, for a more detailed discussion of this topic, including a comprehensive list of references.

may have greater problems integrating an altered body image. Persons who are dissatisfied with many body parts rather than just those affected by the illness also tend to have difficulty integrating an altered body image. This negative feeling toward the whole body can be related to high levels of emotional distress.

Women with gynecologic surgery for cancer, who are frequently used as a comparison group in studies of women with mastectomies, experience much greater difficulty integrating an altered body image than women with mastectomies. Although the appearance of the body does not change after gynecologic surgery, its functioning may have changed in ways that are important to these people. Alopecia also has been associated with negative scores on body image scales.

HEALTH CONSEQUENCES OF ALTERATIONS IN BODY IMAGE

An alteration in body image occurs over time, to some extent is an unconscious process, and needs to be integrated within the self system. This process requires emotional energy that otherwise could be invested in other pursuits. Reality, for that person, has changed, and uncertainty has increased. To some, it must seem as if their personal world is being torn asunder. The process of restructuring the body image may involve changing (1) the image of the body contained within the brain, (2) body posture, (3) body movement, and (4) body function. The person must then determine the personal meaning of the body alteration and evaluate the reaction of members of his or her social support system to the body change. All of these changes must then be integrated within the self structure, with an image of, acceptance of and love of "this is who I am."

It is clear that failure to integrate a changed body image is associated with long-term depression, difficulty with interpersonal interactions, withdrawal from social interaction, and, overall, a lower quality of life. This outcome can be life threatening for persons with cancer in that these persons may choose not to continue treatment. The body image change seems to be even more important than life itself. The depression, lack of energy, and overwhelming changes in view of self leave little strength for participating in the fight for life. From the research, it would appear that these consequences are experienced to some degree by about 25% of persons who have a major body alteration.

NURSING ACTIONS RELATED TO PERSONS EXPERIENCING ALTERED BODY IMAGE

It would appear that nurses could influence the outcome of altered body image at two points: (1) during the process of the initial body image-changing event and (2) during the process of integrating the body image into the self structure. The nurse could influence the changing body image through helping the patient think through the meaning of the change, through proposing alternative meanings not considered by the patient, through role modeling healthy responses to the change, through providing positive feedback as a person in the environment reacting to the change, by helping family members and social support system members to examine the meaning of the changes, and by communicating acceptance of the changes to the patient. Because this process seems to occur over a 2- to 6-month period, ideally, availability of nursing care should extend over this period of time at least.

CANCER SITUATIONS IN WHICH BODY IMAGE MAY BE ALTERED

The knowledge that a person has cancer affects body image before the initiation of treatment or the obvious changes caused by progression of the disease. The person feels a higher degree of vulnerability, a decreased awareness of what is happening within his or her body, and a decreased power to control these little understood changes. An anticipation of overwhelming changes in the body, which no personal action can prevent, affects the patient. Following this realization, the person is confronted with major assaults to body image as the consequence of necessary treatments for the cancer and of progression of the disease. Although some body image changes are related to total body function, others differ with the cancer site and treatment choice.

Side effects of current treatment methods used in care of the cancer patient also can produce body image changes. The most obvious of these are the mutilating effects of surgery, such as experienced by breast and gynecologic cancer patients. However, any cancer that requires surgery will affect body image. Radiotherapy often leads to such consequences as skin changes, alopecia, vaginal stenosis, changes in bowel habits, changes in urinary frequency, pain, fatigue, nausea and vomiting, and infection. Each of these has an effect on body image. Chemotherapy also produces severe adverse reactions, including stomatitis, nausea and vomiting, alopecia, neurotoxicity, hemorrhaging, infection, fatigue, skin changes, diarrhea, sexual dysfunction, and respiratory dysfunction, all of which alter body image.

The cancer process itself produces body image changes as the patient copes with pain, fatigue, weakness, susceptibility to infection, spinal cord compression, septic shock, weight gain, and weight loss. The person may be more distressed over the body changes caused by the cancer than by the threat to survival. Because of the nurse's more immediate concern with the patient's survival and comfort, patient difficulties related to body image changes may not be noted or may be discounted. The nurse may not be able to understand how the patient could focus on body image in the midst of a life-threatening crisis when, for the patient, it may be the most important concern. The focusing of the patient on body image change may be due to denial of impending death, a need for control, or simply that body image is truly the most pressing concern at that time. Although the nurse must continue to address survival and comfort, additional nursing measures must be implemented concurrently to help the patient in managing the alteration in body image.

DETECTING ALTERATIONS IN BODY IMAGE

Because changes in body image apparently do not occur until 2 to 6 months after the actual change in the body, it is not realistic to assess for changes in the body image immediately after diagnosis or surgery. However, it is important for the nurse to make a judgment about the patient's capacity for effectively integrating the body image change when it occurs. Therefore, the initial assessment will be of such factors as self-esteem, self-concept, general coping skills, family dynamics, and social support systems. One purpose of the assessment is to identify patients who are at high risk of experiencing difficulty in managing a body image change. Another purpose is to gather information that can be used to provide guidance to the patient in planning strategies to facilitate effective management of the body image change when it occurs.

The body image change generally occurs at a time in which accessibility to nursing care is diminished. If the patient is receiving adjuvant therapy, the nurses in the outpatient clinic or physician's office will have the most contact during this critical period. If the patient does not have contact with the nurse, ideally the patient should have been given a source of referral for nursing care before discharge. Then, if problems related to body image emerge, a source of nursing care will be available. The clinical nurse specialist on the oncology unit would be a logical source for this nursing care or for further referral.

In assessing body image changes or risk, the nurse must be aware of both verbal and nonverbal messages the patient is communicating. Cues that patients are experiencing difficulties in dealing with body image changes include changes in patient approaches to their bodies, avoidance of discussion of any possible changes, emphatically discussing the positive aspects while denying or ignoring the negative aspects, displaced anger at staff members or family, depression, and overcompensation, indicated by a desire to help other patients with similar problems when they have not yet resolved their own problems. It is also important to gather information about the patient from other health professionals.

Generally, the period from 2 to 6 months after diagnosis of cancer is a time of ongoing treatment or follow-up. It is during this time that patient concerns regarding body image changes emerge. Although sometimes the patient expresses concern during interaction with the nurse, it may be necessary for the nurse to reintroduce the topic of body image changes. The nurse also can obtain information about the patient's previous coping strategies.

Open-ended questions can be used to determine the patient's perception of the impact of the cancer experience on his or her life. This can lead to questioning that can stimulate the patient to evaluate the effectiveness of current coping techniques. Questions that have been found to be useful include the following: "What does this diagnosis of cancer mean to you?" "How is it affecting your life?" "How do you feel you are coping with it?" Concurrently with questioning the patient, the nurse can judge whether the patient is avoiding conversation about the impact of the cancer or, conversely, is intellectualizing the impact. In some cases, the patient may expend more energy in wanting to help other patients with similar concerns than in discussing personal concerns.

The types of questions asked of the patient depend on the quality of the nurse–patient relationship. If a working therapeutic relationship has been established, the nurse can proceed with more probing questions. Otherwise, relationship-establishing strategies must precede questioning. The nurse begins by providing factual information, followed by asking questions that require cognition on the part of the patient. Only then does the nurse progress to questions requiring an emotional response on the part of the patient.

Comments and questions that focus directly on the body image changes can be used at this time. These should relate to the patient's particular situation and may include such comments as the following: "Frequently patients are hesitant to resume social relationships after a mastectomy [or colostomy or head and neck surgery]. Although I see you as being the same person you were, how are you feeling about these changes in your life?" The nurse may share examples of questions previously asked by other patients with the patient. These may include "Will my husband still want me?" "Should I keep my scar covered during intimate times?" "Should I encourage my spouse to touch the altered part?" "What do I tell my children?"

Body image changes that affect internal organs, excluding the reproductive organs, or that are caused by such symptoms as fatigue, pain, and so forth frequently are ignored because they are not directly associated with a visual change in the patient's body. In assessing the patient, these aspects must be included. The nurse should question the patient about thoughts or feelings related to the removal of internal organs, such as fears that the patient may have about the removal of the pancreas. Feelings about the self may be influenced by experiences such as fatigue, pain, or hemorrhaging. Patients may express feelings of lowered self-esteem because of inability to perform tasks in the previous manner.

INTERVENTIONS THAT FACILITATE HEALTHY RESPONSE TO BODY IMAGE CHANGES

Immediately after the body-changing event, the patient usually is not concerned with body image changes. This time is more consumed with task-oriented concerns, such as physical healing and the struggle for survival. Only after these immediate concerns are addressed will the patient turn toward the threat to body image initiated by these changes in his or her body.

The first and most important element for effective interventions for managing body image changes is the establishment of a trust relationship between the nurse and the patient. Maximum effectiveness can be achieved through a nurse–patient relationship that is initiated at the time of diagnosis and continues through the period of integration of the altered body image, which, if successful, can be expected to occur between 1 and 2 years later. Effective nursing interventions focus on education, support, counseling, and referral. Within a trust relationship, the more delicate issues of body image changes can be explored.

Initial interventions with a patient in the early stages of treatment for cancer should include educational preparation for the impending body image change. The nurse needs to be knowledgeable about the specific body image changes associated with the patient's situation. Explanation of impending events related to the cancer process and its treatment and the expected impact on body image can be helpful. The nurse should emphasize that reactions to these changes are commonly experienced by patients with the particular diagnosis. Providing information about these changes will set the groundwork for further nurse–patient discussions at a later time.

This also is an ideal time to inform the patient of the availability of peer support groups. The patient needs reinforcement that his or her concerns are normal. To provide effective referral, the nurse must be aware of community resources for peer support. The American Cancer Society, local cancer treatment centers, and local hospitals usually have information about these groups. In some areas of the country, the American Cancer Society's Reach to Recovery and Dialogue programs have peer support groups as part of their services. The United Ostomy Association and the Lost Chord Club also may provide peer support groups.

If the patient does not respond to the nurse's introduction of the topic, the nurse needs to let the patient know that it is permissible to initiate the topic any time he or she chooses. Also, the nurse should reintroduce the topic periodically to provide the patient with many opportunities to discuss concerns. It is important to give permission implicitly to discuss the topic but not to force discussion. The patient's not responding to the nurse's cues does not necessarily imply lack of integration of body image changes. Some patients are able to integrate the body image changes from their own mental health base and personal resources. This is confirmed by observation of healthy adaptation to the alteration (i.e., touching the altered site, open discussion about the altered body part).

The nurse also must act as advocate in ensuring that the best possible care is given to the alteration site itself to minimize the severity of the body image change. This includes input regarding proper use of equipment (correct bagging techniques of ostomies, correct wound care) and observation of early breakdown of the healing process (early signs of infection, improper suture care, drainage amounts). The knowledgeable, experienced nurse cannot assume that these potential problems will be managed effectively by the physician or the other members of the health care team.

Body image changes frequently are not addressed by the nurse because of time constraints. Dealing with body image changes requires additional time commitment on the part of the nurse that usually is not reflected in the amount of nursing care hours designated in patient classification systems. With a shortage of qualified nurses doing patient care, this aspect frequently gets put on the back burner in favor of "measurable" nursing tasks. A nurse functioning in an expanded role is more likely to have the time necessary for providing these interventions. However, the cost effectiveness of these interventions needs to be documented before institutions or agencies will commit the time required for the care.

Frequently, the alteration is so obvious that the nurse assumes that the patient is dealing with it. For example, so much information about breast disease and alteration has been published in the lay press that the nurse may assume that the patient is educated about the potential emotional responses to loss of a major body organ.

Body image changes are sometimes not addressed because of the nurse's personal discomfort in dealing with the situation. In addition to knowledge about body image theory, the nurse must have worked through personal dilemmas related to body image.

Besides expediting assessment, open-ended questions can be used as an intervention. The questioning also serves as permission granting to the patient to talk about the subject. It can be a starting point for family intervention. The inclusion of the family or significant others in assessment and intervention should be decided on in conjunction with the patient. The patient should be allowed to determine when the family is brought into the discussions about the alteration and may need assistance from the nurse in sharing fears or hopes with the family.

If numerous opportunities for the patient to ask questions are provided, repeated explanations of body function changes are possible. This often leads to discussion involving problem-solving techniques, coping options, and evaluation.

EVALUATING THE INTEGRATION OF BODY IMAGE CHANGES

From clinical practice we know that there are some patients who are unable or unwilling to incorporate the body image change and thus could be classified as a high-risk group. Within this high-risk group will be some persons who, because of their mental health status, are unable to incorporate the body image change and other persons who prefer the secondary gains of a poor body image to the benefits of successfully integrating the body image change. We would like to propose some outcomes that from our clinical experience, seem to be associated with effective integration of an altered body image.

- Resumption of former lifestyle, including relationships, employment, style of dress
- Verbalization of concerns about body image changes
- Manifestation of healthy coping ability
- Ability to touch, look at, reveal altered body site
- Ability to incorporate necessary changes to allow activity (work, play, sex) to be satisfying
- Change in dream content to reflect reintegration of altered body image
- Incorporation of altered body part as part of the "me" identity
- Evidence of high self-esteem
- Ability to discuss and consider reconstruction
- Willingness to resume sexual relations

Alteration in body images, if not effectively integrated within the self system, can greatly diminish the quality of life.

26 Alterations in Sexuality and Sexual Functioning

MARGARET A. LAMB

Cancer affects all aspects of a person's life. Most people diagnosed with cancer have concerns about the sexual ramifications of their illness as well as the proposed treatment for their disease. Often, health professionals focus on the disease process and its treatment. They may neglect the issue of sexuality because of a lack of information regarding

---

See the corresponding chapter in *Cancer Nursing: A Comprehensive Textbook*, by Baird, McCorkle, and Grant, pp 831–849, for a more detailed discussion of this topic, including a comprehensive list of references.

the impact of the disease and its treatment on sexual functioning as well as a generalized feeling of discomfort discussing these issues with clients. This chapter outlines current knowledge about the impact of cancer and its treatment on sexual functioning, discusses the psychosocial factors that affect sexual functioning, enhances the practitioner's skills in the assessment and management of alterations in sexual functioning, addresses the special problems associated with alterations in sexual functioning, and presents related issues and concerns.

SEXUAL FUNCTIONING
General Considerations

Sexuality is a multidimensional, complex phenomenon involving biologic, psychologic, interpersonal, and behavioral dimensions. The World Health Organization's Report on Education and Treatment in Human Sexuality asserts that sexual health is the integration of the somatic, emotional, intellectual, and social aspects of sexual being in ways that are positively enriching and that enhance personality, communication, and love. A wide range of normal sexual functioning exists within the population. This spectrum could include the ability to maintain interpersonal relationships to the ability to sustain the closeness of an intimate, sexually active relationship.

Psychosocial aspects of sexuality

Optimal sexual functioning relies on the integration of key biopsychosocial components. The psychosocial elements involved in sexual functioning vary, depending on the developmental stage of the individuals involved. The young adult faces an array of intimacy issues, including learning to give and receive love, choosing whether or not to marry, and choosing a marital or sexual partner or partners. In adulthood, the majority of clients will focus on the capacity to give and receive gratification in a stable relationship. This capacity is centered not only around the physiologic aspects of sexuality, to be discussed subsequently, but also around the individual's concept of self as a sexual being and his or her sex role. Older adults often focus on the critical task of resolving feelings of self-esteem and despair. This task includes acceptance of one's life cycle and the social factors that accompanied it. These include emancipating adolescent children, achieving a career peak, and accommodating aging parents. During the later years, from retirement to death, sexual activity and interest persist. Sexual functioning is dependent on relatively good health and an interested and interesting partner. Aging persons may find it necessary to nurture one another, to cope with bereavement and widowhood, and to find new meaning in life.

Physiologic aspects of sexuality

The psychosocial aspects of sexual functioning are complemented by the biologic components. The human sexual response cycle comprises two principal physiologic changes: vasocongestion and myotonia. Vasocongestion is the congestion of blood vessels, usually venous, and myotonia refers to increased muscular tension. These physiologic changes are dependent on an intact neurologic system and an appropriate hormonal milieu.

An accurate assessment of sexual dysfunctions is based on a basic understanding of the normal occurrences in the sexual response cycle. Interventions are used to alleviate or minimize the identified causes of sexual dysfunctions.

Many dysfunctions can be caused by physiologic, psychologic, or social variables or a combination of several factors. The discussion of physiologic factors is followed here by the psychosocial implications of cancer and its treatment.

The four major stages in the human sexual response cycle are excitement, plateau, orgasm, and resolution. Excitement is characterized by the onset of erotic feelings and the attainment of erection in men and vaginal lubrication in women. Plateau is a more advanced stage of excitement in which the sex glands become more engorged and undergo positional changes. A number of extragenital conditions also occur, including color change, respiration shifts, and generalized increase in arousal. Orgasm is experienced as the most intense and pleasurable aspect of the sexual response cycle. The male experiences expulsive contractions of the entire length of the penile urethra. Semen is rhythmically expelled from the erect penis. At the onset of ejaculation, the internal bladder sphincter closes, preventing retrograde ejaculation into the bladder. Women experience orgasm as rhythmic contractions of the circumvaginal and perineal muscles and of the swollen tissues of the orgasmic platform. The *orgasmic platform* refers to the vasocongestion of the outer third of the vagina and the labia minora. Resolution is marked by a return to normal of the genital and extragenital responses to sexual stimulation.

Sexual dysfunction occurs in the areas of desire (interest), arousal (excitement), and orgasm (tension release). The fourth stage, resolution, is not associated with sexual dysfunction because it refers to the gradual return to the prearousal state. Physical, psychologic, social, and environmental factors may cause these dysfunctions. Neoplastic disease can cause both biologic alterations and psychosocial sequelae that can affect sexuality negatively. The remaining sections of this chapter address (1) the biologic effects of cancer and its treatment that may interfere with sexual expression, (2) the psychosocial effects that the diagnosis of cancer may have on the client and partner, (3) the assessment and management of sexual dysfunctions related to neoplastic disease, and (4) the special problems associated with alterations in sexual functioning.

PATHOPHYSIOLOGIC FACTORS LEADING TO ALTERATIONS IN SEXUAL FUNCTIONING
Cancers of the Genitourinary Tract: Female
Endometrial cancer

Abnormal vaginal bleeding is the most common symptom associated with endometrial cancer. Abnormal vaginal bleeding can hinder sexual relations because either the client or the partner may feel that vaginal bleeding is aesthetically unappealing. Fear of increased bleeding, spread of the disease, or pain can also negatively affect sexual relations. Most patients diagnosed with endometrial cancer are in the early stages of the disease. The standard surgical procedure is abdominal hysterectomy with bilateral salpingo-oophorectomy. Zussman and colleagues found that 33% to 46% of women reported decreased sexual response after hysterectomy-oophorectomy. Pelvic radiation for endometrial cancer may be employed in both early and late stages of the disease. Pelvic radiation can cause vaginal thinning, dryness, and stenosis. All of these side effects can occur and may persist as chronic problems.

Cancer of the cervix

Cancer of the cervix is the second most common form of gynecologic cancer. Women who have early cervical cancer generally are asymptomatic, whereas those with advanced disease often experience postcoital bleeding, pelvic or sciatic pain, and a thin watery discharge. All of these symptoms are likely to inhibit sexual relations. The treatment options employed for women diagnosed with cervical cancer vary, depending on the stage of the disease. Radical hysterectomy has been associated with diminished or completely disrupted sexuality in the range of 6% to 19%. Pelvic radiation for cancer of the cervix has been associated with a 66% rate of sexual dysfunction. Pelvic exenteration may be employed for the treatment of locally persistent or recurrent cervical cancer. Because of the removal of the vaginal canal as well as the introduction of other major anatomic changes, sexual activity is profoundly affected by this surgery.

Pelvic exenteration may be accompanied by vaginal reconstruction to facilitate healing and continued sexual intercourse. Women who have undergone creation of a neovagina following exenteration have reported two outcomes related to sexual functioning: 57% stated that the reconstruction had been a success and they were able to continue satisfactory sexual relations, and 43% reported disruption in the frequency of sexual activity, dissatisfaction with the variety of the activity or with their ability to become aroused, or dissatisfaction with the neovagina itself (the length was too short, the cavity was too large, there was a chronic discharge, intercourse was painful). Continued surgical adaptations accompanied by better sexual counseling and follow-up are needed to improve the positive response rates.

Cancer of the ovary

Ovarian cancer is the third most frequently diagnosed gynecologic malignancy. The symptoms most commonly associated with cancer of the ovary are anorexia, weight loss, increased abdominal girth, change in bowel function, and vague abdominal pain. These symptoms may affect sexual activity but are commonly insidious in onset and are often associated with late-stage disease. Although no studies of the sexual functioning of patients with ovarian cancer have been done to date, one can extrapolate data from studies done with women who have undergone abdominal hysterectomy and bilateral salpingo-oophorectomy. Adjuvant chemotherapy is prescribed routinely after surgery for women with ovarian cancer. This chemotherapy can have devastating effects on body image, self-image, and sexuality. Side effects include alopecia, anorexia, weight loss, lethargy, and bone marrow depression. Patients with end-stage ovarian cancer often experience a prolonged terminal stage. Many experience repeated bouts of intestinal obstruction, abdominal ascites, cachexia, pleural effusion, and sepsis. Any one of these late-stage symptoms can profoundly affect the ability to express physical love.

Cancer of the vulva

Vulvar cancer most commonly is treated with radical vulvectomy and bilateral groin node dissection. This procedure has a tremendous impact on body image and sexual functioning. Fifty percent of women no longer attempted coitus after the operation, and more than two thirds of the women who did make coital attempts experienced pain and some degree of sexual dysfunction. Andersen and Hacker found that despite the fact that intercourse remained possible, sexual functioning underwent a major disruption after radical vulvectomy.

Cancer of the bladder

Bladder carcinoma is the most frequent malignant tumor of the urinary tract. This disease occurs more commonly in the male population with a ratio of 2:1, males to females. One of the more commonly prescribed treatment options for cancer of the bladder is radical cystectomy. Little information has been reported regarding female sexual functioning after radical cystectomy. Schrover et al. found that women who are sexually active before undergoing radical cystectomy can resume a satisfying sex life with appropriate counseling. Vaginal dryness, tightness, and pain were experienced by all women on initial coital attempts. Most couples were able to overcome these difficulties with the use of vaginal hormone cream, vaginal dilation, and Kegal exercises to help the women become aware of muscle tension in the pelvic floor that may contribute to coital pain. All women who made the effort to resume sexual activity experienced a complete recovery in their ability to achieve orgasm.

Cancers of the Genitourinary Tract: Male

Men who have been diagnosed with genitourinary tract cancer often have sexual difficulties related to the disease itself as well as to the treatments prescribed. Sexual disturbances can result in an inability to attain an erection, an ejaculation, or both. These disturbances can result from both physiologic and psychologic sequelae.

Prostate cancer

The sexual dysfunctions associated with cancer of the prostate have been studied widely. Sexual difficulties may arise from even a diagnostic biopsy of the prostate gland. Approximately 24% of open perineal biopsy patients and 32% of the transurethral resection patients reported erectile failure. The treatment for cancer of the prostate varies with the age of the patient, the extent of the disease, and the patient's preference. The current treatment options include radiation (both external and interstitial implant), radical prostatectomy, oral estrogens, or bilateral orchiectomy. Radiation therapy to the prostate and surrounding tissues can result in erectile difficulties in 37% of the population. Fibrosis of the pelvic vasculature or damage to the pelvic nerves is believed to be the cause of these difficulties. The impotence associated with definitive radiation for cancer of the prostate is usually insidious in onset and permanent in nature. The incidence of sexual dysfunction is much higher in patients who undergo a radical prostatectomy. Diminished or complete erectile failure is seen in up to 90% of this population, whereas ejaculation difficulties, with or without some degree of erectile failure, are seen in 78% of the population. Postoperative impotency has been diminished recently by a nerve-sparing technique described by Shapiro. Oral estrogens, bilateral orchiectomy, or both are currently used to treat metastatic or extensive disease. Of patients who reported erectile difficulties, 47% were treated with orchiectomy alone, 22% with estrogen alone, and 73% with the combined treatment. Gynecomastia is a common occurrence in men treated with estrogen, but this side effect has not been directly correlated with sexual dysfunctions.

Cancer of the bladder

Sexual dysfunction related to the treatment of bladder cancer is dependent on the stage and subsequent treatment of the disease. The treatment of superficial bladder cancer (transurethral resection, intravesicle chemotherapy, or fulguration) usually does not result in organic dysfunction. However, repeated cystoscopies can result in a temporarily diminished desire for sex and transient pain during erection and ejaculation. More advanced bladder cancer is treated with either definitive radiation or radical cystectomy, which usually results in sexual dysfunctions similar to those reported for the surgery and radiation used to treat cancer of the prostate. However, an additional consideration for patients undergoing cystectomy is the necessary formation of an ostomy. Self-esteem and body image can be profoundly affected by the presence of the appliance. Enterostomal therapists play a crucial role in the couple's adaptation to this surgery.

Cancer of the testes

Testicular cancer, although rare, is the number one cause of death from cancer in men between the ages of 20 and 40. A unilateral inguinal orchiectomy, with the preservation of the disease-free testicle, maintains both organic sexual function and fertility. However, the loss of a testis can be devastating to a young man's self-image. Retroperitoneal lymphadenectomy may be used as both a diagnostic and a therapeutic tool. This surgical procedure can sever the nerves that are necessary for seminal emissions, thus decreasing the amount of ejaculate during orgasm. Patients who require bilateral orchiectomy experience a decrease in sexual desire because of lowered levels of serum testosterone as well as an alteration in secondary sex characteristics. The effect of combined chemotherapy and surgery on the sexuality of men with testicular cancer was studied by Brenner et al. Only 11% of the patients sampled reported normal ejaculation following combined treatment. However, no long-term effects on sexual desire were observed. Schrover et al. studied the sexual difficulties experienced by men who had received radiotherapy for testicular cancer. Low rates of sexual activity were reported by 19% of the respondents, low sexual desire by 12%, erectile dysfunction by 15%, difficulty reaching orgasm by 10%, and premature ejaculation by 14%. The two most frequently reported problems were reduced intensity of orgasm (33%) and decrease in seminal volume (49%).

Cancers of Other Related Systems
Breast cancer

The diagnosis of breast cancer and the subsequent surgical removal of a breast are major fears among American women. Although the trend in recent years has been to offer alternative forms of treatment, any therapy involving the breasts is often viewed as disfiguring. The type of treatment options available are dependent on the histologic type of lesion and the extent of the disease. Treatments for breast cancer include mastectomy (either simple, modified radical, or radical), lumpectomy, radiation therapy, and chemotherapy. General disruption of sexual activity, reduced frequency of intercourse, or orgasmic difficulties are estimated to occur in 21% to 39% of all breast cancer patients regardless of the treatment employed. Body image disruption is believed to be the major factor involved in the sexual difficulties of breast cancer patients.

Reconstructive surgery following mastectomy is done on a much more frequent basis today. Little research to date has evaluated the effectiveness of reconstructive surgery in lessening the sexual disruptions previously reported. Sexual dysfunction following mastectomy has been reported in the range of 23% to 37%. In addition, 36% of the partners of mastectomy patients have noted a negative impact on sexuality related to the disease and subsequent treatment. Breast conservation through lumpectomy and adjuvant radiation is becoming a more common practice, when feasible. The impact of this form of treatment on sexual functioning has not been studied extensively. Schain is examining the effect of this form of treatment on the partner. Clinical impressions to date have revealed some dysfunctions immediately after therapy, with a gradual return to near normal function over time. Chemotherapy often is used adjuvantly and palliatively in the treatment of breast cancer. The side effects of chemotherapy can themselves cause disruptions in sexual relationships. Hormonal manipulations, as a result of either chemotherapy or oophorectomy, can cause menopausal symptoms, which also can interfere with sexual expression.

The overall psychologic impact of breast cancer on relationships is considerable. Both the patient and her sexual partner can experience temporary or permanent sexual difficulties. Wellisch described five important variables that influence the impact of breast cancer on a marital relationship: (1) the status of the relationship before the cancer developed, (2) the longevity of the marriage, (3) the stage of the breast cancer, especially as this influences the treatment required, (4) the point in the course of the illness, and (5) the interpersonal skills of the partners. Nursing care directed toward the impact of the treatment for breast cancer on sexuality should include educational information, support, and counseling.

Cancer of the head and neck

Head and neck cancer does not directly affect the sexual functioning of the client. Rather, the disease and its treatment are often severely disfiguring and thus cause a dramatic alteration in body image. Facial disfigurement can cause sexual difficulties for both the patient and the sexual partner. The only known direct effect of radiation therapy is a decrease in sexual desire. The indirect effects include sore, dry mouth, drooling, nausea and vomiting, loss of taste and smell, hoarseness, and malaise. Chemotherapeutic agents have been associated with side effects that inhibit sexual functioning. These include alopecia, nausea and vomiting, diarrhea, constipation, mucositis, altered sense of taste and smell, and erectile problems. In addition, many men report fever, weakness, and fatigue associated with bone marrow suppression. Permanent or temporary sterility, a decrease in sex drive, and alterations in secondary sex characteristics, such as hair distribution, voice changes, and breast development, have been noted.

Cancers Affecting the Nervous System
Colorectal cancers

Colorectal cancers and their treatment can produce major effects related to sexual dysfunction. Sexual ramifications of colorectal cancer include those related to the formation of an ostomy or those related to neurologic deficits. Nursing assessment and interventions related to ostomy and possible sexual dysfunction are discussed under "Special Problems Associated with Alterations in Sexual Functioning." The neural disruption is associated with anterior and posterior resection. The parasympathetic nerve damage associated with abdominoperineal resection for cancer of the rectum results in erectile impotence in 50% to 100% of the patients. Ejaculation is lost in 50% to 75% of patients who undergo abdominoperineal resection and 25% report an inability to penetrate the vagina. Reduction in sexual desire has been reported for both men (32% to 59%) and women (28%) who have undergone surgical resection for colorectal cancer. Twenty-one percent of this same female population reported genital numbness and dyspareunia. In addition to the pathophysiologic basis for sexual disruptions, altered body image and self-esteem on the part of the patient can affect sexuality negatively. The partner may harbor fears and misconceptions that will result in sexual difficulties.

Central nervous system tumors

Both primary and metastatic lesions arising in the CNS can affect sexual desire and functioning. Sexual function is dependent on cortical influences, peripheral nerves, autonomic pathways, spinal cord pathways, and reflex centers. Thus, pathologic lesions involving any of these structures may lead to sexual dysfunction. Scant research has been done on the impact of CNS tumors and sexual function. It is possible, however, to extrapolate from the immense body of knowledge on patients with spinal cord injuries and with lesions involving the brain. Much of this literature has involved male patients, probably because more males have spinal cord injuries and because women are assumed to accept more readily a passive sexual role. An intact pathway from the cortex to the sex organ is not necessary for certain components of the human sexual response cycle, for example, attainment of erection and ejaculation. Rather, these functions are mediated by spinal cord reflexes. The important factor to consider is the level of the injury and the degree of interruption of nerve impulses. Sexual gratification can be experienced from feelings other than those emanating from the sex organs. A thorough assessment followed by individualized interventions can optimize sexual functioning in the client with tumors of the nervous system.

Table 26-1 contains a summary of the effects of various cancers on sexuality, including sexual function, fertility, body image, and partners.

Changes in Hormonal Environment and Vasculature

An appropriate hormonal milieu and adequate vasculature to the sex organs are necessary for sexual functioning. Many cancers and treatments affect either or both of these components. A decrease in the amount of circulating estrogen, through surgical removal of the ovaries or chemical suppression by chemotherapy, can result in vaginal dryness, thinning, and other menopausal symptoms. Men treated with estrogen experience gynecomastia and a decrease in libido. A decrease in the amount of circulating androgens, through surgical removal or chemical suppression, also can result in a decrease in sexual drive and feminization in males. Hormonal replacement may be indicated or contraindicated, depending on the reason for the suppression. Patients with hormonally dependent tumors may have their systemic hormonal environment intentionally altered, or this alteration may have been an inadvertent effect of therapy. Interventions, therefore, may be either an adaptation to or a correction of the hormonal imbalance.

A decrease in the vasculature to the genitals also can interfere with sexual functioning. In the male, this decrease can result in an inability to attain or maintain an erection. In the female, it will result in vaginal dryness, thinning, and dyspareunia. The etiologic factors associated with an alteration in genital vasculature include (1) direct tumor compression of the vessels supplying the genitals, (2) surgical disruption of the genital vasculature, and (3) vascular fibrosis as a result of radiation therapy. This vascular compromise can be temporary or permanent. Often, the onset is insidious in nature, especially if the cause is tumor compression or radiation fibrosis. Treatments may be employed to correct the deficiency in vascularization, but cor-

Table 26–1. EFFECTS OF CANCER ON SEXUALITY, INCLUDING SEXUAL FUNCTION, FERTILITY, BODY IMAGE, AND PARTNERS

| Site | Dysfunction | | Effect on Fertility | Altered Body Image | Impact on Partner | Comments |
	Organic	Psychologic				
Cervix	Treatment of in situ with cone biopsy will not cause dysfunction; radical hysterectomy will shorten the vagina by one third to one half; this may be appreciable but usually is not	Sometimes	No, with cone biopsy for in situ stages; yes, with hysterectomy, radiotherapy, or both	Sometimes	Sometimes (partner may feel he can "catch" cancer or be affected by its treatment, especially by radiotherapy)	Radiotherapy to the pelvis will cause thickening of the vagina and may cause stenosis, and/or fistula formation, or both

Note: Chemotherapy, radiation, and analgesics are all associated with generalized feelings of malaise. This can have a profound effect on the feelings of self-worth, sexuality, and libido. All these factors should be taken into consideration when assessing the sexual needs and problems of cancer patients and their families.

From Lamb, M., & Woods, N. F. (1981). Sexuality and the cancer patient. *Cancer Nursing, 4,* 137–144. *Continued*

Table 26-1. EFFECTS OF CANCER ON SEXUALITY, INCLUDING SEXUAL FUNCTION, FERTILITY, BODY IMAGE, AND PARTNERS *Continued*

Site	Dysfunction		Effect on Fertility	Altered Body Image	Impact on Partner	Comments
	Organic	Psychologic				
Endometrial	Total abdominal hysterectomy with pelvic node dissection usually causes no dysfunction; radiotherapy to the pelvis will cause thickening of the vagina if it is included in the fields	Sometimes	Yes, with either radiotherapy or surgery	Sometimes	Sometimes	Because of lack of literature on female sexual response, it is very difficult to determine difference between physical and emotional dysfunction

Ovary	In premenopausal women, bilateral oophorectomy will result in menopausal symptoms	Sometimes	Yes (except with cases with unilateral oophorectomy)	Sometimes	Sometimes	
Vulva	Simple vulvectomy can result in introital stenosis; radical vulvectomy includes removal of the clitoris	Usually	No, patient is often postmenopausal	Most often	Usually	Radical vulvectomy can cause a decrease in range of motion of lower extremities
Breast	The absence of foreplay using nipple stimulation for arousal may cause some difficulties	Usually	None	Usually	Usually	If oophorectomy and hormonal manipulations are used, this can affect all aspects of sexuality

Continued

417

Table 26–1. EFFECTS OF CANCER ON SEXUALITY, INCLUDING SEXUAL FUNCTION, FERTILITY, BODY IMAGE, AND PARTNERS *Continued*

Site	Dysfunction		Effect on Fertility	Altered Body Image	Impact on Partner	Comments
	Organic	Psychologic				
Prostate	Total prostatectomy results in impotence; simple prostatectomy usually results in retrograde ejaculation	Usually	Usually	Usually	Usually	Bilateral orchiectomy or hormonal manipulations can result in decreased libido and sexual responsiveness; if estrogen treatment is initiated, gynecomastia may result

Testicular	Nerve damage due to retroperitoneal lymph node dissection usually results in retrograde ejaculation and can cause impotence	Usually	Sometimes, if unilateral; always, if bilateral; suggest use of sperm bank before chemotherapy and retroperitoneal lymph node dissection	Yes	Usually	Hormonal aberration (especially decrease in androgen) will cause a decrease in libido and may cause impotence, retarded ejaculation, and a decrease in sexual responsiveness
Bladder	Local — seldom; in males, radical cystectomy involves removal of bladder, urethra, and prostate — therefore, he is impotent. In	Usually	Always with radiotherapy; this cancer is most common in older men	Yes (patients usually have urinary conduit with a stoma)	Usually	

Continued

Table 26–1. EFFECTS OF CANCER ON SEXUALITY, INCLUDING SEXUAL FUNCTION, FERTILITY, BODY IMAGE, AND PARTNERS *Continued*

| Site | Dysfunction | | Effect on Fertility | Altered Body Image | Impact on Partner | Comments |
	Organic	Psychologic				
Bladder *cont'd*	females, cystectomy usually includes urethra, uterus, and anterior vagina					
Colon and rectum	Usually; nerve damage in males negatively effects erectile ability	Usually; especially with formation of an ostomy	None, except with radiotherapy and chemotherapy	Yes (if colostomy formed)	Sometimes	Women sometimes have a hysterectomy with the operative procedure
Leukemia	The disease process and associated blood counts with chemotherapy may affect ability to have an erection	Sometimes	Chemotherapy affects sperm count and ova maturation rebound after cessation of treatment	Usually	Usually	Extensive fatigue often diminishes sex drive and function

Hodgkin's disease	Sometimes	Usually	Usually	
	The disease process and the effects of the therapy may decrease sexual drive and ability		Yes, with radiotherapy to the pelvis without shielding of the gonads; chemotherapy will decrease sperm and ova maturation	Patients on chemotherapy alone should be using some form of contraception; the effect on the sperm counts and ova maturation by chemotherapy is not totally understood

Note: Chemotherapy, radiation, and analgesics are all associated with generalized feelings of malaise. This can have a profound effect on the feelings of self-esteem, self-worth, sexuality, and libido. All these factors should be taken into consideration when assessing the sexual needs and problems of cancer patients and their families.
From Lamb, M., & Woods, N. F. (1981). Sexuality and the cancer patient. *Cancer Nursing, 4*, 137–144.

rection is not always possible. Interventions aimed at adaptation to the resulting dysfunction may be the option of choice. These interventions may include use of a watersoluble lubricant if vaginal dryness is a problem or insertion of a penile implant if erection disruption is the resulting problem.

PSYCHOSOCIAL FACTORS INFLUENCING SEXUAL FUNCTIONING
Psychologic Factors

The psychologic factors that often affect sexuality include (1) alteration in body image, (2) diminished self-esteem, (3) role change, (4) attitudes, (5) beliefs and misconceptions, and (6) anxiety or depression. Any one or combination of these factors can affect the sexual functioning of the patient with cancer. Difficulties can occur at any point in the continuum of cancer care: during diagnosis, workup, treatment, or follow-up or during the stage of progressive or terminal disease, should this be the outcome. The client with cancer, the partner, or both can manifest sexual difficulties that are related to their psychologic responses. The emphasis of this section is on the direct effect of these psychologic responses on sexual functioning.

Body image and self-esteem

Body image can be viewed as a component of self-esteem. Living with cancer produces changes in self-esteem, some transient, some permanent. Self-esteem can be affected negatively by cancer, with or without apparent changes in body image, which, in turn, may contribute to feelings of sexual inadequacy. If in addition to altered self-esteem, the patient must adjust to changes in physical appearance, sexual functioning can be compromised further.

The identification and remediation of the patient's impoverished self-esteem, body-image disturbance, and sexual disruption are key goals of cancer care. An assessment of self-esteem can be achieved during an informal discussion and should be conducted at repeated intervals throughout the cancer continuum. This information will be essential in identifying and correcting sexual dysfunctions related to alterations in self-esteem. Efforts should be made directly, through counseling and behavior modification, to build self-esteem to a level compatible with a feeling of being worthwhile.

Anxiety and depression

Anxiety and depression are the two most common affective disruptions among patients with cancer. Clinical depression can be diagnosed in 17% to 25% of the hospitalized cancer population. Anxiety about the future occurs at critical periods for patients with cancer: at diagnosis, at evidence of recurrence, and during the side effects of therapy. Both anxiety and depression have profound effects on sexual functioning.

A decrease in sexual interest, libido, and activity are all results of depressive and anxious states. Depression and anxiety both have been associated with erectile dysfunctions; anxiety has been associated with premature ejaculation. Interventions are aimed at alleviating the anxiety and depression.

Role changes

Social role refers to the patterns of behavior shared by individuals who occupy a certain position or fulfill a certain function in society. Each individual may occupy a variety of social and cultural roles. During illness, some roles are relinquished and assumed by others. Role reversals are sometimes necessary. A person's identity and sense of worth may be threatened when role changes occur. The shifting roles within families of cancer patients should be taken into account when considering the possible etiologic factors associated with sexual dysfunction.

Attitudes, beliefs, and misconceptions

The attitudes and beliefs of a person with cancer regarding cancer and its treatment often affect sexual functioning. Cancer often is viewed as a punishment for past deeds, either real or fantasized. Some patients may harbor misconceptions regarding the etiology of cancer and the impact that it may have on their own as well as their partner's sexual functioning. Fear of contagion is another misconception of some patients.

Social Factors

Social factors that affect the sexual functioning of the patient with cancer include (1) availability of a sexual partner, (2) evidence of anxiety or depression on the part of the partner, (3) effect of role changes on the partner, and (4) partner's attitudes, beliefs, and misconceptions.

Environmental Factors

Two main environmental factors that may impede sexual expression are (1) hospitalization, with its inherent lack of privacy and traditional views of the patient as an asexual being, and (2) alterations in the home environment that often lead to a decrease in the privacy necessary for intimate relations to occur. Nurses can take an active role in policy setting to allow for intimate time in the hospital setting. This will serve to validate the humanness of their patients as well as to offer holistic care.

The home setting is sometimes altered to allow for convalescent, progressive, or terminal care. This alteration is rarely conducive to intimate relationships. Couples should be encouraged to negotiate with family members, friends, and members of the health care team for private time on a regular basis. Whether or not they choose to use this time for sexual activity is not an issue. The availability of this time will allow for some degree of spontaneity and closeness otherwise lost owing to the hectic surroundings.

ASSESSMENT AND MANAGEMENT OF ALTERATIONS IN SEXUAL FUNCTIONING
Sexual Assessment

Assessment of sexual health begins with a sexual history and is supplemented by data regarding the person's general health, such as that obtained from a physical examination or a general health history. The following is a brief sexual assessment that can be incorporated easily into a more general nursing assessment.

Has being ill interfered with your being a (husband, father, wife, mother)?
Has your illness changed the way you see yourself as a man/woman?
Has your illness affected your sexual function?

A physical examination, not necessarily specific to sexual function, will shed light on potential sexual problems. Dyspnea on exertion, range of motion difficulties, vaginal stenosis detected during an internal pelvic examination are all examples of physical limitations that may impede sexual functioning.

To assess the sexual health of oncology patients effectively, the nurse must first be comfortable with the topic of sexuality. Comfort with self as a sexually expressive human being will convey comfort to others. The ease of obtaining a sexual history can be enhanced by using several simple techniques: ensuring privacy and confidentiality, allowing ample, uninterrupted time, and maintaining a nonjudgmental attitude. A discussion of sexuality early in one's association with the client will legitimize sexuality as an important aspect of health care and ensure that it is an appropriate topic for concern in the nurse–client relationship. Anxiety will be reduced by moving from less sensitive to more sensitive topics. Use of language that is understandable to the client is essential. However, the use of slang or street language may be uncomfortable for the professional nurse. Therefore, defining terms early in the discussion will alleviate this potential problem.

Certain communication techniques incorporated into the interview may be helpful. Using open-ended questions, questions referring to frequency rather than occurrence, and "unloading" questions are specific examples of such techniques. An example of an open-ended question might be,

"Some women are concerned that the removal of the uterus will decrease their sexual pleasure. Do you have this concern?" A question that refers to frequency rather than occurrence is, "How often do you have sexual intercourse" as opposed to "Do you have sexual intercourse?" "Unloading" the question refers to such statements as, "Some men masturbate on a regular basis, whereas others seldom or never masturbate. How often do you masturbate?" Finally, asking the client if he or she has any questions at the end of the assessment will convey a willingness to explore further those issues that were brought up during the assessment.

Interventions

The specific sexual needs or concerns of the client dictate the approach and content of the discussion. These needs and concerns can be either current or anticipated. The American Cancer Society has published two comprehensive booklets to assist cancer patients to adapt to the sexual changes that take place during cancer therapy: *Sexuality and Cancer: For the Woman Who Has Cancer, and Her Partner* and *Sexuality and Cancer: For the Man Who Has Cancer, and His Partner*.

Intervention can be approached in many fashions. The P-LI-SS-IT model provides four levels of intervention. P-LI-SS-IT is an acronym for permission, limited information, specific suggestion, and intensive therapy. The first three levels are considered brief therapy and the fourth is intensive therapy.

Permission. Permission to discuss sexual concerns and problems is the initial step of intervention. Open communication regarding sexuality is essential for the subsequent components of the intervention process. Often patients want to know whether their sexual practices are normal or acceptable. This includes both actual sexual behaviors and thoughts, desires, and dreams. Concerns may develop about becoming sexually aroused at what is thought to be inappropriate times, for example, while the partner is hospitalized. Permission includes reassuring the patient and partner regarding all components of sexuality.

Limited Information. The second level of treatment is referred to as limited information. This level includes the first level, permission, but, in addition, gives specific information that addresses sexual concerns, myths, misconceptions, and questions that have arisen. Included in this level are basic facts on the appropriateness of sexual activity at this point and on the possibility of contagion or exacerbation of the malignancy. False assumptions about loss of sexual function and concerns about fertility are addressed. Providing anticipatory guidance regarding what to expect as a result of disease and treatment is included in this discussion.

Specific Suggestions. If the problem requires more than permission and information, the third level, specific suggestions, is initiated. This level of counseling attempts to help the couple directly to change behavior to reach a stated goal. Before embarking, the professional should have obtained a sexual problem history, as outlined previously. A clearly stated goal also is a requisite for the third level. The resultant plan will include specific activities for the couple. Usually, the couple is seen on several occasions. The subsequent sessions are used to assess progress and address related concerns. Specific suggestions usually pertain to the areas of communication, symptom management, and alternate physical expression.

Communication between partners should be fostered. This includes candid discussions regarding their emotional response to the disease and treatments, their fears and concerns, and their development of active listening skills. Symptom management is essential to optimize sexual expression. Cancer and its associated treatments often cause nausea and vomiting, weight loss, pain, fatigue, shortness of breath, and range of motion difficulties. The management of all of these symptoms may be necessary. Alternate physical expression is necessary if sexual disruption is due to organic changes. If intercourse is difficult or impossible, the couple will have to explore or expand alternate forms of expressing physical love. A thorough discussion of the couple's values and attitudes should be conducted before initiating alternative suggestions. There are many ways of stimulating and giving sexual pleasure: hugging, fondling, caressing, cuddling, kissing, and handholding. Genital intercourse is only one way of expressing physical love. Sexual gratification may be derived from manual, digital, and oral stimulation. Intrathigh, anal, and intramammary intercourse are also options if the female partner is unable to continue to experience vaginal penetration.

Intensive Therapy. Intensive therapy can be instituted if adequate progress is not being made or if the couple has long-standing sexual or marital problems. At this point, the couple is referred to a professional who has received advanced training in sex therapy. This person may be a nurse, social worker, psychiatrist, psychologist, or sex therapist.

SPECIAL PROBLEMS ASSOCIATED WITH ALTERATIONS IN SEXUAL FUNCTIONING

Cancer and cancer care often have symptoms or side effects that can negatively affect sexual functioning.

Fertility Concerns

Clients diagnosed with cancer during their childbearing years often have concerns regarding their future ability to parent children. Surgery, radiation, and chemotherapy all have been demonstrated to cause sterility. The topic of permanent or temporary sterility should be discussed before the onset of treatment. The client or couple's attitudes and values regarding future childbearing should be explored thoroughly. Once the assessment has been completed, preventive measures and procreative alternatives should be discussed and planned. Examples of preventive measures are surgical relocation of the ovaries before pelvic radiation or shielding of the gonads during radiation therapy. If preventive measures are not feasible, procreative alternatives can be suggested, such as contributing sperm to a sperm bank before treatment, artificial insemination, in vitro fertilization and embryo transfer, or adoption.

Storing sperm in a sperm bank is a reproductive option that should be considered when counseling male cancer patients. The banking of sperm offers the client protection from the mutagenic and antifertility effects of cancer therapy. The preserved sperm can then potentially be used in subsequent artificial insemination or in vitro fertilization, as indicated. The issues related to this procedure for male cancer patients are still evolving. These issues include appropriateness of the candidate, costs, collection and storage procedures, legal considerations, and ethical issues. The American Fertility Society (1608 13th Avenue South, Birmingham, AL 35256) provides publications pertaining to infertility and lists of human semen cryobanks in the United States and facilities involved in in vitro fertilization and embryo transfer.

Artificial insemination is the next logical step after banking sperm and determining the appropriate time for conception. Artificial insemination is a procedure that usually occurs in an outpatient setting. Once the approximate date of ovulation is determined, usually via recording of basal body temperature and monitoring of cervical mucosa characteristics, the insemination is scheduled. Two inseminations are done per ovulation cycle. Six to 12 cycles of insemination often are required before pregnancy occurs.

In vitro fertilization and embryo transfer is yet another evolving option for couples who anticipate or are actually experiencing infertility problems. An in-depth discussion of this procedure is unwarranted in this text. Briefly, the ovaries are continually monitored via periodic ultrasound to determine the appropriate time for laparoscopic attainment of the ovum. Once the ripe follicles are obtained, they are mixed with the partner's semen in a culture dish, which is then incubated for 36 to 40 hours. The resultant embryo is then transferred into the uterus, and, if pregnancy occurs, it is established within 2 weeks. A number of issues must be considered by the couple considering this procreative alternative. The overall success rate of in vitro fertilization and embryo transfer is quite low. The costs of the procedure, which is not customarily covered by insurance, are exorbitant. The cost factor alone often leaves this option available to a very few. Finally, this procedure has been found to be quite emotionally taxing. Often an exploration of the couple's coping abilities is determined before initiation into the program. All of these factors should be taken into account by the couple considering this option.

Range of Motion Difficulties

The progression of the cancer as well as the surgical procedures used to treat it may leave the patient with limited range of motion. The emphasis of this discussion is on interventions to optimize the sexual functioning of clients with range of motion difficulties. Suggestions to minimize these effects are to (1) experiment with different positions, (2) use pillows to support body weight, (3) employ relaxation techniques or massage, (4) use warm baths or hot or cold soaks to affected areas before intercourse, (5) use medications (sparingly), and (6) explore alternate ways of expressing physical love.

Ostomy

The presence of an ostomy may affect sexual expression. Education, both before and after surgery, can prevent or minimize the detrimental effects that the presence of an ostomy may have on sexuality. Specific interventions are dependent on the patient's particular type of ostomy. Patients with continent ostomies can plan their sexual activity, remove the appliance, and cover the stoma before initiating sexual relations. If the appliance cannot be removed safely, the patient can empty the appliance before initiating intercourse, use a cover or a body stocking to conceal the appliance, or turn the appliance to the side (if the ostomate is in the dependent position). If the appliance is in the way, explore alternate positions. If a leak occurs, continue sexual play in the shower. The United Ostomy Association (36 Executive Park, Suite 120, Irvine, CA 92714; (714)660-8624) has published several booklets that deal specifically with the sexual concerns of ostomates: *Sex, Courtships and the Single Ostomate; Sex, Pregnancy and the Female Ostomate;* and *Sex and the Male Ostomate.*

Nausea and Vomiting

Nausea and vomiting are frequently associated with cancer treatments. These side effects can interfere directly with sexual functioning. Numerous drug and nondrug approaches have been recommended for control of nausea and vomiting. Antiemetics often are used but they may interfere with sexual function because of their sedative effects. Articles have been published on patient control of nausea and vomiting. If this can be done, alternate nondrug methods to control these symptoms should be explored. These include (1) recalling past strategies that were successful in controlling nausea and vomiting, (2) eating foods that are cold or at room temperature, (3) eating small, frequent meals (especially refraining from large meals before sexual play), (4) avoiding foods with strong odors, (5) avoiding sights, sounds, and smells that stimulate nausea, (6) using relaxation or distraction techniques, (7) providing for fresh air (an open window), and (8) timing sexual activities around periods of nausea (if known).

Pain

Sexual arousal is often impaired by the presence of pain. The goal of pain therapy is to relieve pain or discomfort without hindering sexual responsiveness. The use of pain medication may decrease libido or interfere with erectile ability. Experimenting with alternate forms of pain management, other than medication, should be explored. Relaxation techniques, such as guided imagery, may be helpful. Romantic music can be employed both for mood setting and for distraction and relaxation. Sexual activity itself is a form of distraction. Biofeedback, self-hypnosis, and application of hot and cold packs to the affected areas may substantially alleviate discomfort. The couple should be encouraged to experiment: to discover and use the most comfortable positions. The creative use of pillows should be suggested. Massage can be both therapeutic in reducing pain and an arousal technique. Pain medication should be used sparingly, if at all. Finally, alternate ways of expressing physical love should be explored if the couple's traditional methods of sexual gratification are no longer feasible because of discomfort.

Fatigue

Methods to minimize exertion are necessary if fatigue is a limiting factor in sexual activity. Providing time for rest before and after intercourse often is sufficient to minimize the detrimental effects of a decrease in available energy. Other suggestions include (1) avoid the stress of consuming heavy meals or alcohol before intercourse, (2) avoid extremes in temperature, (3) experiment with positions that require minimal exertion (male client-female astride, female client-male astride, side lying), (4) take timing into consideration (intercourse in the morning rather than at night), and (5) periodically delegate or delay household tasks, such as child care and meal preparation, to conserve energy for intimate relations.

Shortness of Breath

Sexual activity can be directly impaired by dyspnea. The fear of potential dyspnea itself is often a deterrent to initiating sexual play. The use of a water bed to accentuate physical movements during sexual activity can be suggested. In addition, keeping the affected partner's head and upper torso raised (via the use of pillows) will also encourage adequate oxygenation. Pulmonary hygiene before sexual activity may be of benefit. Finally, the affected partner should be encouraged to assume a more passive role and a dependent position during sexual activity.

27 Alterations in Mobility

KARIN DUFAULT
SHARON CANNELL FIRSICH

Alterations in mobility present some challenging problems to the nurse caring for the person with cancer. Although they are less obvious than such problems as nutrition and pain, alterations in mobility may profoundly affect the quality of life for the person and family as they deal with the disease and its treatment.

See the corresponding chapter in *Cancer Nursing: A Comprehensive Textbook*, by Baird, McCorkle, and Grant, pp. 850–863, for a more detailed discussion of this topic, including a comprehensive list of references.

THE INTERACTION OF NORMAL PHYSIOLOGY AND MOBILITY

Effects of Position and Weightbearing

The maintenance of normal muscle and bone strength and structure is partially dependent on weightbearing and normal levels of activity. Both weightbearing and normal mobility help to maintain the balance between bone formation and resorption and muscle mass and strength. The effect of position on mobility is usually produced by limitation of position, which prevents weightbearing or full muscle use, thereby decreasing joint motion and muscle strength.

The direct effect of position and weightbearing is of greatest importance for mobility of the musculoskeletal system, but it is also important to keep in mind the other physical functions that are influenced by mobility: metabolic, respiratory, cardiovascular, integumentary, and eliminative (Table 27–1).

Metabolic functions undergo changes as the metabolic rate is decreased. Tissue atrophies and protein catabolism increases, bone demineralization begins, alteration in the exchange of nutrients occurs, and gastrointestinal disturbances develop. *Respiratory* changes then occur, partly as a direct effect of the immobility, partly as an effect of the metabolic changes. Hemoglobin decreases, lung expansion decreases, and generalized muscle weakness and stasis of secretions develop. The major changes in cardiovascular functioning are orthostatic hypotension, increased cardiac workload, and thrombus formation. Immobility has its greatest effects on the integrity of the *skin* of elderly people with altered sensory or motor function and nutritional or metabolic changes—a fair description of many persons with cancer. Any one of these factors puts the person at risk for alterations in skin integrity. In the *eliminative* processes, several changes relate to altered mobility: urine retention, renal calculi, and urinary tract infections may result, and constipation becomes a common problem.

Effects of Muscle and Joint Movement

The general body effects of position and weightbearing on immobility have been discussed, but the specific effects of decreased muscle and joint use also need to be considered. Normal range of motion can be maintained only with full use and normal activity. With increasing age, range of motion, particularly in the spine, tends to decrease even in persons without actual disease conditions, although these changes are extremely variable from person to person.

The mechanical effect of muscle and, indirectly, joint movement is part of the body's mechanism for maintaining adequate venous return. Alterations result in increased venous stasis and increase the threat of thrombus formation.

Table 27–1. POTENTIAL EFFECTS OF IMMOBILITY

Physiologic

Metabolic
  Reduced metabolic rate
  Reduced adrenal corticoids
  Stress reactions
Cardiovascular
  Orthostatic hypotension
  Increased workload
  Thrombus formation
Skin
  Decubitus ulcers
Respiratory
  Decreased respiratory movement
  Stasis of secretions
  Oxygen–carbon dioxide imbalance
Musculoskeletal
  Osteoporosis
  Contractures
Urinary
  Urinary tract stones
Gastrointestinal
  Ingestion
  Elimination
    Suppression of defecation
    Constipation

Psychosocial

Altered perceptions
Altered social roles
Altered mood states

Developmental

Delayed achievement of developmental tasks
Regression to previous developmental level

Skin integrity is protected indirectly with normal mobility of the muscles and joints, as the maintenance of venous return helps prevent stasis and edema. In addition, normal movement prevents undue pressure on any particular area of the skin, again helping to guard against the dangers that pressure and ischemia present to the skin.

PATHOPHYSIOLOGIC FACTORS THAT INTERFERE WITH MOBILITY IN THE PERSON WITH CANCER
Effect of Disease Process and Treatment

Alterations in mobility stemming from the disease process may be categorized as either structural or functional. In structural effects there is actual disease involvement of the mobilizing body parts themselves (e.g., bones, muscle, nerves, or connective tissue). These structural changes may be due to destruction of tissue, or they may be a result of pain or edema in the body part, which then leads to alterations in the mobilizing structures themselves. In functional effects, the altered mobility is an indirect effect, such as fatigue or altered mental status, that has been produced by the disease process. The alteration means that, initially at least, there is no damage to the mobilizing structures, but because the person is unable to use those structures normally, owing to the absence of strength, coordination, and so forth, the lack of use results in structural changes.

The disease process may have a direct effect on mobility, but an equal problem may be the effect of the treatment. Again this may be structural: surgery, radiation, and even chemotherapy may cause actual changes in the body parts that are necessary for mobility. In addition, these same treatment methods may cause various effects that indirectly produce a functional loss of mobility: pain, fatigue, and weakness all may at some time be part of the person's daily life and have a profound effect on the ability to be normally mobile.

Effect of Lymphedema

Lymphedema may be produced in the person with cancer by the disease itself, with malignant involvement of lymph nodes or surrounding structures causing obstruction of lymph flow and preventing the movement of these osmotically active materials back into the systemic circulation. This same effect may be produced by surgery or radiation during or subsequent to the treatment process as healing and fibrosis occur. Obviously, the location of the alteration will be the most important determinant of the effect on mobility. Lymphedema, although a less common cause of lower extremity immobility in cancer survivors, is still a relatively common problem in the arms of women with radical or modified radical mastectomies. Even with less extensive breast surgery, both discomfort and decreased mobility may result in the affected arm when the patient undergoes lymph node dissection or radiation. It is important to keep in mind that in chronic edema, the tissue spaces become stretched so that less filtration pressure is needed to maintain the edema. This stretching then makes permanent correction of the edema difficult. Prevention of extensive edema that may threaten mobility of any body part then becomes an important goal of posttreatment nursing care. Treatment with radiation or surgery is sometimes helpful in relieving the obstruction that is causing the edema.

Effect of Tumor Involvement of the Bone

Characteristically, the person with a primary bone tumor has a painful mass. This pain often is not actually of immobilizing degree at the outset but may cause alteration in normal mobility as the person's usual activities begin to be curtailed owing to pain. Because primary lesions of the bone most commonly occur in children and young people, often in the bones of the extremities, the effect of increasing disease and subsequent treatment on mobility is likely to be profound. As pain increases, mobility becomes much more limited.

Treatment is most commonly surgical and is certain to produce some modification in mobility. In addition, some alteration will be permanent. Cryosurgery, radiotherapy, and chemotherapy may be used at some stages of treatment and may produce either temporary or permanent alteration in mobility of the affected part. Again, treatment may cause additional pain and fatigue, which compound the total physical impact and further decrease the person's mobility. Secondary use of radiation therapy, chemotherapy, or surgery may be helpful in reducing pain and, therefore, increasing mobility. Both the presence of metastatic tumor and its treatment have some of the same effects on mobility as those of primary bone tumor in that bone pain probably will occur, with its immobilizing effect, and again treatment may produce side effects that compound the immobilization.

Additional threats to mobility often are present for the person with bony metastasis. The population with metastatic disease is likely to be an older group than that of patients with primary disease, so that mobility is already threatened, either from the aging process itself or from other systemic disease. Usually, these people have been treated, or the disease itself may have resulted in immobilizing residual effects. Treatment options may be limited because of the previous treatment. In metastatic disease, the extremities are less likely to be affected, and the bones of the spine, ribcage, and pelvis are more commonly involved. Tumor in these locations often has a profound effect on the person's ability to be normally mobile, whether because of pain at the site or because of weakened bone structure, which may result in pathologic fractures.

Effect of Spinal Cord Compression

Some primary spinal cord tumors may cause alteration in CNS function. These are often relatively slowly progressive, and the neurologic deficits appear later in the course of disease because the spinal cord is able to adapt to the compression. With metastatic lesions, however, neurologic change is often rapid and progressive. Because of the anatomic structure of the spine, symptoms generally begin well below the site of the lesion, and the level of impairment ascends as the compression increases and deeper cord levels are affected. Cord compressions can disturb the patient's sense of position, producing ataxia with its resultant disturbance of mobility. Metastatic tumors are likely to be extradural, and pain—either localized or radicular—is often the first symptom. The localized pain tends to be increased by movement and is particularly immobilizing. Actual compression of the spine may come from encroachment of the tumor, collapse of the vertebral column, or hemorrhage from the tumor. Once the compression begins, it rapidly becomes total. Paresthesia and sensory loss progress to irreversible paraplegia unless decompression can be accomplished. Decompression is most likely to be surgical, although radiation and chemotherapy also may be employed in this urgent situation. Fortunately, early recognition and management of the problem can prevent these serious effects. This makes the nursing responsibilities of assessment and rapid diagnosis of altered sensation and functioning critical.

Effect of Central Nervous System Involvement

Because of the diversity of brain tumors, it is difficult to generalize about their effect on mobility. Altered mobility observed in persons with brain tumors most often is related to treatment effects occurring after the surgery, radiation therapy, or chemotherapy used to treat the primary lesion. This treatment may cause alteration in mobility because of sided weakness or seizures, just as the disease itself may.

PSYCHOSOCIAL FACTORS THAT INTERFERE WITH MOBILITY IN THE PERSON WITH CANCER

Besides the pathophysiologic features that alter the ability of a person with cancer to be freely mobile, numerous psychosocial factors influence mobility (Table 27–1).

Patterns of Activities of Daily Living

The degree of functional independence experienced by a person may influence both the responses to changes in mobility and the changes themselves. Functional independence encompasses the wide range of activities engaged in by persons during the course of a 24-hour day and are often described as activities of daily living and self-care. Activities of daily living capabilities often are considered in the light of whether the person is independent in bed, in the home, or in the community.

Among the activities that are examined to determine functional independence are (1) bathing, (2) communicating, (3) exercising, (4) grooming, (5) dressing, (6) eating, (7) bed and hygiene activities, (8) mobility, (9) transferring, (10) recreation, (11) socializing, (12) homemaking, (13) sexual activities, (14) avocational activities, and (15) vocational activities. A study by Chiou and Burnett indicated the importance of patients' values as they relate to specific activities of daily living. The value placed on the activity was an important factor to consider in identifying rehabilitation goals in this study, which involved stroke patients. The relative value of the activities that indicated functional independence for the person with cancer may also have a bearing on the response of the person to alteration in self-care and, more specifically, to alterations in mobility. Awareness of the degree to which alterations in mobility interfere with the functional independence activities of greatest value to the person can provide insights into understanding the real impact of the changes. The understanding can guide nursing interventions as they relate both to mobility and to enhancement of the other significantly valued activities of daily living. Among the most highly valued activities of daily living are those related to mobility.

General Lifestyle Patterns

Lifestyle patterns represent a complex outcome of many personal, interpersonal, environmental, and societal factors, which arise not only from the person's present situation but also from his or her history and heredity. Carnevali and Patrick defined lifestyle as the totality of a person's approach to living. It incorporates such characteristics as preferences for independence or dependence, high or low stress levels, spontaneity and change or structure and regularity, extroversion or introversion, rapid or slow pace, and high or low physical activity. The preferences translate into observable behaviors in approaching routine as well as unusual events.

PROCESS OF ASSESSMENT IN THE DIAGNOSTIC PROCESS
Assessment of the Problem

Nursing data need to be gathered regarding both the level of mobility and the potential for sequelae related to immobility. The data collected must be both objective and subjective.

The two aspects of data gathering—history and physical assessment—must be attended to. There are many indexes for measuring the activities of daily living—probably the most useful way to examine the alteration in mobility. Because more than 43 different indexes have been developed, few of which have been documented empirically, it is difficult for the nurse to find a generally accepted means of evaluating the patient's level of activity. Probably the two most commonly used scales are the Karnofsky Scale and the Barthel Index. Although few scales have been developed specifically for oncology patients, the existing scales often have useful approaches for the nurse's consideration in assessment of the patient with a problem of immobility.

Having developed the initial database that allows assessment of the person's present level of mobility and the potential for sequelae secondary to that level of mobility, the nurse is ready to move on to the identification of actual or potential health problems and formulate the nursing diagnoses on which the care plan can be built (Table 27-2).

Defining the Characteristics of the Problem

The accepted nursing diagnosis for alterations in mobility is Mobility, impaired physical—related to alterations in lower limbs or alterations in upper limbs. The major characteristics that must be present are the inability to move purposefully within the environment, including bed mobility, transfers, and ambulation, or the inability to move because of imposed restrictions (e.g., bedrest, mechanical devices). Minor characteristics that may be present are range of motion limitations, limited muscle strength or control, and impaired coordination. Information gathered from the assessment process should allow the nurse to identify which of these defining characteristics are present or are realistic potentials for a given client.

Etiologic and Risk Factors Related to the Problem

Because the diagnostic process allows the nurse to put in rational order the quantities of information accumulated in the database, it is necessary to look beyond the major and minor characteristics of the problem to examine etiologic and contributing factors, since it is toward these factors that nursing interventions are likely to be addressed. For impaired physical mobility, these factors fall into four categories: pathophysiologic, treatment related, situational, and maturational. The *pathophysiologic* factors may relate to neuromuscular impairment or to musculoskeletal factors. The *treatment-related* factors may be associated with activity restrictions such as bedrest, physical changes such as amputation, or mechanical devices. *Situational* factors are personal or environmental and may consist of such things as pain or trauma. Finally, *maturational* developmental factors involve primarily the very young or the very elderly and their limitations, such as lack of balance in the toddler or cautious gait in the elderly with failing eyesight (Table 27-1).

MANAGING SPECIFIC PROBLEMS OF MOBILITY
Activity Intolerance

Activity intolerance (the state in which the person experiences an inability, physiologically and psychologically, to endure or tolerate an increase in activity) is a commonly occurring problem for the person experiencing cancer or cancer treatment and is directly related to the impairment of physical mobility. The causative factors may relate to fatigue or problems with oxygen transport. When these factors have been adequately identified for the patient, nursing action can be taken. In focusing the assessment data (both subjective and objective), it is helpful first to examine factors that increase fatigue, then to examine the effects of fatigue on the activity level, and then to examine the actual response to activity. It is here that the use of an activity index, such as the Karnofsky Scale or Barthel Index, can be useful.

After the assessment data are focused, it is possible to examine the results and decide which contributing factors (such as inadequate sleep or rest periods, pain, medications, daily schedule, and lack of incentive) are variably amenable to nursing action. The daily schedule and rest periods require creative problem solving with client, family, and caregivers all involved so that a satisfactory schedule can be developed. Pain management is not discussed here because it is covered

Table 27-2. FOCUSED ASSESSMENT CRITERIA

Subjective Data

History of systemic disorders
   Neurologic
   Cardiovascular
   Musculoskeletal
   Respiratory
   Debilitating diseases
History of symptoms that interfere with mobility
   Symptoms
      Pain
      Muscle weakness
      Fatigue
   Criteria
      Onset
      Duration
      Location
      Description
      Frequency
      Precipitated by what?
      Relieved by what?
      Aggravated by what?
History of recent trauma or surgery
Current drug therapy
   Pain
   Sedative
   Laxatives
   Chemotherapy

Continued

Table 27-2. FOCUSED ASSESSMENT CRITERIA *Continued*

Objective Data

Dominant hand
Motor function
  Right arm
  Left arm
  Right leg
  Left leg
Mobility
  Ability to turn self
  Ability to sit
  Ability to stand
  Ability to transfer
  Ability to ambulate
Weightbearing (assess right and left sides)
  Gait
  Assistive devices
  Restrictive devices
  Range of motion (shoulders, elbows, arms, hips, legs)
Endurance
  Assess
    Resting pulse, blood pressure, respirations
    Blood pressure, respirations, and pulse after activity
    After activity, assess for the presence of indicators of
      hypoxia
Peripheral circulation
  Capillary refill time
  Skin color, temperature, and turgor
  Peripheral pulses

extensively elsewhere in this book (Chapter 23), but it is crucial to the achievement of optimal activity levels for the person. Further treatment, such as surgery, radiation therapy, and chemotherapy, will at times be indicated to reduce pain and allow increased mobility. Medications sometimes interfere with sleep management for the person with activity intolerance, either because side effects of medication make adequate sleep difficult or because the scheduling of medications interferes with the sleep cycle. Usually with consideration of the goal (to increase sleep and rest, thereby increasing activity tolerance), it is possible to modify medication schedules to reduce, if not eliminate, the negative effect of the medication regimen on sleep pattern.

The lack of incentive may present the greatest challenge to the nurse in motivating the client to increased levels of activity. Although it is difficult to find research documentation for many of the nursing interventions used in this challenging problem, empirically it has been found helpful to make contracts with the client about activity, identify progress, and consider concrete incentives, such as behavioral or physical rewards.

Alteration in Activities of Daily Living and Self-Care

The success of persons in maintaining functional independence while coping with cancer depends in part on the effectiveness and efficiency of their mobility. When the ability to move around is compromised, so too may be initiative, self-confidence, and motivation to be involved in the activities that had significance to daily life. An essential step in caring for the cancer patient with alterations in mobility is to learn from the patient what the status of his or her mobility is in relation to usual activities of daily living and customary lifestyle. What activities can or cannot be done independently? Which activities require assistance? Which activities are of greatest significance to the person, and which do the family consider most important? Has the patient given up some activities and at what price? Have frequency, duration, and regularity of the activities been changed because of mobility alterations? How is the family affected by the changes? What are the safety concerns related both to the alteration in mobility and the alteration in activities of daily living? One of the most obvious associations between altered mobility and activities of daily living is the fact that most activities of daily living ordinarily occur in certain places within the home, workplace, or community. If a person is unable to walk to the usual setting for whatever reason, independently or with assistance, other modes of getting there must be used, such as wheelchair or lift. Otherwise, the activity must be performed wherever the person might be spending the majority of time, such as in bed. The extent to which this is a significant deviation from what has been normal to the person's lifestyle may indicate the difficulty of adapting to the change. Limitations of physical movement of the upper extremities, such as with lymphedema or pathologic fractures, also affect the ability to perform self-care activities.

Another factor to be assessed is whether the process leading to the alteration in mobility is the same process directly affecting alteration in the self-care ability. For example, if spinal cord compression damage is the cause of the alteration in mobility, it may also be the direct cause of deficits in other personal self-care abilities, such as toileting, depending on the level of spinal cord involved. Compensating for the mobility change would not necessarily correct the self-care deficit and would call for additional nursing interventions that targeted the neurologic problems. Pain may be another type of limitation on both mobility and self-care ability. The assessment also includes objective data in the form of observing mobility factors in relationship to performance of specific activities of daily living.

Alteration in Bowel Elimination

Probably the most significant interaction between mobility and bowel elimination is the tendency to constipation when mobility is seriously limited. If the person reports hard stools fewer than three times weekly and complains of difficulty moving the bowels and also is immobile, it is likely that the two are at least partially related. A therapeutic bowel regimen will need to be instituted until or unless the immobility problem can be resolved. Corrective measures should include evaluation of the diet, with an attempt to increase the fiber. Bran should be used moderately at first, but fresh fruits and vegetables can be encouraged to an amount equal to 800 g per day (4 to 5 servings). Encourage the client to identify fruits and foods that have laxative effects. Fluid intake should total at least 2 L daily, with the emphasis on water or fruit juices, not on caffeine drinks. Warm water should be drunk in the morning to stimulate the gastrocolic reflex. Activity or even range of motion exercises are often helpful. Establish a regular time for elimination using the client's normal pattern as much as possible with relation to time, place, position, and equipment. Privacy is extremely important to many people. It may be necessary to use suppositories, stool softeners, or mild laxatives. Constipation should be treated early and consistently for the immobilized person so that it can be managed with the most physiologic and least irritating measures. When the patient is neutropenic or thrombocytopenic, it is particularly important to use care in managing constipation to prevent trauma to the rectal area. Diarrhea as an alteration in bowel elimination may present a problem for the client in that immobility may be increased by the fear of increasing diarrhea ("Every time I move, I have another stool"). This is obviously best dealt with by managing the diarrhea effectively, to allow mobility to return to optimal levels.

Alteration in Peripheral Tissue Perfusion

One of the classic problems associated with immobility is the development of peripheral thromboses, which present the nursing problem of altered peripheral tissue perfusion. The primary nursing concern here is a preventive one to keep this a potential problem rather than an actual one. When immobility is added to the tendency toward increased clotting often present in persons with cancer, the person is at considerable risk for development of thromboses. Having established that the potential for this problem exists, the nurse will be watchful that blood pressure is maintained at optimum levels to allow adequate tissue perfusion—

whether this is a problem of cardiac output or of peripheral circulation—especially as it is affected by the sympathetic nervous system. In addition, cellular perfusion, which is vulnerable to obstruction and changes in oxygen level of the circulating blood, must be maintained. Position and mobility have important effects on the optimal maintenance of tissue perfusion. Antiembolic stockings should be used by these patients. Range of motion exercises at least every shift with arm and leg exercises every 1 to 2 hours should be a part of the plan of care. If the person has a problem of immobility that decreases general activity or promotes obstruction of circulation, it is incumbent on the nurse to be alert to means of minimizing the circulatory compromise that may result, thereby minimizing the potential problem. It is also important to realize that the thrombocytopenic patient may need guidance in the kind and amount of activity that is safe.

Impairment of Skin Integrity

The major defining characteristics of the nursing diagnosis relating to the potential impairment of skin integrity are that the person reports fatigue and inability to move or turn and is on imposed bedrest or is immobile. Obviously, the person with cancer who has altered physical mobility is at high risk for this nursing diagnosis. When the contributing factors of impaired oxygen are added, the risk becomes even greater. In assessing clients for particular risk, the oncology nurse will watch for skin deficits such as dryness, edema, thinness, or obesity and for impaired oxygen transport as in anemia or edema. Irritants such as radiation therapy, incontinence, nutritional deficits, systemic problems such as infection or liver failure, and sensory deficits present particular hazards as well.

Alteration in Meaningfulness—Powerlessness

Alterations in mobility and the subsequent experience of dependence can lead to a perceived lack of personal control over one's life, accompanied by apathy, anger, or depression. Each change that threatens the patient's normal life-style, creates dependence, threatens adequacy and competence, and removes the person from the decision-making process at any level can bring varying degrees of helplessness and powerlessness and the sense that external forces are controlling. The powerlessness may be manifested by physical findings, such as facial flushing or pallor, rapid or bounding pulse, increased blood pressure, sweating, trembling, restlessness, sleep disturbances, changes in eating habits, irritability, demanding behavior, or avoiding or leaving situations.

Powerlessness is a subjective state and, therefore, requires validation on the part of the person experiencing it.

An assessment should include the person's usual level of control and decision making and the effects that losing control produces. By asking the patient questions related to decision-making patterns, role responsibilities, perceptions of control, and personal fears, subjective data will be obtained that will contribute to the nursing assessment of the patient's sense of potential or actual powerlessness. By observing the patient's manner of participation in activities of daily living or information seeking and responses to limits placed on decision making and self-control, the nurse can identify the factors contributing to the sense of powerlessness and provide opportunities for patient involvement in decision making that can be followed consistently by all caregivers.

Alteration in Emotional Integrity—Grieving

The grieving process is a normal and expected response to a significant loss of something valued. Losing one's ability to be mobile is in itself a significant loss of freedom and control, which may precipitate yet other losses for the person with cancer. Becoming unable to move may result in loss of ability to perform other activities of daily living independently: loss of body image, self-esteem, and self-identity, loss of social contacts, loss of employment, loss of stable income, and loss of ability to perform usual roles, to name a few. Altered mobility also may herald for the person with cancer the progression of disease and with it the anticipated loss of a personal future and of life itself, with all its associated grief. The family experiences the grieving process along with the patient.

Nursing interventions are directed toward helping the patient and family to express the grief, to describe the meaning of the losses, to competently move through the grieving process with a sense of realistic hope, and to experience the losses as a potential for personal growth.

Although most persons are successful in completing grief work, some exhibit signs that the normal grief process has been seriously delayed or disrupted. Psychiatric intervention is required when one or more of the following characteristics are present: (1) extreme depressive reaction, (2) psychotic break with reality, (3) suicidal tendencies, and (4) substance abuse.

Sensory-Perceptual Alteration—Visual, Kinesthetic

Alterations in mobility can result in a decrease in the amount, pattern, and interpretation of incoming stimuli of a physiologic, sensory, motor, and environmental nature, particularly if the person is bedbound. Lack of communication and lack of touch contact may occur when the person affected by restrictions on mobility has relied on relationships outside the home as the primary source of input. Loved ones and acquaintances may be reluctant to maintain contact because of their own sense of helplessness, not knowing what to say or do to be of assistance in the situation.

Decreased mobility also may result in decreased physiologic function of the respiratory, renal, cerebral, circulatory, and sensory systems, which alter sensory-perceptual function. Immobility may interfere with sleep–rest cycles and with fluid, electrolyte, and nutritional balances, all of which may influence the ways in which the environment is sensed and perceived. In addition, all of these changes may be accompanied by fear of the unknown and potential and actual losses of control, income, familiar persons, objects, and surroundings. Heightened anxiety, depression, fatigue, and boredom contribute to a dulling of sensory responses.

Nursing action can be directed toward manipulating the environment to provide adequate and significant sensory stimulation and toward teaching the patient and family to do likewise. Attention needs to be paid to identifying stimulation, activity, and diversion that are meaningful to the patient.

MANAGING SPECIAL PROBLEMS OF MOBILITY
Lymphedema

The woman with axillary lymph node dissection for breast cancer and the man with prostate cancer or penectomy and groin node dissection most commonly experience this problem. Any time lymph node dissection has occurred or tumor has interfered with lymphatic circulation, the patient has a potential problem. Physically, the problem in mobility usually occurs because of tissue edema that is secondary to obstruction, whether it is caused by scar tissue or by tumor. The edema must be minimized because it tends to become chronic once it is established in the tissue. Ironically, some of the measures used to reduce edema, such as elevation of the part or elastic bandaging, also tend to reduce mobility, so it is important to strike a balance between one treatment and another to maintain maximum range of motion.

Collateral lymphatic drainage usually develops throughout the first 3 to 4 weeks after surgery. Prevention of edema by elevation of the part, massage and exercise to encourage circulation and maintenance of function, and prevention of infection are particularly important during the first 3 months after surgery. If a problem with edema continues despite these conservative measures, an elastic sleeve or stocking may be used. A pneumatic pump attached to such a support may be useful in reducing edema and allow the client to be more comfortable and more mobile. The physical therapist may be an important resource at this point. Client teaching should include avoiding blood pressure measurement, injections, blood drawing, contact with abrasive or irritating materials, and lifting or carrying heavy objects with the affected limb.

Bone Tumors

Because two major symptoms of bone tumors—pain and impairment of function—directly affect mobility, it is not surprising that these tumors present a particular challenge to nursing care with respect to mobility.

Management of pain is obviously a high priority if the person is to increase mobility successfully. The nurse should keep in mind that the nonsteroidal anti-inflammatory drugs (NSAIDs) alone or with narcotic pain medications may be most helpful for the person with bone involvement. Additionally, radiation therapy may be necessary to reduce tumor bulk and pain. Nonchemical means of pain management, such as diversion and imaging, may be of particular significance, and activity itself may be an adjunct in pain management.

Pathologic fractures present a special problem for mobility in the person with bone tumors. In most cases, the fracture treatment methods are similar to those for other fractures, but the complexity of managing pathologic fractures is greater because of the underlying disease process. The effect of the fracture and its treatment will depend largely on the location of the tumor. Sometimes, amputation is necessary and presents its own problems for mobility.

The treatment of bone tumors, whether by surgery, radiation therapy, or chemotherapy, usually will increase mobility and decrease pain. At times, these treatments negatively affect mobility by increasing pain, fatigue, and strength. Because primary bone tumors are more likely to occur in young people, often these patients have the advantage of youthful resiliency of tissue and spirit. Conversely, the management of metastatic bone tumor often presents real challenges because the person is likely to be older, has other disease or treatments as part of the history, and may focus on many other things besides regaining mobility.

Spinal Cord Compression

Spinal cord and nerve root compression of whatever cause (primary spinal cord tumors, metastases from lung, breast, prostate, and kidney, or lymphoma and multiple myeloma) constitutes an oncologic emergency. The characteristic initial symptom in 90% of patients is pain and discomfort in the form of thoracolumbar back pain, often in a beltlike distribution and frequently extending to the groin or legs. Lower extremity weakness is evident is approximately 76% of patients. The weakness, reflex alterations, or paralysis results from upper or lower motor neuron damage.

Unfortunately, the condition often is not recognized until paraplegia is established. The symptoms of muscular weakness, tiredness, and heaviness of the extremities and sensory paresthesia are too often ignored by the patient, physicians, and nurses. When paraplegia or quadriplegia becomes manifest, recovery to a good level of function is unusual.

To prevent devastating complications, it is essential to provide careful nursing assessment and patient teaching, emphasizing timely reporting of signs and symptoms related to potential spinal cord compression for those at risk. Other symptoms related to spinal cord compression include constipation and urinary retention with overflow incontinence, altered gait, ataxia, loss of muscle tone, and decreased sensation in the extremities. Early diagnosis and treatment can lead to complete restoration of function.

Amputation

Lower extremity amputations have a more direct effect on general mobility than do upper extremity amputations, but the general problems are similar: adapting to a prosthesis, making necessary modifications in activities of daily living, and maintaining a positive attitude toward the rehabilitation process. Because of the belief of some health care personnel as well as lay people that rehabilitation is pointless in cancer, particularly metastatic cancer, this process may be particularly challenging for the oncology nurse. If the nursing care of the person with an amputation secondary to malignancy is to be effective, this challenge must be met. It is important to keep in mind that amputation is rarely used alone and the person is almost always treated with some combination of chemotherapy or radiation therapy. These treatments may have other implications for the client's mobility.

Central Nervous System Tumors

The final special problem of mobility to be discussed is that of CNS tumors, another potential oncologic complication that can result in a neurologic emergency. Space-occupying brain malignancies can be primary tumors, but most often they result from arterial metastases from cancers of the lung, breast, prostate, and colon, malignant melanoma, lymphoma, and leukemia. Neurologic symptoms are related to the location and size of the cancer, the extent of local compression and destruction of brain tissue by the mass and edema, and the degree of increased intracranial pressure or obstruction to the normal flow of cerebrospinal fluid.

Mobility may be particularly affected with parietal lobe involvement because sensorimotor function is under parietal control and may be manifested by weakness, atrophy, clumsiness, dysdiadochokinesis, and independent movements unrecognized by the patient. Cerebellar dysfunction can decrease mobility by reducing muscle coordination and ataxia resulting from compression of motor tracts. Frontal (precentral) lobe involvement may result in weakness, hemiparesis, disturbed gait, automatism, rigidity, tonic spasms of toes, and seizures, all of which can affect mobility. Occipital lobe damage may cause visual damage that likewise influences mobility.

The initial treatment of primary tumors often is surgical excision, with removal limited by the location and invasiveness of the cancer. Because most of the malignant brain tumors, both primary and metastatic, are radiosensitive, radiation therapy generally is indicated. Researchers are hopeful that radiation therapy of metastatic disease to the brain may be improved through using radiosensitizers and improved use of computed tomography (CT) and magnetic resonance imaging (MRI) to guide therapy. Local or systemic chemotherapy has been more effective for metastatic tumors than for primary tumors, although continued clinical investigations hold greater promise.

Ultmann and Phillips identified factors that must be considered when determining appropriate treatment for patients with brain metastasis. When the general condition of the patient seems to indicate treatment of the CNS lesion, these investigators consider the following factors to determine the type of local treatment to be employed (namely, surgery, radiation therapy, chemotherapy, or a combination).

1. Number of lesions
2. Location of lesions
3. Primary site
4. Patient age and general functional condition
5. Status of other metastatic disease and the primary tumor
6. Relative radioresponsiveness and radiocontrollability
7. Interval between treatment of the primary lesion and development of brain metastases

Nursing care of the patient with alterations in mobility related to CNS tumors and their treatment includes careful monitoring and reporting of existing or new symptoms, helping with mobility, and intervening to protect from injury. Assessment includes observations of any evidence of increased intracranial pressure and sensory changes as well as motor function and muscular strength of extremities. Activity tolerance and unsteady gait also need to be assessed with each contact, recording ataxia and subjective indications of weakness and fatigue.

28 Complications of Advanced Disease

CYNTHIA CHERNECKY
RUTH L. KRECH

ANATOMIC AND PHYSIOLOGIC FEATURES
Definition of Advanced Disease

Advanced disease is defined as at least one acute organ dysfunction caused by either metastasis or cancer treatment that results in a client's need for comprehensive management in an intensive care environment.

See the corresponding chapter in *Cancer Nursing: A Comprehensive Textbook,* by Baird, McCorkle, and Grant, pp. 864–874, for a more detailed discussion of this topic, including a comprehensive list of references.

PATHOPHYSIOLOGY AND INTERFERING FACTORS LEADING TO ADVANCED DISEASE

Dysfunctions in one vital organ generally lead to subsequent dysfunctions in other vital organs because the vital organs function interdependently.

Vital Organ Metastasis
Brain

Two percent of all cancers are primary brain tumors, and 15% of all cancer clients develop neurologic symptoms from advanced disease. The most common site of metastasis in the brain occurs in the frontal lobe. Although less common, metastases to the temporal, parietal, and occipital lobes occur with similar frequency. The brainstem is the least likely site for metastasis.

Generalized signs and symptoms of brain metastasis include headache, loss of motor function, impaired mentation with lethargy, seizures, sensory loss, and increased intracranial pressure (Table 28–1). These signs and symptoms result in deficits in the following four areas: cognition, mobility, activities of daily living, and bladder and bowel control. The latter three areas are quite manageable on a general medical-surgical division. However, a deficit in cognition, known as neuropsychiatric syndrome, presents an acute situation in which the need for nursing care is greatly increased.

Neuropsychiatric syndrome can be manifested in several ways, ranging from acute anxiety disorders and personality changes to depressed consciousness, stupor, and coma.

Heart

Another facet of advanced disease is heart involvement. Metastases to the heart, specifically the pericardium, occur in 5% to 10% of all clients with cancer. Although cardiac

Table 28–1. SIGNS AND SYMPTOMS OF INCREASED INTRACRANIAL PRESSURE (ICP)

1. Decreased level of consciousness
2. Pupil dilation; occurs on the same side as the tumor
3. Increased systolic blood pressure and widening pulse pressure followed by sharp drop in blood pressure
4. Bradycardia followed by sharp tachycardia
5. Simultaneous bradycardia and increased systolic blood pressure*
6. Decreased respiratory rate
7. Papilledema only when increased ICP develops slowly
8. Hyperreflexia
9. Gait impairment

*Early significant finding.

metastasis can occur through any of the defined modes of metastases, bloodborne and lymphatic metastases are most common. These two patterns of metastases probably account for the fact that cardiac metastasis is almost always accompanied by metastasis to other organs.

Metastasis to the pericardium results in the accumulation of fluid in the pericardial sac. This sac is elastic and may stretch to accommodate as much as 1 L of fluid before cardiac decompensation occurs. This results in a syndrome known as pericardial effusion, which, if ignored, can progress rapidly into cardiac tamponade. If cardiac tamponade can be avoided, the mean survival rate of clients with pericardial effusion alone is 9 to 13 months. A thorough knowledge of the signs and symptoms is imperative. These include dyspnea, cough, nausea, vomiting, epigastric abdominal pain, hepatomegaly, leg edema, and neck vein distention.

Management of undiagnosed pericardial effusion includes treatment of the symptoms, such as providing oxygen for dyspnea, and direct bolstering of the body's hemodynamic compensatory responses with IV fluids and vasopressors. Once a definitive diagnosis has been made, pericardial effusion can be treated with a pericardiocentesis, chemotherapy to the pericardial cavity, or external beam radiation to the heart.

Bone

The third vital organ identified in advanced disease is the skeletal system or bones. Metastasis to the bone occurs in 70% of all clients with cancer. One of the most sensitive diagnostic tests in the determination of bone metastasis is the bone scan. Bone metastasis, which deossifies and softens bones, itself is not lethal. However, the resulting pain, neurologic deficits, and immobility can significantly decrease a client's quality of life. The quality of life can be further compromised by the occurrence of a pathologic fracture.

Pathologic fractures occur in 8% of all clients with cancer. Symptoms may vary according to the location of the fracture. More specifically, pathologic fractures occur most commonly in the spine, ribs, long bones, and sternum. Metastases primarily affect the thoracic and lumbar regions of the spine.

Management of pathologic fractures generally focuses on pain control, palliative chemotherapy, and localized radiation therapy. Localized radiation is either partially or completely effective in the treatment of bone pain in 73% to 96% of clients.

Lung

Lung metastasis, which is the second most common site of metastasis, occurs in 29% of all clients with cancer. The most frequent complication of advanced disease in the lungs is malignant pleural effusion. In fact, almost 50% of all pleural effusions are caused by cancer. Pleural effusion is an exudative process in which irritation of the pleural membrane by cancer cells results in an increased production of fluid in the interpleural space. Normally, the space between the visceral and parietal pleura contains 5 to 15 ml of fluid. However, when cancer cells create overproduction and underabsorption, the interpleural space can contain more than 500 ml of fluid. Although approximately 25% of clients with pleural effusion have no symptoms, signs and symptoms for those with as much as 300 ml of interpleural fluid include dyspnea, pain, and hypoxia. For those with more than 300 ml of fluid in the interpleural space, signs and symptoms become more severe. These include tachycardia, tachypnea, asymmetric bulging of the intercostal spaces, diminished or absent breath sounds, and mediastinal shift.

Goals of management of malignant pleural effusion include treatment of both the symptoms and the cause (metastasis). Selection of the treatment depends on the prognosis and the present condition of the client. Surgical pleurectomy is reserved for clients who are good surgical risks because the procedure has a 10% mortality rate. Needle thoracentesis and chest tube insertion relieve symptoms, but additional procedures, such as sclerosis or pleurodesis, are required for control of pleural effusion. Once treatment for pleural effusion has been implemented, ongoing nursing assessment of respiratory status is imperative.

Liver

One of the most common phenomena of advanced disease is metastatic liver involvement. This has a most profound impact on survival rates. For example, mean survival rates of clients with liver metastasis range from 1.4 months for clients with widespread metastasis to 16.7 months for clients with minimal disease.

A complication of advanced disease to the liver that may decrease the length of survival time is malignant ascites.

Malignant chylous ascites occurs because of an obstruction in the lymphatics. Consequently, the fluid is turbid milky or creamy due to the presence of lymph. This type of ascites occurs most frequently as a result of lymphoma.

Malignant clear ascites occurs as a result of a hypoalbuminemia-induced reduction in the plasma oncotic pressure. In this situation, the protein in the ascitic fluid is greater than the serum protein, and additional fluid is drawn into the abdominal cavity.

General signs and symptoms of malignant ascites include abdominal distention, shortness of breath, and nausea.

Sequelae of Therapies
Drug toxicities

Drug toxicities affect four major organs: heart, lung, liver, and kidney. For example, chemotherapy-induced heart toxicities cause heart enlargement, which develops into congestive heart failure and pulmonary hypertension. In the lungs, antineoplastic agents damage the alveolar epithelium and the basement membrane, which decreases the amount of collagen secreted. The result is fibrosis with impaired gas exchange. The effects of chemotherapy on the liver range from increased level of hepatic enzymes seen with high doses of the drugs to hepatic fibrosis associated with long-term therapy, although the etiology is unknown. Each of the aforementioned types of toxicities is not uncommon in cancer therapy, but kidney toxicity is a more common cause of advanced disease and is discussed in more detail.

Drug-related kidney toxicity occurs when the chemotherapeutic agents cause direct damage to the glomerulus, tubules, or both. In addition, drugs can cause indirect damage through vascular changes. The risk of such damage increases when combination drug regimens are used.

The signs and symptoms of kidney toxicity mimic those of renal failure. They include increased blood urea nitrogen and creatinine values, decreased urinary output, fluid retention, pulmonary rales, nausea, vomiting, edema, and pruritus. In addition, the client should be monitored for metabolic acidosis and cardiac dysrhythmias.

Management of chemotherapy-induced kidney toxicity should include efforts to prevent renal toxicity, such as to administer diuretics and hydration before, during, and after drug administration. Of course, even though prevention efforts are employed, it is not always possible to avoid renal failure, and the client may progress into chronic renal failure. In this instance, dialysis would be indicated.

Radiation

Unlike systemic chemotherapy, external radiation-induced advanced disease is site specific. That is, the areas of the body receiving the radiation will be the areas in which potential complications can occur. For example, radiation to the head and neck area may cause nausea, taste changes, and stomatitis. Although symptoms such as these are quite manageable, the consequences of radiation to the bowel are potentially fatal.

For clients whose cancer extends through the bowel wall, surgery alone is insufficient. Initially, radiation offers further control of the cancer with minimal danger of complications. However, with 5000 rad or greater, the client has a 10% chance of developing bowel adhesions, bowel obstruction, or fistulization. Six to twelve months after therapy, the bowel may become increasingly friable, eliminating the possibility of further surgical intervention. The outcome is malabsorption and paralytic ileus with concomitant bowel necrosis.

Bone marrow transplantation

The third therapeutic sequela that is likely to cause advanced disease is bone marrow transplantation. This therapy generally is used to treat leukemias, although it is being used experimentally on some solid tumors, such as lung cancer, breast cancer, and melanoma. Bone marrow transplantation has one major complication: graft-versus-host disease (GVHD).

Graft-versus-host disease occurs when the donor T cells proliferate and attack various cells in the already compromised host. The four grades of GVHD are distinguished by the degree of organ involvement, with grade 1 involving only a skin rash and grade 4 involving multiorgan failure and extreme decrease in clinical performance. In addition, GVHD can be either acute, with an onset of 7 to 14 days, or chronic, with an onset of 2 to 12 months after bone marrow transplantation.

Unfortunately, GVHD occurs to some degree in 50% to 70% of all bone marrow transplantation clients. Management includes symptom control only.

PROCESS OF ASSESSMENT AND MANAGEMENT OF ADVANCED DISEASE

Assessment and management of advanced disease is a complex process. Taking into account the anatomic and pathophysiologic factors and therapeutic sequelae already presented, the nurse has a basis on which to assess and care for clients with advanced disease.

Physical Assessment, Laboratory Values, and Diagnostic Tests of Vital Organs

Physical assessment serves as a device for detecting abnormalities that may be life threatening and for identifying signs that may suggest complications of advanced disease. Additional sources of data are necessary to complete the process of assessment, including laboratory values and diagnostic tests.

Nursing Diagnoses and Interventions for Advanced Disease

The establishment of a database leads to the next phase of the nursing process: formulation of the nursing care plan. Care plans should serve only as guidelines for care plan formulation of clients with advanced disease.

Brain: Alteration in thought processes

The client shows evidence of impaired thought processes related to decreased level of consciousness and impaired judgment resulting from neuropsychiatric syndrome.

Nursing interventions
1. Assess level of consciousness every 2 to 4 hours.
2. Assess for increased intracranial pressure every hour or with each client contact.
3. Check vital signs every 1 to 2 hours.
4. Take safety precautions: padded siderails, soft restraints, bed in lowest position, call light within easy reach.
5. Reorient the client to time, place, and reason for hospitalization with each client contact.
6. Explain the client's condition to the client and the client's family with each contact. Assist them in asking questions and expressing concerns about the present and future.

Heart: Decreased cardiac output

The client experiences altered cardiac output (decreased) that is related to dyspnea, tachycardia, neck vein distention, and epigastric or abdominal pain that results from pericardial effusion.

Nursing interventions
1. Assess respiratory rate, heart rate, and blood pressure every 15 to 30 minutes and record pulse pressure.
2. Assess neck vein distention with head of bed elevated up to 60 degrees every hour.
3. Assess electrocardiogram for a decrease in QRS voltage, electrical alternans, and dysrhythmias.
4. Monitor intake and output every hour.
5. Auscultate heart and lung sounds every 2 hours.
6. Administer oxygen as prescribed.

Bone: Impaired physical mobility

The client has impaired physical mobility related to pain, numbness, weakness, and bladder and bowel incontinence resulting from pathologic fractures.

Nursing interventions
1. Palpate bones for tenderness and crepitus every 4 hours.
2. Assess alignment of bones every hour.
3. Position the client using techniques of proper body alignment associated with comfort and support of wasted limbs.
4. Measure respiratory rate and quality every 4 hours.
5. Monitor intake and output every 8 hours, noting continence.
6. Splint the client within the draw sheet when transferring.

7. Medicate around the clock for pain.
8. Schedule passive and active range of motion exercises, taking into account a client's pain and ability.
9. Encourage isometric exercises when range of motion exercises are contraindicated.

Lung: Impaired gas exchange

The client experiences impaired gas exchange related to dyspnea, hypoxia, absent breath sounds, and altered arterial blood gases resulting from pleural effusion.

Nursing interventions
1. Auscultate breath sounds every 2 hours. Do not expect to hear a friction rub because fluid separates the pleura.
2. Inspect thorax for symmetry of respiratory movement, use of accessory muscles, and tracheal position every 2 hours.
3. Measure blood pressure and heart rate every 2 hours.
4. Monitor intake and output every 4 hours.
5. Elevate head of bed to 60 degrees for comfort.
6. Assess respiratory rate every 30 minutes.
7. Administer oxygen as prescribed.
8. Medicate for pain, anxiety, or both.

Liver: Altered nutrition

The client shows effects of altered nutrition—less than body requirements—related to abdominal distention, hypoalbuminemia, shortness of breath, and nausea resulting from malignant ascites.

Nursing interventions
1. Monitor intake and output every 4 hours.
2. Measure abdominal girth daily.
3. Record blood pressure, heart rate, and respirations every 2 hours.
4. Monitor serum albumin levels and serum and urine osmolality.
5. Restrict sodium intake.
6. Restrict fluids to less than 1500 ml per day.
7. Weigh daily.
8. Assist the client to a high Fowler's position to ease respirations.
9. Perform skin care every 4 hours.

Kidney: Impaired skin integrity

The client experiences alteration in skin integrity related to fluid retention, edema, and increased blood urea nitrogen level resulting from chemotherapy-induced renal failure.

Nursing interventions
1. Monitor intake and output every hour.
2. Weigh the client at the same time every day.
3. Record blood pressure, heart rate, and respiratory rate every 2 hours.
4. Turn and position the client every 2 hours.

5. Massage bony prominences and apply lotion to skin every 4 hours.
6. Provide hyperalimentation as prescribed.
7. Restrict dietary protein intake.

Drainage Odor

In advanced disease in which metastases are extensive, it is not unusual to encounter direct invasion of cancer cells into the epithelium. This type of metastasis causes loss of vascularity, with ultimate necrosis and infection. The result is a purulent, friable, malodorous lesion.

Management of these odors offers relief of one of the many problems a client with advanced disease must face. Initial management should always include wound cleansing and debridement. However, these measures alone are rarely effective. One of the most effective methods of odor control is irrigation with room-temperature yogurt or buttermilk and normal saline. Odiferous wounds, irrigated with these products at least four times a day on a regular basis, become nonproblematic within 4 days. A second effective method is to mix a 6-g packet of Bard absorptive dressing with 10 ml of sterile water and 10 ml of Puri-Clens (Sween Co.) and place this mixture in the wound, followed by a sterile dressing, twice a day. Although aerosols should not be used exclusively, commercial room deodorizers, such as Hexon odor antagonist, may be helpful.

Hope

According to DuFault and Martocchio, "Hope is a multidimensional dynamic life force characterized by a confident yet uncertain expectation of achieving a future good which, to the hoping person, is realistically possible and personally significant." For any client with cancer, hope is an important concept. Usually, the hope is for a cure or remission so that a normal lifestyle can be resumed. However, when a complication occurs, whether it is the first indication or a later indication of advanced disease, the hope for cure is shattered.

It is the responsibility of nurses to help such clients and their families understand that hope is not lost. Although nurses must acknowledge the fact that cure is no longer a realistic possibility, other hopes may be kept alive. Nurses can encourage a hopeful attitude by helping clients and their families develop an awareness of life, identify reasons for living, establish support systems, incorporate religion or humor, and set realistic goals. Nurses must emphasize that although hopes may change in focus and direction, there is never "no hope."

Suicidal Ideation

The final special problem associated with advanced disease is suicidal ideation. Suicide is 1.3 times higher in men with cancer and 1.9 times higher in women with cancer than in the general population.

Suicide attempts arise in an effort to gain control over a situation in which there is no perceived control. Signs and symptoms include verbalization of the intention and the means with which to act on that intention, loss of hope, and loss of interest in any specific aspect of life.

Nursing management of the client with suicidal ideation includes constant assessment and observation because clients generally leave clues. The nurse should be available to assist in channeling aggressive feelings into constructive behaviors, fostering feelings of control, and finding hope and meaning in life. It is appropriate when such a situation arises to consult a psychiatric mental health clinical nurse specialist.

SUMMARY

Advanced disease is a complex phenomenon, and it often mandates decisions that will result directly in life or death. Advanced disease is not curable, and management of its complications has limitations. It is vital for caregivers to consider the goals of the client and family as well as the goals of aggressive management when complications are imminent. Potential risks and benefits of interventions should always be examined carefully to ensure the client maximum quality of life as he or she defines it. When there is agreement among all parties that aggressive management is no longer appropriate, invasive, disturbing interventions should be minimized or eliminated, and palliative management should be implemented.

29 Supportive Care of the Dying Patient

JOYCE ZERWEKH

TRANSITION

The transition from active treatment to supportive care of the dying patient involves a major turning point in philosophy and action. On ceasing to try to rescue the perishing, one is then free to care for the dying.

Nurses can promote up-front decision making in that transition between living and dying. As colleagues on the health care team, it is vital to insist on open discussion and decisions regarding the continuance of active treatment and the relief of suffering. In oncology, the move from active treatment that can significantly prolong life or offer a cure to palliative treatment that comforts the terminally ill is often a continuum, so that there is not a definite point when a patient is treated as living one day and dying the next. The fully informed patient lives with a foot in each world—that of the living and that of those preparing to die.

PATHOPHYSIOLOGY OF MULTIPLE ORGAN FAILURE

Many changes near the time of death are predictable, and anticipating them can help prepare the dying person and family to manage. Infection, organ failure, pulmonary or myocardial infarction, hemorrhage, or extensive carcino-

---

See the corresponding chapter in *Cancer Nursing: A Comprehensive Textbook,* by Baird, McCorkle, and Grant, pp. 875–884, for a more detailed discussion of this topic, including a comprehensive list of references.

matosis have been identified as major processes underlying cancer death. The closer the moment of death, the more likely are common pathophysiologic events. The progression from innumerable preterminal disease processes to final cardiopulmonary arrest can be conceptualized as a journey down a tunnel that is wide at the top but becomes steeper and narrower, with "a gradually diminishing number of possible conditions, any and all of which will lead to a relatively limited pathophysiologic 'common pathway of death.'" This terminal common pathway will eventually include cardiopulmonary failure and often renal or hepatic failure, or both. The human responses to this predictable multisystem failure include nursing diagnostic focus on impaired physical mobility, nutrition and fluid balance, thought processes, comfort, gas exchange and airway clearance, and then impending death.

The heart may fail because of myocardial damage or the workload imposed by preterminal pathologic conditions, such as pulmonary lesions, pericardial or myocardial metastases, anemia, sepsis, or brain herniation onto the medulla. Common causes of pulmonary failure include pulmonary lesions, pneumonia, pulmonary infarct, pulmonary edema, pulmonary effusion, or brain herniation. The hypoxemia and reduced perfusion of vital organs that accompany cardiopulmonary failure cause marked loss of capacity for mobility, eating or drinking, and mentation or consciousness. Comfort is impaired because of edema or ascites, acute air hunger due to impaired gas exchange or ineffective airway clearance, and feeling apprehensive until consciousness is lost. Death is impending as the blood pressure drops, peripheral cyanosis deepens, periods of apnea lengthen, and accumulating pulmonary and pharyngeal secretions produce a death rattle.

Hepatic and renal failure frequently are associated events in death due to cancer. Hepatic metastases may eventually diminish liver function so that ammonia and other metabolites correlated with the development of hepatic encephalopathy are not detoxified. Reduced synthesis of albumin and reduced detoxification of aldosterone and antidiuretic hormone produce extravascular fluid accumulation, and resistance to blood flow into the liver forces fluid into the peritoneal cavity. Renal failure occurs with hypovolemia reducing renal perfusion with renal malignancy. Retention of sodium causes peripheral and pulmonary edema. Azotemia and metabolic acidosis occur owing to failure to excrete nitrogenous waste and hydrogen ions. These pathophysiologic events contribute to a remarkably common nursing diagnostic pattern. Again, capacity for mobility, nutrition absorption, and thought are impaired by accumulating toxic metabolites. Comfort is threatened by fluid buildup in the lungs, abdomen, and periphery.

HUMAN MORTALITY
Human Process

Institutional dying has only recently become the norm in Western society. In contrast, throughout human history, death occurred in one's own bed at home. Death in the past was a familiar crisis that people learned early *to face and to survive*. The sanitized and invisible contemporary pattern of dying does not permit the development of emotional and cognitive coping skills that until recently were a given in human experience. Nursing dying people and their loved ones involves recapturing the best of the past by helping people see death as a normal part of the life cycle, a phase that is extremely difficult but over which they have choices and some control.

Humanization instead of medicalization of dying involves a major shift in paradigm in which primary attention is given to the human experiences and choices of the person who is dying. Open communication and participation are facilitated in contrast to withholding of information and withdrawal that result when dying is perceived as unspeakable defeat.

Switching Goals

Even when the expected outcome is death, nursing and medical practices too often continue unchanged, as if the expected outcome were life. It is essential that the nurse take the lead in setting *conscious,* deliberate goals to comfort individual and family members and respect their choices.

Dying as an Individual Process

A person copes with dying as he or she has coped with living; the wise will be wise and the difficult stay difficult. "Those who are not informed about their life-threatening situation are wrongly denied their right to choose the way they will end their lifetime." Given adequate information appropriate to their individual circumstances, people's responses to news of a limited life expectancy are as varied as people themselves. People who have been living with cancer and multiple treatment methods have already been living with a cloud over their heads. They have experienced many discomforts and inconveniences as their life has been increasingly medicalized. Body appearance and functions have changed. Roles and relationships have been altered. In short, they have already grieved many losses in grieving for the death of their familiar selves.

When the decision is made that no further treatment will stop the spread of cancer, normal coping mechanisms include initial shock and denial, which then are followed by varying degrees and expressions of denial, bargaining, sadness, and raging. The process is not linear but cyclic along a continuum. People cope with this final loss as they have coped with other losses and changes in their lives. Coping patterns are predicted by these past events as well as by cultural heritage. To understand individual reaction, also remember that the grieving process is superimposed on normal development tasks.

Normalizing is a basic strategy for individuals and families facing a terminal illness. People do not wish to live every moment around the reality of dying. They normalize by discounting seriousness, drawing attention away from the disease, and trying to live life as usual. Some may do this until symptoms flood all activity and interaction.

Nursing diagnoses focus first on identifying individual strengths and then building on them. Nurses should anticipate that the patient will face progressive impairments with anxiety, fear, anticipatory grieving, hopelessness, powerlessness, deficient knowledge, disturbance in self-concept, altered sexuality, and impaired social interaction.

Interventions to support the dying person are never standardized and are always relevant to specific nursing diagnoses. However, generic approaches for all people who are losing themselves include a strong affirmation of their personhood: strengthening and validating their identity, translating medical and nursing information to whatever is relevant for their everyday living and planning, and fostering choices about how to live and die. Family caregivers and hospice nurses have identified the paramount needs of the dying person to be respect for their wishes, control of discomfort, open communication with professional caregivers, and normal family relationships.

Dying as a Family Process

Dying persons need age-appropriate information, opportunities to express their feelings and thoughts, chances to be involved without inappropriate responsibility, chances to be playful and carefree at times, and knowledge of how their life in the family will continue.

A history of open family communication, skill in problem solving, and ability to accept help from others and plan ahead enable the smoothest transitions. All families face the same tasks. All must witness their loved one's physical and emotional suffering, grieve in their own way, manage everyday life, and learn to function without the loved one. Central family members must assume the caregiver role and gradually assume the responsibilities of the dying person.

As with the individual, generic interventions with the family foster strengths and family identity, provide information, and advocate the making of choices. The nurse synthesizes client goals, individual family member goals, and the whole range of possible nursing goals to develop a working focus.

Children in families in which a member is dying need special attention. Assessment should consider development stage and family roles.

For some people, pets are important members of the family system, perhaps the most significant other in the person's life. Those with close attachments to their beloved animals should be given every opportunity to have them present and placed comfortably on the bed, chair, or nearby floor.

A wide repertoire of nursing interventions is needed to support family coping: these include active listening, resource identification, problem solving, advocacy, networking, coordination of health team and helpers, participation in family conferences, negotiation, values clarification, conflict resolution, referral, assistance with realistic limit setting, and grief counseling. Small realistic goals and structured expectations are vital.

The strategy for nurses must be to assess the family system, set therapeutic boundaries, mediate conflicts, and help patients and family members to identify and build on their own strengths.

Dying as a Spiritual Process

The spirit might be described as the central vitality in a person's soul. It is the nonphysical force that gives meaning and integrity to life and can be expressed in religious beliefs or anything that provides transcendent meaning. The spiritual comprises a person's relations to things larger than the self—causes, principles, art, history, higher forces, values, or the supernatural.

As death draws near, the ordinary material preoccupations of everyday living and conventional medicine become irrelevant. Nurses who are busy with medical and nursing rituals should ask themselves about the relevance of their agendas. Facing the loss of self, loved ones, and known reality, the patient is struggling to find meaning and hope. Take time to discover this person's story and struggles. The language of spiritual distress may include themes of estrangement from others and from God, blame of self and others, hatred of self and others, expression of anguish, wish for more faith and experience of God, or desire for specific religious practices.

The nurse's paramount responsibility is to listen, diagnose distress of the human spirit, and affirm the ultimate importance of spiritual concerns at the end of life. If the nurse can remain present beside a dying person, that compassionate presence converts the experience into a triumph of love and human community.

Where Death Will Occur

People should die where they choose, where they feel secure and comforted. For those with loving families whose members are capable of caregiving, that place will generally be home. Home is familiar, life can be normalized, loved ones can actively participate, and closure of relationships is possible.

The absolute components of adequate home care include available health professionals who support home care and possess palliative care expertise, available homemaking and personal care assistance, and loved ones who can respond to basic needs when the dying person can no longer manage alone. Home hospice programs focus on the quality of life of the whole family. Psychosocial and spiritual dimensions of care are actively included. The terminal course of events is anticipated, and preparations are made for expert management of terminal symptoms.

Decisions about the place of death should be discussed as early as possible. The public and health professionals need to understand the present constraints of hospital and home health services. A family needs to plan ahead by examining carefully all possible financial resources: individual and family assets, provisions and limitations of Medicare, and private insurance. Decisions should be determined by client and family wishes, known financial resources, and available community services. To maximize autonomy, every effort should be made for the person to live the last moments in a place of choice.

ASSESSMENT AND MANAGEMENT OF THE PERSON FACING IMMINENT DEATH
Assessment: Focusing on Comfort

When the desired outcome is comfort and death according to the patient's own preferences, the focus of nursing assessment is attention to the expression of subjective experience. Our clients are the only experts in what they are experiencing and desiring. Nurses are tempted to focus priorities on the "real" problems we want first to solve rather than the lived experience our client needs to share. Thoughtful assessment attends first to the client's expression of distress, validating it as a first priority for action. Occasionally, a client's need for control will be stronger than the desire for comforting intervention. This wish is seldom expressed directly but can be discovered through repeated failure to adhere to palliative measures.

Assessment of persons who are dying systematically considers physical, psychosocial, and spiritual dimensions. The question should always be asked: How will having this information assist in providing comfort and meeting the client's expressed wishes? In general, new discomforts should be investigated to determine any cause that could be reversed.

Anticipatory Guidance

An essential strategy is to prevent the recurrent physical and emotional crises that can be anticipated with progressive loss of function and likely complications of the disease course. Families of persons who are dying at home should be similarly ready to manage predictable problems. Anticipatory guidance is most likely to succeed when it matches a family style that copes by problem solving and planning ahead. It will be least successful with people who have lived their lives from crisis to crisis.

Managing Common Physical Responses to Dying

Mobility and Progressive Self-Care Deficits. Client and family need to prepare for the day when the person is first chairbound and then bedbound. Goals focus on client choice. Anticipation of increasing dependency is highly threatening, and acceptance of it is tantamount to accepting defeat, so intense grieving is to be expected.

Alterations in Nutrition, Fluid Balance, and Elimination. Every effort should be made to provide adequate nutritional intake for the dying person who wishes to eat. However, food and fluid are essential when the anticipated outcome is living, but they are not essential for a comfortable dying. Food and fluid are so closely linked with love and sustenance that well-meaning loved ones and professionals often *force* them on dying people against their wishes.

Hydrating a person with cardiopulmonary, renal, or hepatic failure can contribute to pulmonary edema and accumulating pharyngeal secretions, increase peripheral edema and ascites, increase the edema layer around tumors, result in vomiting of the increased gastric fluid volume when the intestine is blocked, and increase urine volume that requires catheterization because of patient weakness. The main complaint of dehydrated hospice patients who are near death is dry mouth, which can be relieved by good oral hygiene.

Nausea and Vomiting. Comfort and not better nutrition is the goal. Scheduled antiemetics used in combination are the most effective. In contrast to the parenteral route employed during chemotherapy, the person dying at home or in a nursing home is medicated using the rectal and oral routes, which require higher doses. Vomiting due to an inoperable malignant bowel obstruction is managed with stool softeners and metoclopramide to promote stomach emptying and small bowel peristalsis when obstruction is incomplete. Complete obstruction is managed with narcotics to slow the cramping of peristalsis and with antiemetics.

Impending Death

Death is impending as fluid intake becomes minimal, urine output is scant or absent, level of consciousness drops, blood pressure slides, peripheral cyanosis deepens, apneic periods lengthen, and pulmonary and pharyngeal secretions rattle. The nurse assists in the labor before death by explaining and normalizing each occurrence, offering comfort measures, and enhancing the humanity of the participants. Although the dying person is usually no longer able to participate, the nurse constantly reminds those gathered that everything spoken may be heard by the dying person. The timing of death remains uncertain, which is exhausting for family and those who would like to be present at the time of death. Nurses can try to help loved ones recognize that it is the lifelong relationship rather than the presence at the actual moment of death that is important. If any of life's unfinished business can be resolved by loved ones saying what remains unsaid, asking for or offering forgiveness and love, such expressions should be fostered. Resolution of specific business matters or spiritual reconciliation may be needed.

When death occurs at home, the nurse helps family members prepare for what is ahead by knowing how to diagnose death and whom to call. Physician, coroner, funeral home, and sometimes police will have to be notified. Different regulations prevail in different areas, and the only way to prevent crises is to *negotiate in advance* with the different organizations involved. The family must particularly understand the implications of calling the emergency telephone number 911, which will activate resuscitation procedures. Sometimes, people take such action because of fear or ambivalent goals, but ways should be sought to circumvent the resulting purposeless technologic disaster. At home and in the nursing home and hospital, *do not resuscitate* orders must be clarified and well documented.

Following Death

After death has occurred, the family should be encouraged to do what feels comfortable and appropriate to their beliefs. Some people will choose to touch and speak to their loved one. Through touching and perhaps bathing the body, the nurse present at the time of death can model this as a normal way of working through the finality of death and saying goodbye. Verbal and nonverbal expression will range from silence and withdrawal to wailing and rending of garments. The nurse advocates for the family to stay with the body as long as they wish and intervenes to prevent the rapid removal to morgue or mortuary. In anticipation of death, it is extremely valuable to help the family prepare a checklist of whom to call and what arrangements to make immediately after the death.

Bereavement places survivors at significantly higher risk of physical and emotional dysfunction. Recognizing this, bereavement services have been an essential component of hospice care. The nurse who works with many people who are dying brings a holistic understanding of the family to the assessment of those who may be at risk for dysfunctional grieving. Nurses who see only a few dying people or are especially involved with a family may choose to make bereavement contacts at the funeral or the family home.

LOOKING INTO THE FACE OF DEATH: THE COMPASSIONATE CAREGIVER

A nurse's patients keep dying; how can the nurse continue to care about them? Each person must find a balance. Awareness of self is the fulcrum. This can be a lifelong pursuit of self-discovery and a growing clarity about personal needs and agendas. One challenge is not to impose one's own needs on patients in ways that diminish their well-being. For instance, in situations of great suffering in which nurses face a bottomless pit of needs, they should beware of initiating *rescuing* responses that place them in the position of beneficent givers and the clients in the position of helpless victims.

"Give from your own excess, not from your essence." Consider ways to bring joy into life so that ways can be found to face death and despair. Association with good people and exposure to beauty are important and life-affirming. Explore spiritual teachings and practice. Find meaning in great literature, art, music, nature, and the everyday experience of love. Reexamine the ways in which denial, distancing, and materialism may hinder an authentic existence. Beware of overextension. Set limits on commitments, keep life uncluttered with things and activities, and establish boundaries between personal and public life, as needed. And finally, consider the seasons of life: periods of plunging in to comfort the comfortless and make just the inequities and periods of personal renewal and reintegration. When energy and enthusiasm lessen, practice self-anticipatory guidance by developing a self-care plan before burnout.

30 Oncologic Emergencies

CHRISTINE MIASKOWSKI

Careful assessment of the oncology patient is essential to diagnose emergency conditions early and initiate treatment promptly. This prompt recognition and immediate treatment can halt the progression of the oncologic emergency and often reverse potentially disabling side effects.

OBSTRUCTIVE EMERGENCIES

The major obstructive emergencies associated with malignant disease are superior vena cava (SVC) syndrome, intestinal obstruction, and third space syndrome.

Superior Vena Cava Syndrome

The superior vena cava is a thin-walled, low-pressure blood vessel that lies within the confined, rigid space of the mediastinal cavity. This blood vessel collects blood from the venous vessels that drain the head and neck and the upper thoracic cavity. The growth of a tumor within the mediastinal cavity results in compression of the superior vena cava as well as other blood vessels and organs.

Four mechanisms underlie the development of SVC syndrome: occlusion by an extrinsic mass, occlusion as a result of tumor invasion into the vessel wall, obstruction of the vessel lumen by a neoplastic thrombus, and occlusion of the vessel by thrombus formation on an intravascular catheter. The most common cancers that can cause this syn-

---

See the corresponding chapter in *Cancer Nursing: A Comprehensive Textbook*, by Baird, McCorkle, and Grant, pp. 885–893, for a more detailed discussion of this topic, including a comprehensive list of references.

drome are bronchogenic carcinoma and lymphomas and metastatic disease from the esophagus, colon, testes, and breast.

The primary signs and symptoms result from the obstruction of blood flow in the venous system of the head, neck, and upper trunk. The severity of symptoms depends on the rapidity, degree, and location of the obstruction and whether collateral circulation has developed. Initial symptoms include periorbital and conjunctival edema, facial swelling, and tightness of the shirt collar (Stoke's sign). These symptoms disappear within a few hours when the patient assumes an upright position. Assess for fullness of the arms, swelling of the fingers and hands, difficulty removing rings, erythema of the face, neck, and upper trunk, and epistaxis. Late symptoms include distention of the veins of the thorax and upper extremities, dysphagia, cough, dyspnea, tachypnea, hoarseness, cyanosis, and intracranial hypertension. The acute, emergency situation leads to a decrease in venous return, with a marked reduction in cardiac output and a decrease in cerebral perfusion. Patients experience respiratory difficulty, hypotension, and mental status changes.

The primary treatment for SVC syndrome is radiation therapy. For bronchogenic carcinoma, the usual dose is 4000 to 6000 rad over a 5- to 7-week period; for malignant lymphoma, the dose is approximately 2000 to 4000 rad. Chemotherapy may be administered concurrently. Agents used are cyclophosphamide, methotrexate, and nitrogen mustard.

Supportive care includes maintenance of a patent airway, oxygen therapy, diuretics, steroids, and heparin.

Intestinal Obstruction

Intestinal obstruction can involve either the large or the small intestine. An obstruction to the flow of gastric contents can lead to life-threatening pathophysiologic changes.

Only 10% to 20% of all small bowel obstructions are the result of malignant disease: carcinoid, adenocarcinomas, sarcomas, lymphomas, melanomas, and metastatic tumors of the colon and rectum, ovary, or cervix. The primary cancers that produce large bowel obstructions are adenocarcinomas and metastatic disease arising from ovarian or cervical tumors or from lymphomas.

The signs and symptoms are listed in Table 30–1.

The primary goals of medical therapy are to relieve the distention by inserting a nasogastric or long intestinal tube, correct the fluid imbalance with vigorous hydration, and, if possible, surgically remove the obstruction.

It is especially important to assess the patient for signs and symptoms of strangulation or perforation: changes in the character of the patient's pain or abdominal girth, development of rebound tenderness, and abrupt cessation of bowel sounds.

Table 30-1. ASSESSMENT PARAMETERS FOR SMALL AND LARGE BOWEL OBSTRUCTION

Small Bowel Obstruction	Large Bowel Obstruction
Colicky pain, early in the obstruction	Crampy, lower abdominal pain
As obstruction progresses, pain becomes mild, nonlocalized, and a steady discomfort	
Obstipation	Alternating diarrhea and constipation
Distention	Marked distention
Vomiting begins early	Vomiting occurs late
Fever	
Leukocytosis	
Signs of hypovolemia	
Bowel sounds for both small and large bowel obstruction	
Proximal to the obstruction, they are high-pitched and hyperactive	
Distal to the obstruction they are diminished or absent	

Third Space Syndrome

Third space syndrome is the shift in fluid from the vascular to the interstitial space owing to lowered plasma proteins, increased capillary permeability, or lymphatic blockage secondary to trauma, inflammation, or disease. Changes in pressures at the capillary membrane, increased capillary permeability, lowered plasma proteins, or changes in the integrity of the lymphatic system are the most common etiologic factors.

Generalized third space syndrome is commonly seen in patients who have undergone major surgical procedures (e.g., abdominoperineal resection, pelvic exenteration) or are in septic shock. Third space syndrome is divided into two phases: the loss phase and the reabsorption phase. The loss phase typically occurs immediately after surgery and is usually self-limited to 48 to 72 hours, characterized by a shift in fluid from the vascular space to the interstitial space. Patients show signs and symptoms of hypovolemia. Monitor for hypotension, tachycardia, low central venous pressure, decreased urine output, and an increased urine specific gravity. The patient's fluid intake exceeds total output by a ratio of 3:1. Treatment involves the replacement of fluid and electrolytes as well as plasma proteins.

The reabsorption phase is characterized by a shift in fluid from the interstitial space into the vascular space. The hallmark sign is a marked increase in urine output (i.e., greater than 200 ml/hour). The major problem is hypervolemia. Monitor for hypertension, tachycardia, elevation in central venous pressure, weight gain, rales, dyspnea, and jugular venous distention.

METABOLIC EMERGENCIES
Syndrome of Inappropriate Antidiuretic Hormone Secretion

The SIADH secretion, a syndrome of hypotonicity of plasma and hyponatremia that results from the aberrant production or sustained secretion of ADH (vasopressin), is defined as secretion that continues in the face of hypotonicity of plasma. Cancer is the most frequent cause of the SIADH secretion. Most frequently associated with carcinoma of the lung, these cancers have the ability to synthesize, store, and release ADH. Certain chemotherapeutic agents can produce this syndrome. Vincristine and cyclophosphamide have been shown to stimulate the release of excess amounts of ADH.

This syndrome induces profound neurologic symptoms and should not be mistaken for a psychosis. Treatment depends on the severity of symptoms. Initial treatment may involve water restriction. In severely symptomatic patients, 3% sodium chloride solution will be administered.

Hypercalcemia

Several mechanisms produce hypercalcemia in patients with cancer. It can occur in the presence of bony metastasis. The cancer produces a diffusible substance that causes bone resorption of calcium. Certain tumors are suspected of producing excess amounts of parathyroid hormone.

Neuromuscular symptoms include apathy, depression, malaise, fatigue, and profound muscle weakness. Cardiovascular effects are shortening of the Q-T interval and prolongation of the P-R interval. Symptoms of polyuria and nocturia are present. Anorexia, nausea and vomiting, and abdominal pain can progress to ileus and obstipation.

Treatment is focused on enhancing renal excretion of calcium and decreasing bone resorption of calcium through IV hydration with normal saline and calciuretic diuretics. Mithramycin often is used. Effects are seen within 24 to 48 hours and may last up to 7 days. Major toxicities are thrombocytopenia, hepatocellular necrosis, and hemorrhage. The second drug used is calcitonin, which also inhibits bone resorption of calcium. The major side effect is nausea and vomiting. A third drug is IV phosphate.

Septic Shock

Septic shock, a major form of distributive shock caused by a massive overwhelming infection throughout the entire body, is the major cause of death in patients with cancer, particularly patients with leukemia and lymphoma.

Septic shock is divided into two phases, warm shock and cold shock. In *warm shock,* the release of endotoxin and the subsequent dilation of the arteries and veins result in mental confusion, chills and fever, flushed and warm skin, tachycardia, tachypnea, and decreased PO. In *cold shock,* more endotoxin is released, which stimulates the release of histamine and bradykinin, potent vasodilators that produce an increase in capillary permeability, a decrease in circulating blood volume, and a decrease in tissue perfusion. Signs and symptoms are cold skin, peripheral edema, tachycardia, hypotension, tachypnea, pulmonary congestion, hypoxemia, oliguria, and metabolic acidosis.

The treatment of septic shock is summarized by the acronym VIP. V = Ventilate. I = Infuse. Crystalloid solutions as well as colloid solutions must be infused. P = Perfusion. Dopamine is used most commonly because it will improve cardiac output and maintain renal perfusion. Antibiotics are prescribed empirically in patients with septic shock.

Disseminated Intravascular Coagulation

Disseminated intravascular coagulation (DIC) is an alteration in the normal clotting mechanism that manifests itself as diffuse clotting occurring simultaneously with hemorrhage. DIC has been associated with intravascular hemolysis from transfusion reactions, overwhelming viral or bacterial sepsis and shock, particularly gram-negative, and release of thrombin from malignant cells.

The pathophysiologic mechanisms are excessive conversion of prothrombin to thrombin and the generation of fibrin clots, which result in soluble clot deposition in tissue capillaries. This fibrin deposition impedes blood flow and can result in tissue hypoxia and necrosis. As the excessive clotting proceeds, normal homeostatic controls cannot maintain an adequate supply of platelets, clotting factors, and fibrinogen. Fibrin split products begin to accumulate, and the patient has a tendency to hemorrhage. Observe for bleeding and clotting. Patients develop clots in the microcirculation of organs with the highest blood flow (e.g., kidney, central nervous system, and skin). Assess for hematuria, changes in mental status, and acrocyanosis (i.e., generalized sweating, with cold, mottled fingers and toes). The coagulation profile, including prothrombin time, partial thromboplastin time, fibrinogen level, platelet count, and fibrin split products, must be monitored.

The primary treatment of DIC is to remove the precipitating factor or underlying cause. The major intervention involves the administration of heparin. Heparin inactivates thrombin, which will inhibit the clotting process and thereby inhibit fibrinolysis. This, in effect, stops the DIC cycle.

Remaining interventions include platelet transfusions and prevention of shock and acidosis.

INFILTRATIVE EMERGENCIES
Neoplastic Cardiac Tamponade

Neoplastic cardiac tamponade results from an accumulation of fluid in the pericardial sac, a significant constriction of the pericardium by tumor, or from postirradiation pericarditis. The signs and symptoms are extremely variable: extreme anxiety and agitation, an oppressive feeling over the precordium, dyspnea and tachypnea, cough, dysphagia, hiccups, hoarseness, nausea and vomiting, perfuse perspiration, changes in level of consciousness, tachycardia, jugular venous distention, pulsus paradoxus, or distant or muffled heart sounds. Electrocardiogram may show electrical alternans.

Emergency management of the acutely ill patient involves rapid diagnosis and treatment with a pericardiocentesis to remove the fluid. The patient may require supportive therapy, including oxygen, IV hydration, and administration of pressor therapy. Surgery for a pericardial window or for placement of an indwelling pericardial catheter may follow.

Spinal Cord Compression

Spinal cord compression can occur as a result of direct extension of the tumor from the paravertebral nodes to the spinal cord or from metastatic disease to the vertebral column. Seventy percent of all cord compressions occur in the thoracic area.

The signs and symptoms vary depending on the location and degree of the infiltration. The hallmark symptom is pain, usually located over the site of the compression. It typically worsens when the patient moves, coughs, sneezes, or performs a Valsalva maneuver. Compression progresses to motor weakness, followed by sensory changes. Late signs and symptoms associated with autonomic dysfunction include bowel and bladder dysfunction.

Management includes a laminectomy with rapidly progressing or acutely severe neurologic deficits. Radiation therapy, as a single agent, is used with minimal or slowly progressing symptoms or an incomplete block on myelogram. Emergency management before surgery or radiation therapy includes IV administration of high-dose steroids.

Carotid Artery Rupture

Rupture of the carotid artery occurs most frequently in patients with head and neck cancers. Etiologic factors include invasion of the arterial wall by tumor or erosion of the arterial vessels after surgery or radiation therapy.

Minor oozing is evident at the site of the invasive lesion before the true emergency situation. In the case of a carotid artery blowout, treatment involves direct finger pressure over the bleeding site, adequate hydration, and blood and blood products and stabilization before surgery. Surgery involves ligation of the carotid artery above and below the site of rupture and excision of the necrotic segment.

31 Alterations in Energy: The Sensation of Fatigue

BARBARA F. PIPER

ANATOMIC AND PHYSIOLOGIC FEATURES

Fatigue is a universal experience that is relieved usually by a good night's sleep. However, for many cancer patients, fatigue is not dissipated so easily. It becomes a chronic, unpleasant sensation that no longer protects the individual from overwork or exhaustion. The actual mechanisms that produce fatigue, even at the muscle level, remain controversial. Thus, surprisingly little is known about fatigue that can guide nursing care.

Contributing Factors
Lack of multidisciplinary collaboration

Several factors have contributed to this lack of knowledge about fatigue. One of these relates to the number of different disciplines that have investigated fatigue. This interest of

See the corresponding chapter in *Cancer Nursing: A Comprehensive Textbook,* by Baird, McCorkle, and Grant, pp. 894–908, for a more detailed discussion of this topic, including a comprehensive list of references.

different disciplines has led to many different definitions
and perspectives in the literature that make it difficult to
review findings from various studies and determine what is
useful to nursing practice.

Different types of fatigue

Muscle physiologists consider fatigue to be *central* when
CNS mechanisms are involved and *peripheral* when peripheral nervous system mechanisms are involved. Central
fatigue may be caused by lack of motivation, impaired transmission down the spinal cord, and impaired recruitment of
motor neurons. It also may be caused by "an exhaustion or
malfunctioning of brain cells in the hypothalamic region."
Peripheral fatigue may be due to impaired functioning of
the peripheral nerves, neuromuscular junction transmission,
or fiber activation (Fig. 31–1).

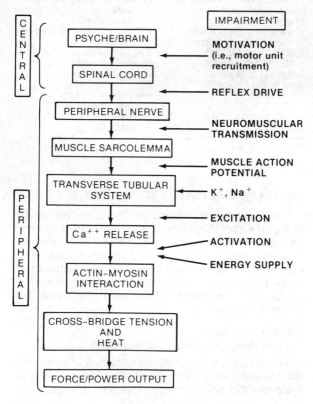

Figure 31–1. Central and peripheral model for fatigue. (Adapted
from Gibson, H., & Edwards, R.H.T. [1985]. Muscular exercise and
fatigue. *Sports Medicine* 2:121.)

Another classification system found in the literature categorizes fatigue as being *normal, pathologic, situational,* or *psychologic* in its origins. None of these classification systems is as helpful to guide nursing practice as is the *acute* and *chronic* model for fatigue that characterizes symptoms by their duration.

Acute fatigue protects the individual from overwork or exhaustion; chronic fatigue may no longer perform this function and may serve no purpose. Its actual function is unknown. Causes of acute fatigue usually are identifiable and involve a single mechanism. Often, acute fatigue is related to some form of exertion or activity. In contrast, chronic fatigue may involve multiple and additive causes that may not be easily identifiable or related to activity.

Acute fatigue is perceived as normal or expected tiredness. Symptoms are localized usually to a specific body region, such as tired eyes, arms, or legs. Chronic fatigue is perceived as abnormal or excessive and is described as a more generalized, whole body response. It is described as a totally overwhelming experience; patients feel that they must give into it when it occurs and hope that it will dissipate soon.

Acute fatigue is rapid in onset, of short duration—days or weeks—and intermittent. Chronic fatigue usually has a longer, more insidious onset that has a cumulative effect. When a threshold point is reached, the person realizes that the fatigue is unusual. It persists over time, lasts for more than 1 month, and is constant or recurrent. Acute fatigue usually is dissipated by a good night's sleep. Chronic fatigue may not be resolved so easily, and a combination of approaches may be needed to lessen the sensation.

Lack of concept clarification

Frequently, concepts such as *malaise* and *weakness* are used interchangeably with fatigue as if they have the same meanings. This lack of distinction hinders knowledge development. Clinically, it is important to distinguish these concepts from one another because nursing management depends on accurate assessment and diagnosis of patient problems, and nursing management may vary.

PATHOPHYSIOLOGIC MECHANISMS OF FATIGUE IN CANCER PATIENTS
Fatigue Framework

In the following sections, a framework is presented that synthesizes the fatigue literature for the purpose of guiding nursing practice and research in this pervasive phenomenon.

Manifestations of fatigue

In the center of the framework are the subjective (perceptual) and the objective (physiologic, biochemical, and behavioral) indicators of fatigue that have been reported. Sign and symptom patterns may vary according to the primary cause of the fatigue, such as stimulation or overwork of a specific muscle group, type of occupational activity, or emotional depression. Currently, the best way to assess and measure fatigue in clinical populations is to determine the person's own perception of the fatigue experience. Fatigue is a subjective feeling of tiredness, influenced by circadian rhythm and other factors and varying in duration, unpleasantness, and intensity.

Mechanisms of fatigue

Accumulation of Metabolites. Accumulation of various metabolites has been associated with fatigue. Whether these products cause fatigue or merely parallel its occurrence remains unknown. In cancer patients, accumulations of lactate, hydrogen ions, and cell destruction end products are likely mechanisms. Continuous muscle work is known to produce an accumulation of lactic acid that can contribute to decreased muscle strength. Another possibility is that fatigue may be associated with changes that result from hydrogen ions that are produced as lactate accumulates.

Fatigue may be caused by the accumulation of cell destruction end products and toxic metabolites in the blood that inhibit normal cell functioning when cells undergo lysis. Increasing fluid intake in these patients may promote more rapid dilution and excretion of these substances and thus prevent fatigue.

Changes in Energy and Energy Substrate Patterns. Changes in energy patterns are common in cancer patients and may result from abnormalities in energy expenditure, cancer cachexia, anorexia, infection, fever, and imbalances in thyroid hormones.

Activity and Rest Patterns. Activity and rest patterns can play significant roles in the prevention, cause, and alleviation of fatigue.

Disease Patterns. Commonly, fatigue precedes, accompanies, or follows many adult and pediatric malignancies. How fatigue patterns vary prospectively by disease type, site, and extent is unknown.

Treatment Patterns. Fatigue is reported to be a pervasive and distressing occurrence in chemotherapy patients. Anemia, cell destruction end products, and nausea and vomiting may be contributing factors. Because fatigue can be caused by disorders in neurotransmission, it is hypothesized that drugs that cross the blood–brain barrier or have neurotoxicities may be more likely to produce fatigue than other agents. Since many agents are used in combination drug protocols, it may be difficult to isolate the fatigue produced by one drug from that produced by another.

Fatigue Patterns. Frequently, fatigue patterns reflect

chemotherapy treatment patterns. Some chemotherapy patients may report a biphasic fatigue pattern. In these patients, fatigue occurs on day 1 of each treatment cycle, may last 1 to 4 days (corresponding to stress, antiemetic, and chemotherapy effects), and recurs during the nadir of each cycle (when bone marrow suppression is anticipated to be the greatest).

Fatigue is common in patients undergoing radiation therapy and seems to coincide with treatment patterns. It is common and often dose limiting in patients treated with biologic response modifiers (BRMs). It is not clear how fatigue may be caused by these agents, but because anorexia, weight loss, and fatigue form a constellation of symptoms in these patients, a combination of mechanisms, particularly central neurophysiologic mechanisms, is likely.

Fatigue may result from surgery and diagnostic testing. Anxiety and test preparation and duration most likely influence fatigue during diagnostic testing.

Symptom Patterns. Other symptoms may precede, accompany, or follow fatigue, such as pain, nausea, or diarrhea.

Oxygenation Patterns. Any factor that alters or interferes with the ability to obtain or maintain adequate oxygen levels in the lungs or blood, such as anemia, can influence fatigue.

Changes in Regulation/Transmission Patterns. Fluid or electrolyte imbalances or changes in neurohormone levels can potentially affect neurotransmission and muscle force, resulting in fatigue, sleep disorders, or altered biorhythms.

PSYCHOSOCIAL FACTORS INFLUENCING FATIGUE
Psychologic Patterns

Several psychologic patterns, such as usual response to stressors (coping strategies), depression, anxiety, degree of motivation, and beliefs and attitudes, may influence fatigue in cancer patients.

Attitudes can influence behaviors. Chronic, unrelenting fatigue can lead to a loss of hope and a desire to escape. Chronic fatigue can prevent the person from engaging in the kinds of valued activities that give meaning to life. As a consequence, the person may lose the desire to go on living.

Other Related Patterns

Other factors that may contribute to fatigue include environmental patterns, such as noise, temperature, and allergens, social patterns, such as perceived social support, cultural beliefs, and economic factors, life-event patterns, such as the common transitional events associated with growth and development, and innate host factors, such as age, sex, genetic makeup (e.g., type of muscle fibers and their predisposition to fatigue), and unique bio-rhythms.

ASSESSMENT AND MANAGEMENT OF FATIGUE
Assessment

To design an effective plan of care, the nurse should perform a thorough assessment of all subjective and objective data that may influence fatigue for that individual. Subjective data should include an assessment of usual patterns of functioning and possible changes that have occurred as a result of illness or treatment. It is important for the nurse to remember the differences that may exist between acute and chronic fatigue states and the multidimensionality of the fatigue experience. Engel and Morgan suggest that the following dimensions of a symptom need to be assessed: symptom location, pattern, intensity, onset, and duration, aggravating and alleviating factors, and associated symptoms. Additional information should be collected about the person's perception of the meaning of fatigue, how distressing it is, and the physical, emotional, and mental symptoms experienced.

Physical examination, laboratory data, and the patient's past and present medical history may reveal coexisting diseases that may be contributing to the fatigue. It is important for the nurse to assess the patient's current medication history. This should include information about prescription and nonprescription drugs, vitamin, caffeine, and alcohol intake (which disrupts rapid eye movement sleep), and other social or recreational drug use.

Behaviorally, the nurse needs to assess for any changes in the patient's physical appearance, performance status, and ways of moving, talking, or interacting that may indicate the presence of fatigue. Environmental factors, such as heat or noise, need to be assessed.

Nursing Diagnoses

Many people assume that fatigue is tied to some form of activity, exertion, or ability to perform. Viewing fatigue from this limited perspective may lead to an ineffective plan of care. Chronically fatigued patients who have cancer may have multiple causes for their fatigue, such as radiation therapy, anxiety about cancer, anorexia, and insomnia. This type of diagnosis will require a more complex intervention plan than if the problem were assessed from an activity dimension alone.

Subjective dimension

Several instruments exist that measure subjective fatigue. The Fatigue Symptom Checklist contains 30 fatigue symptoms arranged in a checklist format so that the presence or absence of the symptom can be indicated.

An instrument that measures subjective fatigue, the Piper

Fatigue Scale (PFS), has been tested and shows good reliability and validity estimates with radiation and chemotherapy populations. The revised scale measures four dimensions of fatigue: temporal (relating to the timing, onset, and duration of the fatigue), severity (relating to intensity, distress, and degree of interference in activities of daily living), sensory (relating to the physical, emotional, and mental symptoms of fatigue), and affective (relating to the emotional meaning of the fatigue).

Objective dimension

A variety of *physiologic indicators* have been used to measure fatigue. These include melatonin, a neurotransmitter, the electromyogram, and heart rate and oxygen consumption. Other indicators that might be studied include rates and degrees of anemia and changes in levels of blood glucose, thyroid hormones, serum electrolytes, and temperature.

Several *biochemical indicators* have been studied. These include hydrogen ions or pH changes, muscle biopsies, magnetic resonance spectroscopy, lactate, and pyruvate.

Nurses have attempted to identify *behavioral indicators* of fatigue. Rhoten developed an observational checklist to measure fatigue in five postoperative patients.

Management of Fatigue
Goals

Balancing energy intake with energy output and believing that "energy can be mobilized for healing" are essential assumptions and beliefs that underlie all nursing care. *Energy conservation* requires assessment of the person's current energy status, the energy-depleting factors that can and cannot be controlled, and the anticipated energy costs of various activities. All decisions about energy-conserving methods must be weighed against the negative consequences of increased patient dependence.

Effective energy utilization is needed to regenerate or maintain energy reserves. Activities should be encouraged to maintain and build on current levels of functioning. It is important for the nurse to teach patients to think about their energy stores as a bank. Deposits and withdrawals must be planned on a daily and weekly basis to ensure participation in valued activities. New goals or activities may need to be considered for those that no longer can be achieved.

Energy restoration can occur through efforts that conserve energy, promote energy expenditure, enhance nutritional status, and reduce the negative impact of physical and emotional stressors.

Interventions

Management of fatigue involves a wide range of nursing activities that span the treatment continuum, from preventing chronic fatigue and screening those who may be at high risk for it to tailoring therapies to fit the different etiologies and initiating referrals on the patient's behalf.

Unfortunately, no fatigue interventions that have been tested in cancer patients can be recommended to guide nursing practice at this time.

Until additional studies can be conducted that test specific interventions in patients with cancer, those who have the disease may be our best teachers. Table 31–1 summarizes preliminary data on patient responses to the question: "What do you believe most directly contributes to or causes your fatigue?" The responses are listed in descending order of frequency.

Table 31–2 summarizes patient responses, again in descending order of frequency, to a question asking what they did to relieve their fatigue.

SPECIAL PROBLEMS RELATED TO FATIGUE
Quality of Life Issues

Fatigue can influence the quality of a person's life negatively by interfering in the ability to perform the kinds of activities and roles that give meaning and value to life.

Decreased Mobility

Fatigue can both result from and lead to decreased mobility and functional status. Prolonged inactivity and fatigue can cause decreased muscle strength, weakness, and loss of endurance.

Decreased Self-Care

A person may become so fatigued and weak that performing the basic activities of daily living, such as bathing, dressing, and eating, becomes too much of an effort without additional assistance from others. Helping people decide what is most important for them to do on their own can assist in maintaining independence and self-respect for as long as possible.

Social Isolation

As a person becomes increasingly more fatigued, the desire to engage in social activities and interactions declines. Increased physical dependence can lead to further declines in social activities, which can result in social isolation for both the patient and the family caregiver.

Role Changes and Family or Caregiver Fatigue

As chronic fatigue begins to alter what patients can do for themselves, family members or caregivers begin to assume many of the roles previously performed by patients. These increased physical and emotional demands on the family member can lead to caregiver role fatigue.

Table 31–1. PERCEIVED CAUSES OF FATIGUE IN CANCER PATIENTS

Psychologic Patterns	Sleep/Wake Patterns
Stress	Insomnia
Worry	
Depression	**Disease Patterns**
Anxiety	Cancer
Emotional strain	Other
Treatment Patterns	**Other Patterns**
Radiation	Symptoms
Surgery	Environment
Chemotherapy	Nutrition
Medical	Innate host factors
Activity/Rest Patterns	
Work	
Everyday activities	
Hospital/RT travel	

From Piper, B. F. (1989). Fatigue: Current bases for practice. In S. G. Funk, E. M. Tornquist, M. T. Champagne, L. A. Copp, & R. A. Weise (Eds.), *Key aspects of comfort: Management of pain, fatigue, and nausea*, p. 196. Used by permission of Springer Publishing Company, Inc., New York 10012.

Table 31–2. MEASURES USED BY CANCER PATIENTS TO RELIEVE FATIGUE

Activity/Rest Patterns	Sleep/Wake Patterns
Rest	Sleep
Nap	
Alter activities	**Other Patterns**
Sit/lie down	Nutritional
Read	Environmental
Walk/exercise	Social
	Symptoms
Psychologic Patterns	
Distraction	
Relaxation	

From Piper, B. F. (1989). Fatigue: Current bases for practice. In S. G. Funk, E. M. Tornquist, M. T. Champagne, L. A. Copp, & R. A. Weise (Eds.), *Key aspects of comfort: Management of pain, fatigue, and nausea*, p. 197. Used by permission of Springer Publishing Company, Inc., New York 10012.

Depression

As a result of the changes mentioned earlier, loss of self-esteem, depression, and loss of hope can occur. A person may not have the desire to fight the disease, participate in treatment, or go on living. Maintaining hope, fighting disease, and participating in treatment protocols take energy. For chronically fatigued individuals, it simply may take too much energy—energy that they may no longer have or want to expend—to go on living.

SUMMARY

Oncology nurses have a major role in recognizing and treating this pervasive, distressing, and perhaps life-threatening sensation. Much work needs to be done to document patterns of fatigue in specific cancer populations and to test various interventions. Only through a collaborative network of oncology nurses and nurse researchers can the care given to the chronically fatigued cancer patient be improved.

A How To Choose A Home Care Agency*

MARILYN D. HARRIS
CAROL ANN PARENTE

Finding the best home care agency for your needs requires research, but it is time well spent. Quality of care and caliber of personnel will be overriding factors, of course. Fortunately, in most communities, families have a wide choice of agencies from which to choose. Some offer sliding-scale fee schedules. Some will accept indigent patients.

Here are some questions to consider when making a decision on what home care agency is best for you.

1. How long has the agency been serving the community?
2. Does my physician know the reputation of the agency?
3. Is it certified by Medicare? Even if your care will not be paid for by Medicare, the fact that an agency is Medicare-certified is one measure of quality. It means that the agency has met certain minimum requirements in financial management and patient care.
4. Is the agency licensed? In most states, a home care agency must be licensed by the state, usually by the state health department.
5. Does the agency provide written statements describing its services, eligibility requirements, fees, and funding sources? Often an annual report will offer helpful guidance on the agency.
6. How does an agency choose its employees? Does it protect its workers with written personnel policies, benefit packages, and malpractice insurance?
7. Does a nurse or therapist conduct an evaluation of your needs in the home? What is included—consultations with family members? with the patient's physician? with other health professionals?

*From National Association for Home Care. (1984) How to choose a home care agency. Washington, DC: Author.

See the chapter on home care services in *Cancer Nursing: A Comprehensive Textbook*, by Baird, McCorkle, and Grant, pp 1023–1032, for a more detailed discussion of this topic, including a comprehensive list of references.

8. Is the plan of care written out? Does it include the specific duties to be performed, by whom, at what intervals, and for how long? Can you review the plan?

9. Does the plan provide for the family to undertake as much of the care as is deemed practical?

10. What are the financial arrangements? Can you get them in writing, including any minimum hour or day requirements the agency may have and any extra charges to be involved in the care program?

11. Does the professional supervising your home care plan visit your home regularly? Are your questions followed up and resolved?

12. What arrangements are made for emergencies?

13. What arrangements are made to ensure patient confidentiality?

14. Will the agency continue service if Medicare or other reimbursement sources are exhausted?

15. Some people feel that accreditation assures quality of service. Accreditation is a voluntary process conducted by nonprofit professional organizations. Visiting nurse associations and other community nursing groups are accredited by the Community Health Accreditation Program (CHAP). The Joint Commission on Accreditation of Hospitals accredits hospitals and their affiliate agencies. And the National Home-Caring Council accredits homemaker–home health aide services.

To locate home care agencies in your community, you might start by asking your doctor, or consult with the hospital discharge planner, if home care will follow hospitalization. Agencies will be listed in the yellow pages under any of several health-related headings. Your county or city will have listings of publicly funded services. If your community has an information and referral service, check with it. Often Information and Referrals (I&Rs) are affiliated with the local United Way (sometimes called United Fund).

Most states have state home care associations that can help you locate a good agency. The National Association for Home Care (NAHC) can help you contact your state association. Their address is 519 C Street, N.E., Stanton Park, Washington, DC 20002.

B How To Find Hospice Care

MADALON AMENTA

If hospice care is desired but not suggested at the time the patient is diagnosed with a terminal condition, the nurse or the family should know that there are several ways to find help. The National Hospice Organization publishes and sells an annual *Guide to the Nation's Hospices* that lists all known hospice organizations by state and town, contact person, phone number, type of hospice, operational status, scope of service, and counties served. The 1988 NHO Guide also lists the names, addresses, and phone numbers of the officers of the 43 state (plus District of Columbia) hospice organizations, most of which also maintain directories of hospices by location, contact person, and scope of services.

Other national organizations that assist families and professionals in the search for satisfactory hospice care through national telephone referral services are the Hospice Association of America (a subsidiary of the National Association for Homecare) and the National Institute for Jewish Hospice.

When choosing a hospice, the family should be alerted to standards of care expressed in national accreditation, certification, and state licensing credentials. In a state that licenses hospices, the state health department will have up-to-date lists of all caregiving organizations that meet this basic standard. The state health department will also have lists of all Medicare-certified hospices, and the Joint Commission on the Accreditation of Healthcare Organizations (JAHCO) lists all those that are accredited.* As a rule, a hospice will provide this information when contacted.

Some communities may have hospices at various levels of operation; some may be providing only referral, volun-

---

*Useful Addresses: National Hospice Organization, Membership Department, 1901 North Fort Myer Drive, Arlington, VA 22209, (703) 243-5900; Hospice Association of America, 210 7th Street, S.E., Washington, DC 20003, (202) 547-5263; Joint Commission on Accreditation of Healthcare Organizations, Hospice Programs, 875 North Michigan Avenue, Chicago, IL 60611, (800) 621-8007; National Institute for Jewish Hospice, 6363 Wilshire Boulevard, Los Angeles, CA, (800) 446-4448.

See the chapter on hospice services in *Cancer Nursing: A Comprehensive Textbook*, by Baird, McCorkle, and Grant, pp 1033–1043, for a more detailed discussion of this topic, including a comprehensive list of references.

teer, and bereavement services, whereas others offer comprehensive programs fully certified, accredited, and licensed if applicable. The family should be assisted in making the decision, if there is a choice, based on their needs and their resources, human as well as financial.

C Cancer Organizations

PATRICIA GREENE
TERESA ADES

NURSING ASSOCIATIONS

1. Association of Pediatric Oncology Nurses (APON)
   11508 Allecingie Parkway
   Suite C
   Richmond, VA 23235
   Telephone: (804) 379-5513

   A national specialty organization for nurses interested in the care of children with cancer.

   Membership dues: $55/year U.S., $75/year foreign

2. International Association of Enterostomal Therapy (IAET)
   2081 Business Center Drive
   Suite 290
   Irvine, CA 92715
   Telephone: (714) 476-0268

   The professional organization for ET nurses and health care professionals involved in the care of patients with stomas, draining wounds, fistulas, pressure ulcers, or incontinence.

   Membership dues: $65/year active, $60/year associate, $32.50/year retired

3. International Society for Nurses in Cancer Care (ISNCC)
   c/o Carol Reed-Ash, RN, EdD, Secretary-Treasurer
   Adelphi University
   School of Nursing
   Box 516
   Garden City, NY 11530
   Telephone: (516) 663-1001

   An organization of cancer nurses worldwide established to advance the knowledge and understanding of cancer nursing and to foster the dissemination of this knowledge.

   Membership dues: $100–250/year based on size of organization

---

See the chapter on cancer organizations in *Cancer Nursing: A Comprehensive Textbook*, by Baird, McCorkle, and Grant, pp 1162–1176, for a more detailed discussion of this topic, including a comprehensive list of references.

4. Oncology Nursing Society (ONS)
   1016 Greentree Road
   Suite 200
   Pittsburgh, PA 15220-3125
   Telephone: (412) 921-7373

   A national specialty organization of registered nurses
   dedicated to excellence in patient care, teaching, research,
   and community service in the field of oncology.

   Membership dues: $53/year active, $26.50/year student,
   $26.50/year retired

MULTIDISCIPLINARY ASSOCIATIONS

1. American Association for Cancer Education (AACE)
   c/o C. Michael Brooks, EdD, Secretary
   401 Community Health Services Building
   Birmingham, AL 35294
   Telephone: (205) 934-3054

   An educational and scientific organization providing a forum
   for those concerned with cancer education.

   Membership dues: $75/year

2. Association of Community Cancer Centers (ACCC)
   11600 Nebel Street
   Suite 201
   Rockville, MD 20852
   Telephone: (301) 984-9496

   An organization of health care professionals committed to
   high-quality care for the cancer patient treated in a
   community setting.

   Membership dues: $650/year delegate, $100/year general

3. International Association of Psychosocial Rehabilitation
   Services (IAPSRS)
   5550 Sterrett Place
   Suite 214
   Columbia, MD 21044
   (303) 730-7190

   An organization to help advance the role, scope, and quality
   of services designed to facilitate the community adjustment of
   psychiatrically disabled persons.

   Membership dues: $55/year individual, $25/year students;
   organization dues based on annual operating budget

4. International Association for the Study of Pain (IASP)
   909 N.E. 43rd Street
   Suite 306
   Seattle, WA 98105-6020
   Telephone: (206) 547-6409

   An international organization of health care professionals
   actively engaged in pain research and those who have a
   special interest in pain syndromes.

   Membership dues: $55–110/year regular, based on income,

$55/year trainee, $250/year contributing affiliate, $1000/year contributing support

5. International Psycho-Oncology Society (IPOS)
   c/o Anthony Marchini
   Executive Committee Assistant
   Memorial Sloan-Kettering Cancer Center
   1275 York Avenue
   New York, NY 10021
   Telephone: (212) 639-7051
   Telex: MSKCC NYKTLX 64-9169

   An international organization to further the development of the psychologic and social aspects of cancer control.

   Membership dues: Extremely low to encourage membership from all parts of the world (approximately $20/year)

6. The National Hospice Organization (NHO)
   1901 North Fort Myer Drive
   Suite 307
   Arlington, VA 22209
   Telephone: (703) 243-5900

   A membership organization made up of hospice providers and professionals that promotes and maintains quality care for terminally ill individuals and their families.

   Membership dues: $40/year individuals, $200–500/year hospice provider membership, based on number of patients served

VOLUNTARY HEALTH ORGANIZATIONS

1. American Cancer Society, Inc.
   1599 Clifton Road, N.E.
   Atlanta, GA 30329
   Telephone: (404) 320-3333

   The nationwide voluntary health agency dedicated to eliminating cancer as a major health problem by preventing cancer, saving lives from cancer, and diminishing suffering from cancer through research, education, and service.

   Each year, volunteers participate in an educational and fund-raising crusade that provides support for developing and conducting the many activities of the society.

   Membership dues: N/A

2. Leukemia Society of America, Inc.
   National Headquarters
   733 Third Avenue
   New York, NY 10017
   Telephone: (212) 573-8484

   A national voluntary health agency dedicated solely to seeking the cause and eventual cure of leukemia and allied diseases.

   All programs are supported by contributions.

   Membership dues: N/A

3. International Union Against Cancer (UICC)
   Rue du Conseil—General 3
   1205 Geneva, Switzerland
   Telephone: (41-22) 20 18 11

   A unique organization of voluntary and professional cancer
   organizations devoted to all aspects of the worldwide fight
   against cancer.

   Membership dues: $1000/year or a share of a national
   subscription calculation based on WHO national assessments

INDEX

Note: Pages in *italics* indicate illustrations; those followed by t refer to tables.